AF903926

GRAPHIC HANDBOOK

IMMUNOLOGY AND INFECTIOUS DISEASES

of the Dog and Cat

For this English edition:

Graphic handbook of immunology and infectious diseases of the dog and cat
Copyright © 2013 Grupo Asís Biomedia, S.L.
Plaza Antonio Beltrán Martínez nº 1, planta 8 - letra I
(Centro empresarial El Trovador)
50002 Zaragoza - Spain

This book has been published originally in Spanish under the title:
Manual gráfico de inmunología y enfermedades infecciosas del perro y el gato
© 2013 Grupo Asís Biomedia, S.L.
ISBN Spanish edition: 978-84-941389-9-7

Translation:
David A. Bruhn
Esperanza Gómez-Lucía Duato

Illustrator:
Jacob Gragera Artal

ISBN: 978-84-941389-0-4
D.L.: Z 1501-2013

Design, layout and printing:
Servet editorial - Grupo Asís Biomedia, S.L.
www.grupoasis.com
info@grupoasis.com

Servet is the publishing house of Grupo Asís

AUTHORS' CVs

The authors of this book are Professors at the Animal Health Department of the Faculty of Veterinary Medicine of the Complutense University of Madrid, where they teach and do research.

Dr. Mª del Mar Blanco Gutiérrez (Coordinator)

She graduated and obtained her PhD in Veterinary Medicine from the Complutense University of Madrid (UCM). During her whole professional career she has focused her teaching and research on the fields of Microbiology and Immunology. She has taught undergraduate and master's students as well as specialised training and postgraduate courses, and completed teaching assignments in Italy, Portugal and France as part of the Erasmus Staff Mobility Programme. She has participated in the writing and translation of several books on Veterinary Medicine and has designed and prepared educational materials as part of projects for innovative teaching. She is the author of numerous scientific publications in specialised international and national journals, as well as review and science popularisation articles. She was a visiting researcher at different institutions in Europe and the USA, where she focused her work on the study of several aspects of the pathogen-host interaction.

Dr. José Antonio Orden Gutiérrez (Coordinator)

He graduated and obtained his PhD in Veterinary Medicine from the UCM. He has focused his research on the fields of Microbiology, Immunology and Infectious Diseases. He has published more than 60 articles in journals listed in the *Journal Citation Reports*, of which he is the primary author of approximately half of them. In addition, he is the author of several research and science popularisation articles published in specialised national journals and has participated in the writing of several books. He was a visiting researcher at the Washington State University (United States), where he worked on lymphocyte differentiation molecules. He teaches undergraduate courses, mainly in the area of Infectious Diseases, as well as postgraduate courses.

Dr. Mª Teresa Cutuli de Simón

She graduated and obtained her PhD in Veterinary Medicine from the UCM. She teaches the subjects of Microbiology and Immunology and Clinical Microbiology at undergraduate level as well as postgraduate courses. She is the Head of the Sub-Service of Mycology, Service of Microbiology and Clinical Parasitology, Veterinary Teaching Hospital, UCM. She is co-author of the *Manual de Microbiología Veterinaria*, *Manual de Inmunología Veterinaria* and *Guía práctica para Identificación y Diagnóstico en Micología Clínica*. She collaborates actively in the Innovative Education Projects of the UCM: "Virtual Laboratory of Veterinary Microbiology", "Basic Immunotrivial Pursuit", "Advanced Immunotrivial Pursuit" and "Viropolis: a game to know more about Virology". In addition, she is the author of several national and international specialised scientific publications and review and science popularisation articles. She carries out her research on the biocontrol of mites and on the study of the pathogen-host interaction in trout lactococcosis.

Dr. Ana Doménech Gómez

She graduated and obtained her PhD in Veterinary Medicine from the UCM. She is Professor of Immunology and Infectious Diseases both at undergraduate and postgraduate level. She is a member of the Spanish Society for Virology, European Society for Virology and European Association of Veterinary Laboratory Diagnosticians. She is co-author of the *Manual de Inmunología Veterinaria* and has participated in several Innovative Education Projects of the UCM such as "Basic Immunotrivial Pursuit" and "Advanced Immunotrivial Pursuit" and "Viropolis: a game to know more about Virology. Her research interest focuses on animal, both feline and ovine, retroviruses, mainly on the study of pathogenesis and immune response, the development of diagnostic methods and new treatments such as interferon. She is the author of numerous scientific publications in specialised international journals and has collaborated in the writing of books and science popularisation and review articles on retroviruses.

Dr. Gustavo Domínguez Bernal

He graduated and obtained his PhD in Veterinary Medicine from the UCM. He currently teaches subjects related to Immunology and Infectious Diseases both at undergraduate and postgraduate level. He participates actively in the popularisation of science by collaborating in initiatives such as Science Week or by developing new digital educational methods as part of Innovative Education Projects. He is the author of numerous scientific publications in international journals and several review articles about the interaction between pathogens and host cells. He was a visiting researcher in several European countries. He currently focuses his research on the design of new vaccine strategies against viruses (Porcine Reproductive and Respiratory Syndrome, PRRS), bacteria (*Salmonella*) and protozoa (*Leishmania*) that affect different animal species.

Dr. Alicia Gibello Prieto

She graduated in Biological Sciences from the UCM and obtained her PhD from the Faculty of Veterinary Medicine of the same university. She has focused her teaching on the subjects of Microbiology and Immunology at undergraduate and master's level and in specialised training seminars. She has participated in the writing and translation of several books on Veterinary Immunology and has designed and prepared educational materials as part of projects for innovative teaching in Microbiology and Immunology. Her research focuses on the use of microorganisms in bioremediation processes and on the pathogen-host relationship in diseases affecting aquaculture, mainly on the study of new diagnostic systems, mechanisms of virulence and/or pathogenicity, and on the immune response of the host. She is the author of numerous scientific publications in specialised international and national journals, in addition to science popularisation articles. She completed her scientific training with research visits at different institutions in the United Kingdom: the University of Leicester and the Institute of Food Research of Reading.

Dr. Esperanza Gómez-Lucía Duato

She is a Full Professor of Animal Health and has taught Microbiology and Immunology since the beginning of her teaching career, almost 30 years ago. She is a member of the Board of Directors of the Spanish Society for Virology (SEV), Group for the History of Virology (GHV) and Group for the Teaching and Diffusion of Microbiology (D+D SEM). She is also a member of the European Society for Virology. She completed her research training with long research visits at the Universities of Madison (Wisconsin), Harvard (Masschusetts), Oregon Health Sciences University, and Davis (California) and a teaching assignment in Munich as part of the Erasmus Staff Mobility Programme. She is the co-author of "Virtual Laboratory of Veterinary Microbiology", "Viropolis: a game to know more about Virology", "Basic Immunotrivial Pursuit", "Advanced Immunotrivial Pursuit" and *Manual de Inmunología Veterinaria*. She focuses her teaching on the subject of Microbiology and Immunology in Veterinary Medicine at undergraduate level. In addition, she is the coordinator of the Official Master's degree in Virology of the UCM. She researches on animal retroviruses, especially in bovids, small ruminants and feline species.

Dr. Guadalupe Miró Corrales

She graduated and obtained her PhD in Veterinary Medicine from the UCM. She is a Diplomate of the European Veterinary Parasitology College. She is a Professor in Parasitology and Parasitic Diseases at the Department of Animal Health of the Faculty of Veterinary Medicine of the UCM. She is the Head of the Service of Infectious and Parasitic Diseases of the Department of Animal Health of the Faculty of Veterinary Medicine of the UCM. She is a founder member and currently President of the European Group of Experts on Canine Leishmaniosis LEISHVET. She is the Spanish Representative at the European Scientific Council of Companion Animal Parasites, and President of the Spanish Delegation (ESCCAP *España*). She is the author of several books and numerous publications and scientific articles on small animal parasitoses and infectious diseases. She has specialised in the health control of cat and dog populations and researches on various zoonoses such as leishmaniosis, toxoplasmosis and parasitic gastroenteritis.

Dr. Isabel Simarro Fernández

She is a Full Professor of Animal Health and focuses her teaching at undergraduate level on the fields of: Infectious Diseases, Preventive Medicine and Enforcement of Public Health laws, and Zoonoses and Public Health. In addition, she participates in the UCM's Master's degree in Virology as a co-coordinator of the specialty of Veterinary Virology. She is an elected Member of the Board of Directors of the Veterinary Teaching Hospital and was the Head of the Service of Microbiology and Parasitology of the Veterinary Teaching Hospital of the UCM from its opening in September 1998 to September 2006. She has published more than 40 articles in journals listed in the *Journal Citation Reports*. She is the author of various research and science popularisation articles in specialised national journals and has participated in the writing of several books.

PREFACE

If people were asked what domestic animals are most important to man, the answer would be without a doubt almost unanimous: dogs and cats, our pets *par excellence*. That is why it is essential for our pets to be healthy, and this is what many veterinary colleagues dedicate their work to.

As the authors of this book, we aimed at creating a practical and manageable handbook, which would also be complete and updated on the essential aspects related to important infectious processes in small animal clinical medicine: the key aspects of the immune response in the dog and cat, the main infectious diseases and their prevention by means of vaccination. The book is thus divided into three separate parts, although consistency has been maintained throughout the work and cross references have been included in the illustrations to facilitate the reading of the different topics that are addressed. One of the most arduous tasks during the creation of this book has actually been the coordination of the contents of the first chapter, in which the key aspects of the immune response are explained; that is why I would like to highlight the fact that each illustration included in this first part is the final result of the work of a whole team, whose aim was to make its understanding easier.

I would like to emphasise the commitment of all the authors of this book, who did not hesitate to participate in this challenge and add one more task to their already busy schedule. I hope their dedication, effort and energy will be reflected in this handbook. I would also like to acknowledge the great work of the staff at the Publishing Company, as regards both the organisation and editing of the contents and the graphic design work; the fact that these aspects have also been developed by veterinary surgeons has contributed to a better communication and coordination between all of us. Finally, I believe I speak for all the authors when I thank our families, friends and colleagues, who have been partly deprived of our company during the preparation of this book. This work is dedicated to all of them.

Mª del Mar Blanco Gutiérrez
Madrid, October 2013

PROLOGUE

As a Professor at a faculty of Veterinary Medicine and president of the Spanish Association of Veterinary Medical Colleges, I am honoured to write the prologue of this handbook, as it contributes in an excellent manner to a better knowledge of basic immunology applied to the understanding, and in particular to the prevention, of the infectious diseases in dogs and cats.

Any text that contributes to the understanding of complex phenomena, as is the pathogen-host relationship, deserves to be considered with great attention, and this handbook fulfils this function a in a very remarkable manner, showing great rigour and precision in the explanation of the different concepts, which are clearly exposed.

In addition to what has previously been said, the excellent quality of the illustrations included in this book is also worth highlighting. This will help readers to understand the mechanisms involved in the pathogenesis of the diseases and the immune responses that are triggered in the organism of the animal with the administration of the vaccines used for their prevention.

This handbook will be of great practical use to students of Veterinary Medicine, who need summarised and schematic representations so as to clearly understand the immunological aspects of animal diseases. But I would like to particularly emphasise the fact that it will also be useful to veterinary professionals who dedicate their work to pet clinical practice, as it will provide them with information that is easy to read, and help them to find an answer to their questions and have a greater knowledge of this area of their work.

For all these reasons, I would like to congratulate and thank the authors, professors and researchers, who are renowned for their solid scientific work and have a wide teaching experience –which supports the quality of their work– for the important contribution they have made with the creation of this handbook.

Juan José Badiola Diez
Professor at the University of Zaragoza and President
of the Spanish Association of Veterinary Medical Colleges

TABLE OF CONTENTS

1 Basic immunology of the dog and cat

2 Main infectious diseases in dogs and cats susceptible to vaccination

3 Vaccination

F FOLDOUT PAGE

LYMPHOID ORGANS AND TISSUES

The immune system comprises a set of organs and structures in which the cells responsible for the immune responses are generated, accumulated and acquire maturity. Lymphocytes develop and mature in the primary lymphoid organs. The secondary lymphoid organs are the places where mature lymphocytes meet and contact with antigens.

1. The bone marrow and the thymus gland are the **primary lymphoid organs** (as well as the ileocecal Peyer's patches in the dog). They are the organs where lymphocytes mature and undergo the selection process which leads to the elimination of the autoreactive ones that would react to self-Ag (see Chart 10). The primary lymphoid organs develop early in fetal life.
2. The bone marrow is a spongy tissue in the interior of the long bones or the flat bones. It contains a common multipotent stem cell progenitor, from which all blood cells are derived through a process known as hematopoiesis (see Chart 2). In addition, it is the site where B cells mature.
3. The thymus is the first lymphoid organ that is formed during fetal development and is fully functional at birth. It persists as a large organ approximately until sexual maturity, when it becomes less functional, and the proliferation and differentiation of T cells decrease. In the thymus, pre-T cells produced by the bone marrow in very early stages mature to T cells.
4. **Secondary lymphoid tissues** and **organs** arise late in fetal life and persist throughout the life of the animal. They include the lymph nodes, spleen and mucosa-associated lymphoid tissue (MALT, which comprises among others the tonsils, Peyer's patches and mesenteric lymph nodes). Their primary function is to facilitate interactions between antigen-presenting cells (APC) and lymphocytes.
5. Secondary lymphoid organs are rich in T and B cells, and APC (macrophages and dendritic cells). They are the sites where specific or acquired immune responses are executed (see Chart 5). Systemic immunity relies mainly on the spleen and lymph nodes, while the local immunity develops in the MALT (see Chart 11).
6. **Lymph nodes** consist of a reticular network filled with immune cells. They are strategically positioned along the lymphatic circulation and the responses against lymph-borne Ag begin in them.
7. In the **spleen** the immune responses develop in the white pulp, which contains the immune cells. The responses against blood-borne Ag initiate here.
8. Immune responses against ingested or inhaled Ag or potentially harmful substances often initiate in the **MALT**. These Ag are captured by specialized cells, inducing a local response (see Chart 11).

LYMPHOID ORGANS AND TISSUES

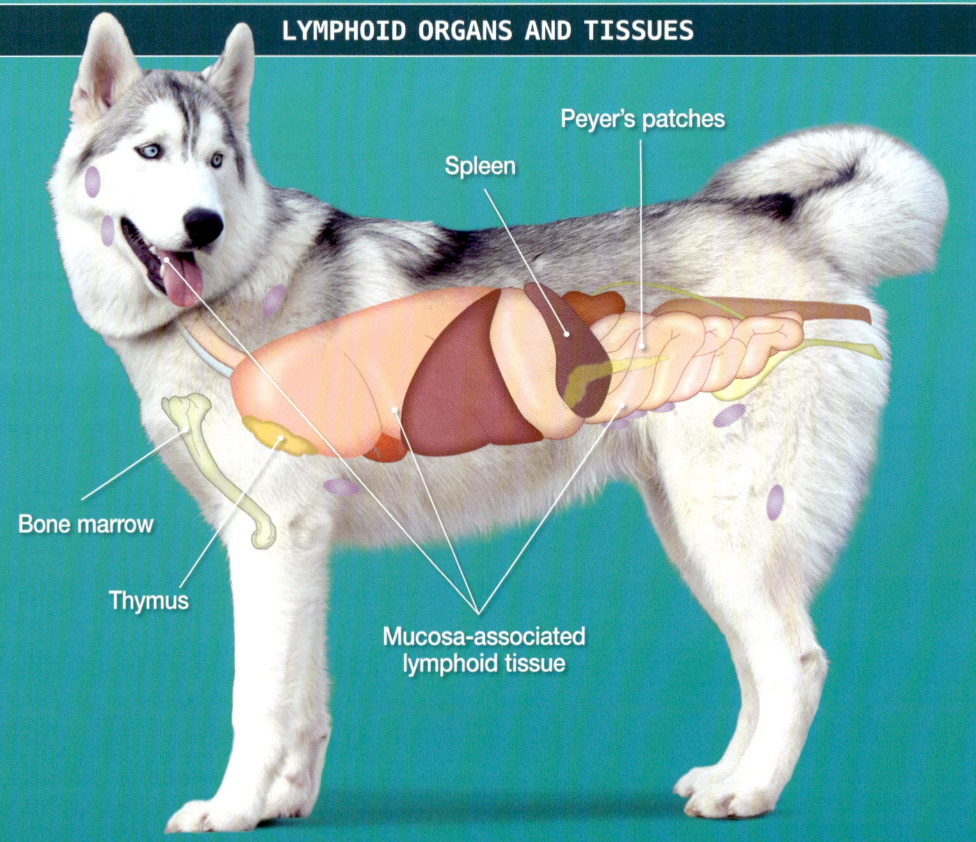

LYMPHOID SYSTEM

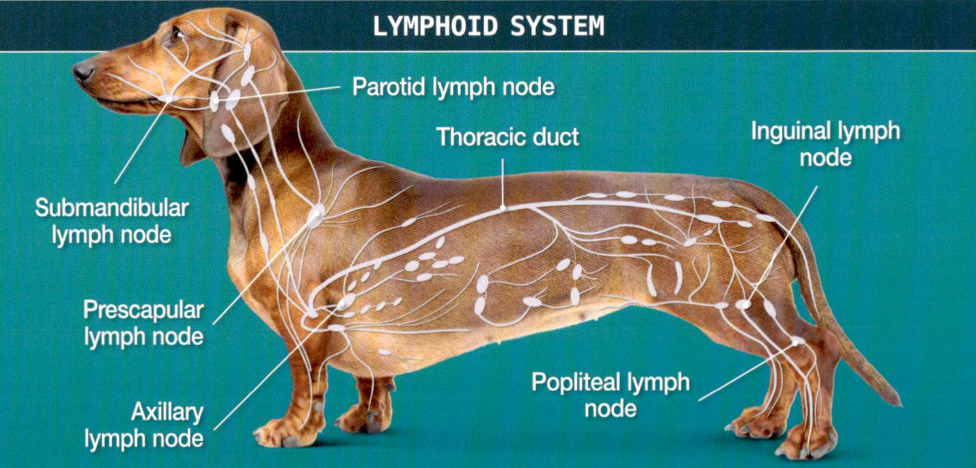

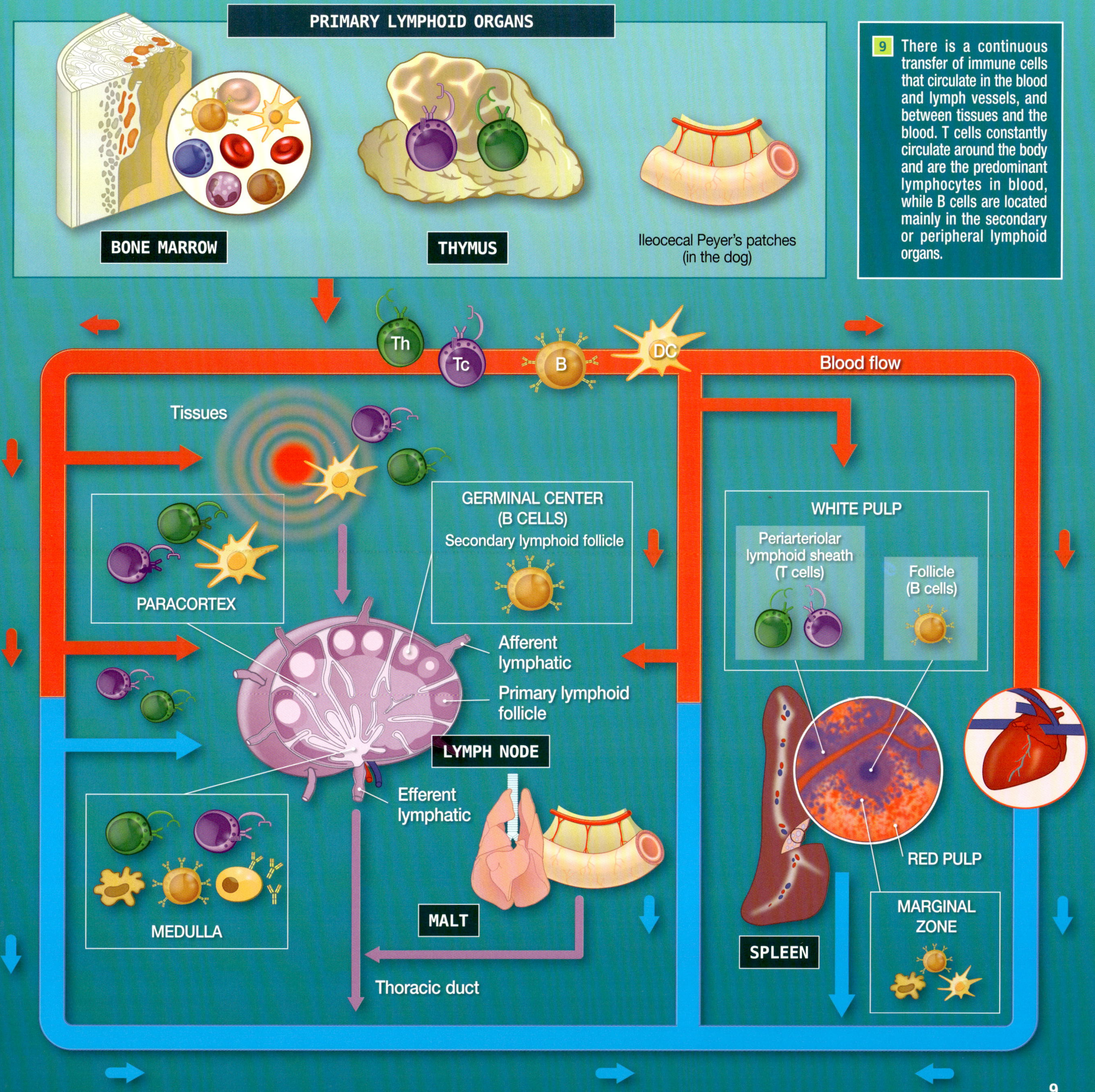

9 There is a continuous transfer of immune cells that circulate in the blood and lymph vessels, and between tissues and the blood. T cells constantly circulate around the body and are the predominant lymphocytes in blood, while B cells are located mainly in the secondary or peripheral lymphoid organs.

CELLS OF THE IMMUNE SYSTEM

After birth, all blood cells and those of the immune system arise from the bone marrow of long bones. Specifically, a hematopoietic stem cell gives rise to a pluripotent stem cell, which originates two cellular lineages: the lymphoid lineage and the myeloid lineage.

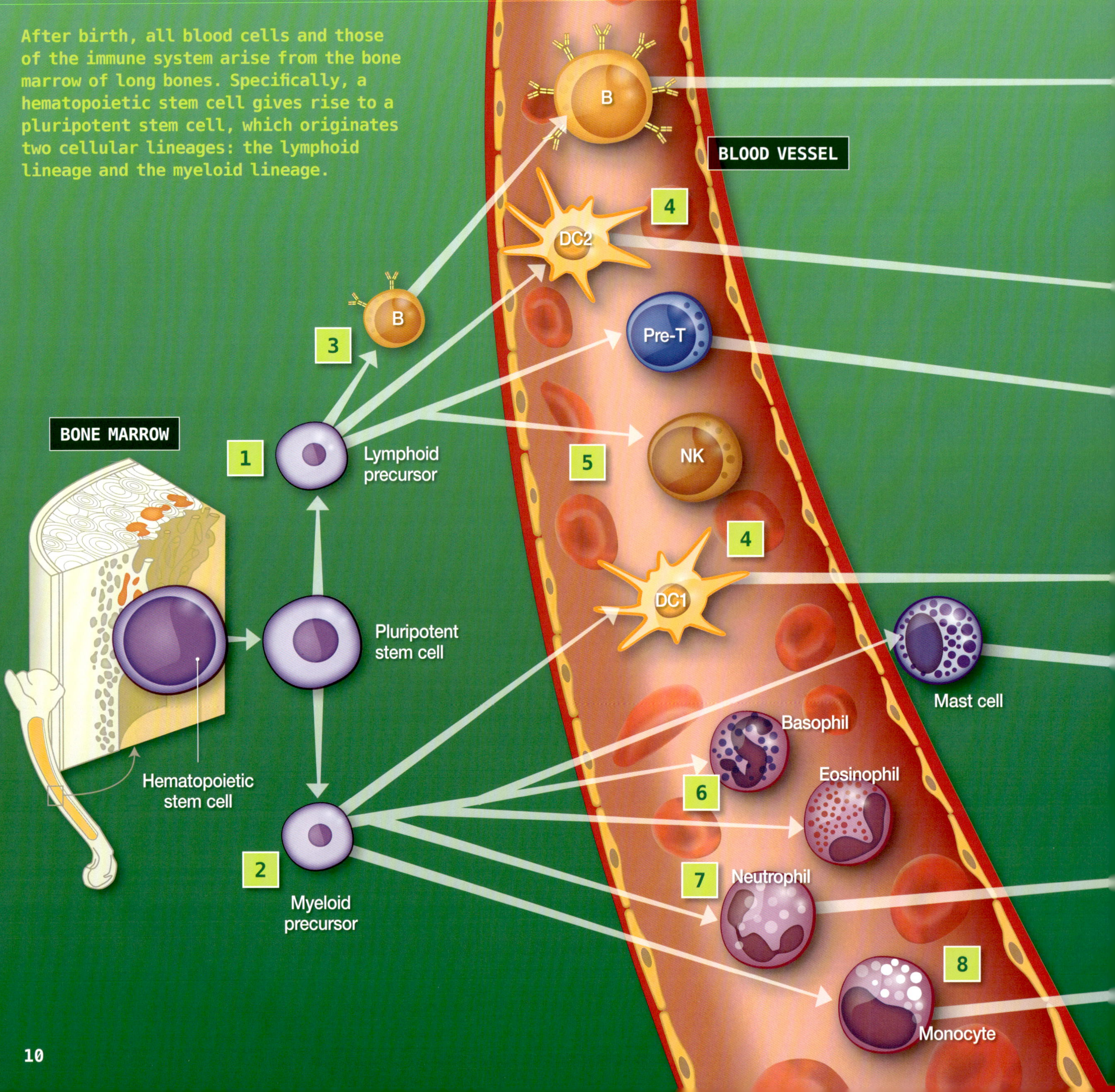

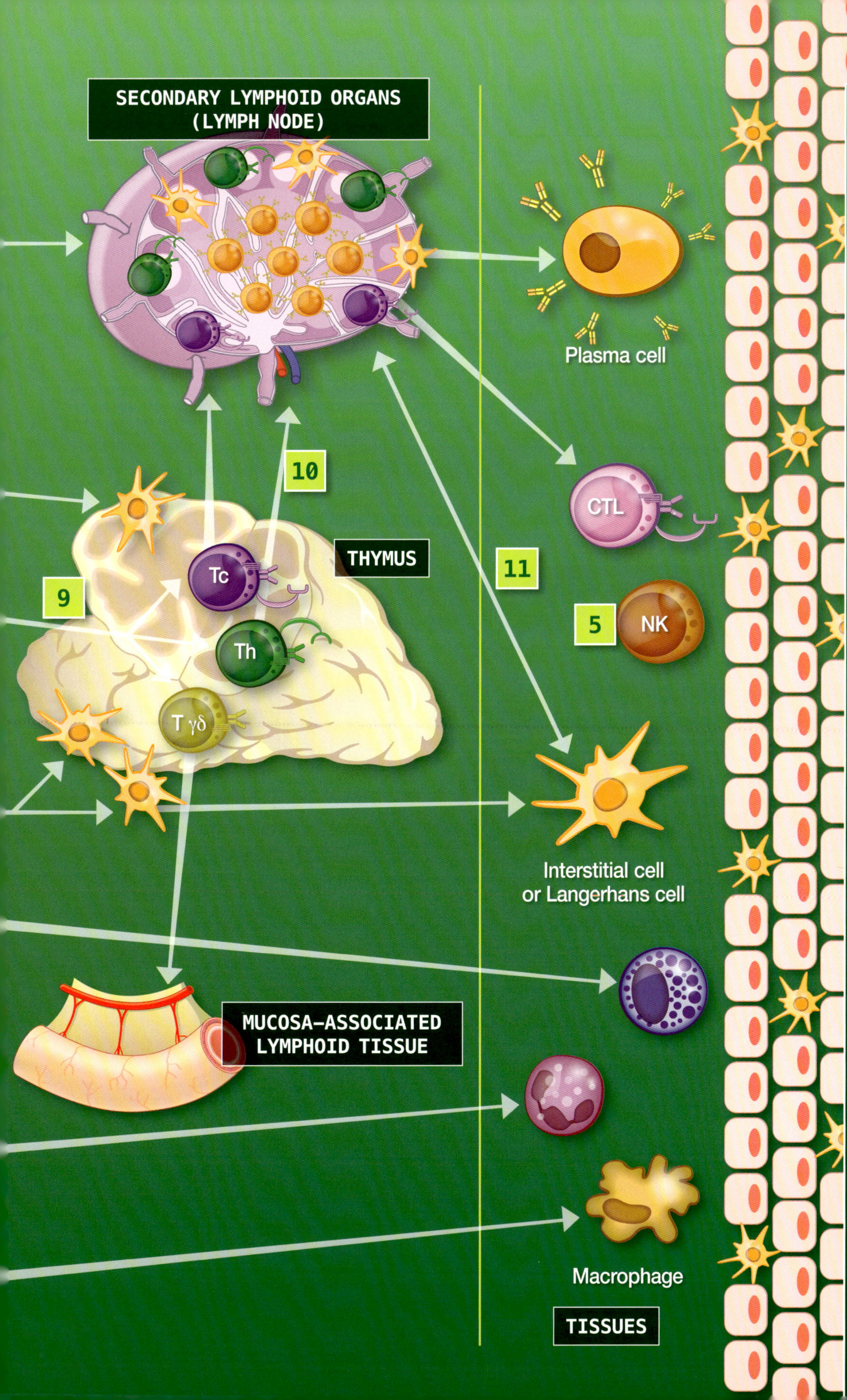

1. The **lymphoid precursor** gives rise to B cells, plasmacytoid dendritic cells (DC2), pre-T cells and NK cells.
2. The **myeloid precursor** gives rise to myeloid dendritic cells (DC1), monocytes and polymorphonuclear granulocytes (basophils, eosinophils, and neutrophils).
3. **B cells** mature in the bone marrow and in the Peyer patches, where they acquire the repertoire of specific receptors for the recognition of Ag (BCR). Mature B cells migrate first to the blood and later to the secondary lymphoid organs (see Chart 1). They are responsible for the specific humoral response.
4. **Dendritic cells** are the most important Ag presenting cells (APC). They are specialized in capturing, processing and presenting Ag to T cells. They are located in the thymus, secondary lymphoid organs and, those of myeloid origin (DC1), also in epidermis and other tissues (interstitial cells).
5. Unlike B cells and T cells, NK cells are quickly activated and they can penetrate tissues to attack tumor and infected cells, by innate mechanisms or by antibody dependent cellular cytotoxicity (ADCC).
6. **Basophils and mast cells** derive from a common progenitor and are similar morphologically. Basophils predominate in blood and mast cells in tissues. Both of them participate in inflammatory and allergic processes.
7. **Eosinophils**, and predominantly **neutrophils**, are phagocytic cells. Neutrophils are the first phagocytes to arrive to the focus of the infection as they quickly migrate from the blood to tissues by diapedesis.
8. Blood carries **monocytes** to the different tissues, such as liver, lungs, bones, secondary lymphoid organs and connective tissue, where they quickly differentiate to **macrophages**. Their main function is to phagocyte and act as APC.
9. In the thymus, T cells mature, acquire the repertoire of specific receptors for Ag recognition (TCR) and become tolerant to self-Ag. Based on the type of TCR, they are classified into two subsets: a) **$\alpha\beta$ T cells**, which acquire the CD4 or CD8 markers, which determine their function, and b) the **$\gamma\delta$ T cells**, which generally do not express differentiation markers (some can express CD8) and abound in mucosal surfaces.
10. Mature T cells leave the thymus and migrate to the secondary lymphoid organs, where they become activated after the recognition of Ag presented by the dendritic cells. Cytotoxic T cells (Tc, or CD8+) are in charge of the cell-mediated adaptive responses, whereas the T helper cells (Th, or CD4+) cooperate in the activation of B cells and Tc cells (see Chart 5).
11. The **interstitial dendritic cells** of tissues (DC1) and Langerhans cells of the skin derive from the myeloid lineage and express a large amount of class II MHC molecules on their surface. Unlike the **plasmacytoid dendritic cells** (DC2), they may recirculate through the blood and the lymph between the tissues and the secondary lymphoid organs.

RECOGNITION MOLECULES IN THE IMMUNE SYSTEM

Cells of the immune system have different molecules on their surface, which perform important immunological functions. Many of these molecules are called by the initials CD followed by a number. They can be surface markers characteristic of a cell lineage, such as CD3 on T cells, or of a state of activation and maturation. In addition, these molecules can be used as immunological markers for diagnostic purposes.

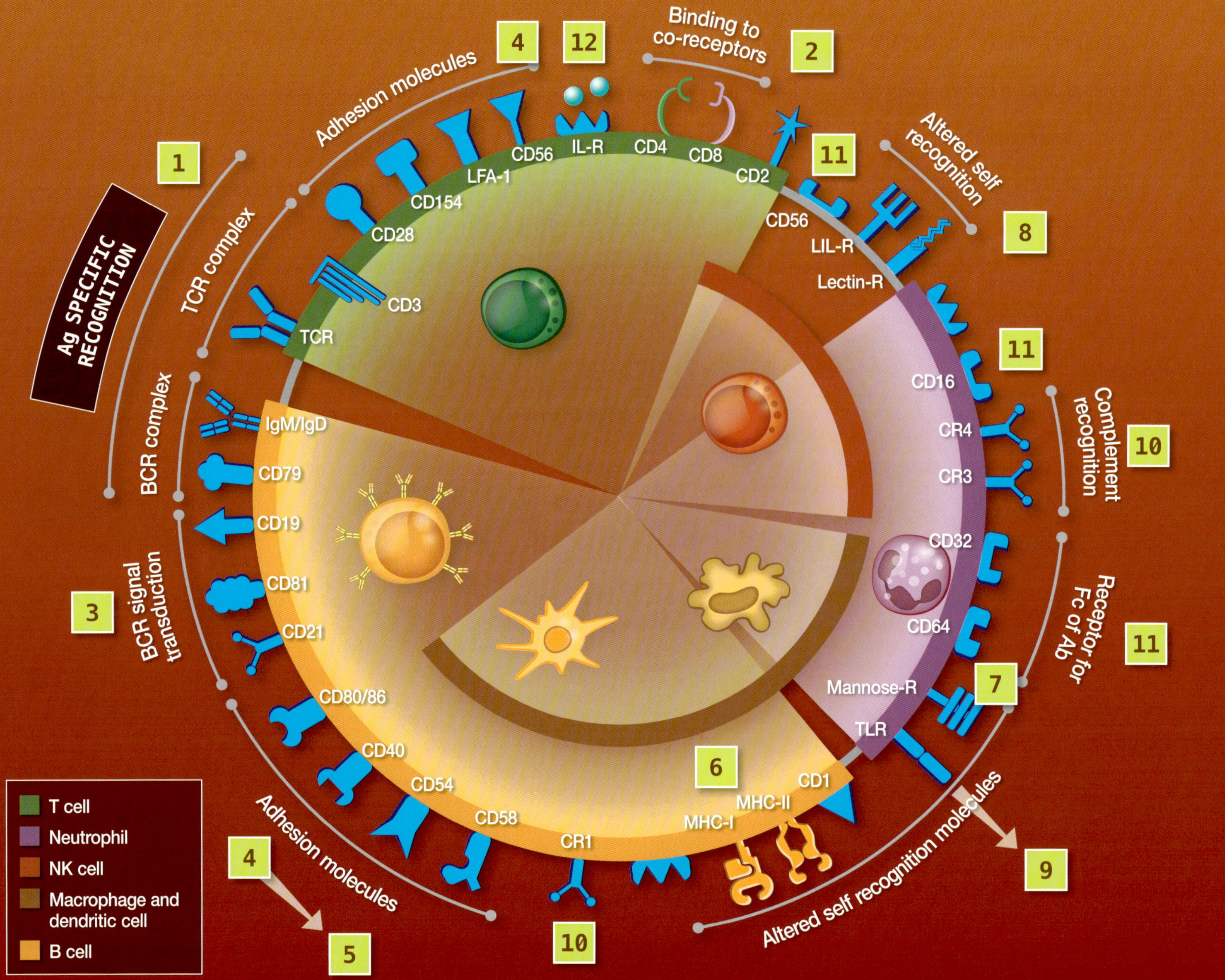

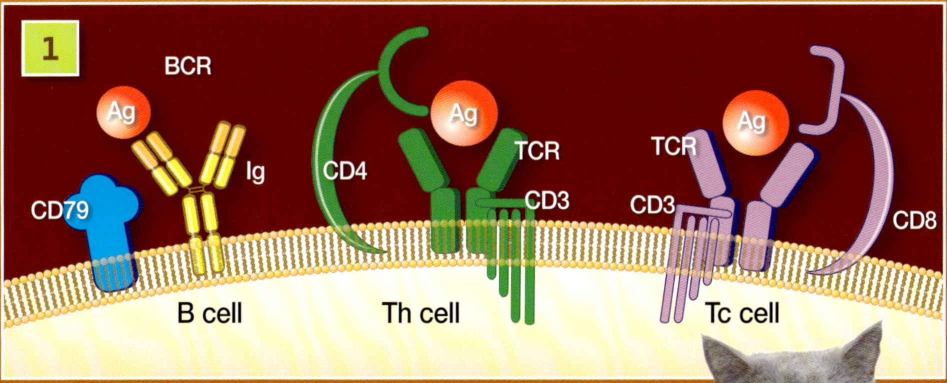

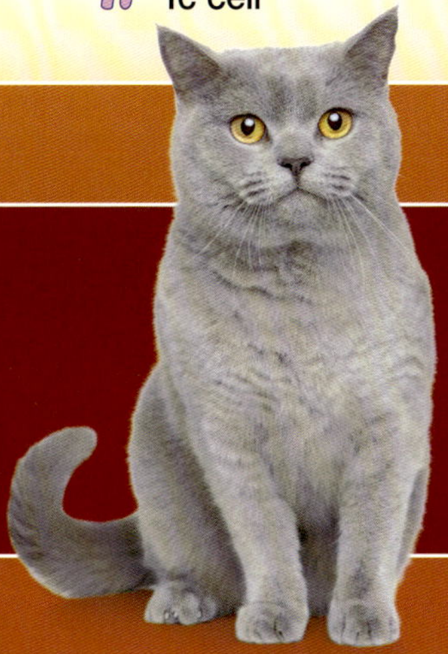

2 **CD4 and CD8 markers can be used to quantify the Th and Tc cells** by flow cytometry, using anti-CD4 and anti-CD8 monoclonal Ab. The CD4/CD8 ratio in healthy cats is above 1.0; a ratio below this value is considered pathological and may be caused by an immune deficiency.

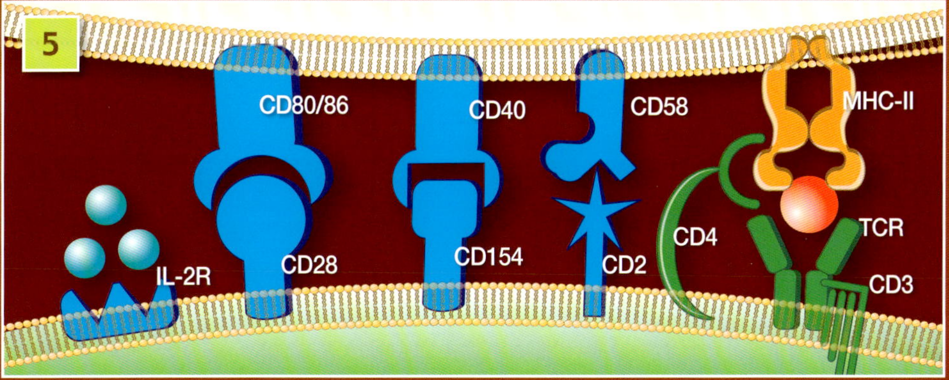

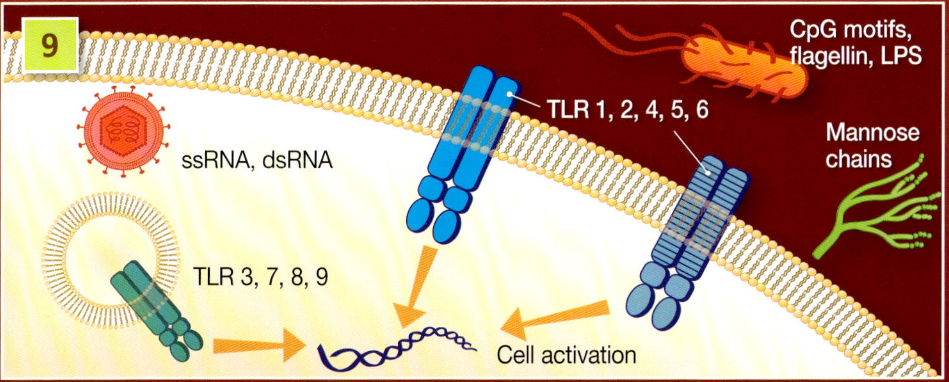

1 **BCR** (membrane Ig-CD79) **and TCR-CD3**, as well as CD4 and CD8 markers on lymphocytes are involved in specific recognition of the Ag.

2 CD4 and CD8 markers act in T cells as co-receptors for recognition of Ag. **CD4 is characteristic of Th and CD8 of Tc.** Unlike other mammals, the CD4 marker in the dog is located also on neutrophils and macrophages.

3 Markers CD19, CD81, and CD21 act as co-receptors on B-cells, participating in cellular activation. CD21 is also the receptor for components C3b and C3d of complement (CR2).

4 There are many adhesion molecules involved in cell interactions at the immunological synapse between the APC and Th cells, and between Th cells and either B cells or Tc cells (CD2, CD28, CD54...). The consequence of these interactions is cell activation.

The immunological synapse

5 The immunological synapse is the contact point of two cells of the immune system. The interaction between cells is established through the adhesion molecules and the cytokines. Such exchange of information between cells is necessary for the activation of lymphocytes.

6 **Type I MHC molecules (MHC-I) are present in virtually all nucleated cells**; on the other hand, **type II MHC molecules are present only on the APC** where they associate with processed peptides. These MHC-peptide complexes are recognized by the TCR of T cells.

7 Some of the molecules involved in the recognition of the "non-self" Ag are the mannose receptor and the toll-like receptor (TLR).

8 NK cells possess other receptors involved in the recognition of self and altered MHC-I: LIL-R (CD85) and the C-type lectin family receptors.

9 The **TLR** are expressed on the APC, neutrophils and NK cells. They are important molecules in the innate immune response (see Chart 4) and they recognize the **PAMP** (pathogen-associated molecular patterns). The TLR can be located on the surface or can be intracellular. The binding of the TLR to their ligands triggers the production of enzymes and cytokines that stimulate phagocytosis and activate lymphocytes.

10 Receptors for the complement fractions C3b and C4b (CR3 and CR4) of neutrophils and macrophages stimulate phagocytosis. Other receptors, in addition, promote the removal of immunocomplexes; for example, CR1 (CD35) present on phagocytes and B-cells. Receptors for C3a, C4a and C5a of phagocytes, mast cells and basophils are involved in chemotaxis and anaphylaxis.

11 **Receptors for the Fc of the Ab** facilitate the removal of the immune complexes and infected cells by phagocytosis or by ADCC (antibody-dependent cellular cytotoxicity). These receptors are found on NK cells, dendritic cells, macrophages and neutrophils (see Charts 5 and 13).

12 Membrane receptors for cytokines are expressed on a variety of cells of the immune system. They are involved in intercellular communication through the transcription of certain genes that mediate a particular cellular function. The receptor for IL-2 (IL-2R) is a characteristic marker of activated T cells.

INNATE IMMUNITY

Innate immunity is the first line of defense against non-self agents. Its characteristics are: immediate response, non-specificity (unable to distinguish subtle differences between Ag), and lack of memory (equal reaction in composition and intensity after repeated exposures to the same Ag).

BARRIERS AT THE BODY SURFACES

1 There are physical, chemical and biological barriers on the body surface and on the respiratory, digestive and urogenital systems, which try to avoid the entry of pathogens. These mechanisms and their components act continually.

- **a** **Eyes:** blinking, flushing action of tears.
- **b** **Respiratory tract:** cough and sneeze, mucociliary elevator of the trachea, surfactant agents, mucus, autochthonous microbiota.
- **c** **Skin and hair:** integrity, desquamation, desiccation, fatty acids, pH, autochthonous microbiota.
- **d** **Gastrointestinal tract:** saliva, vomit, bile acids, peristalsis, mucus, pH, autochthonous microbiota.
- **e** **Genitourinary system:** mucus, pH, autochthonous microbiota.

INTERNAL INNATE IMMUNITY COMPONENTS

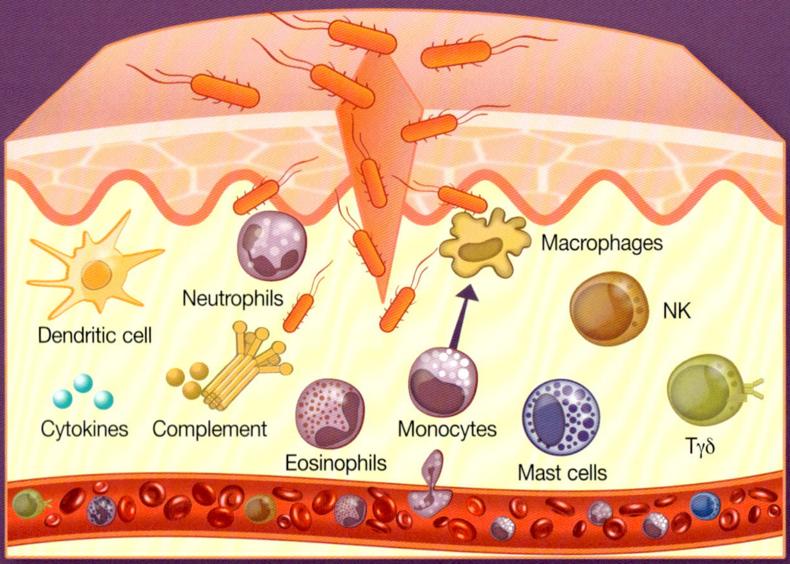

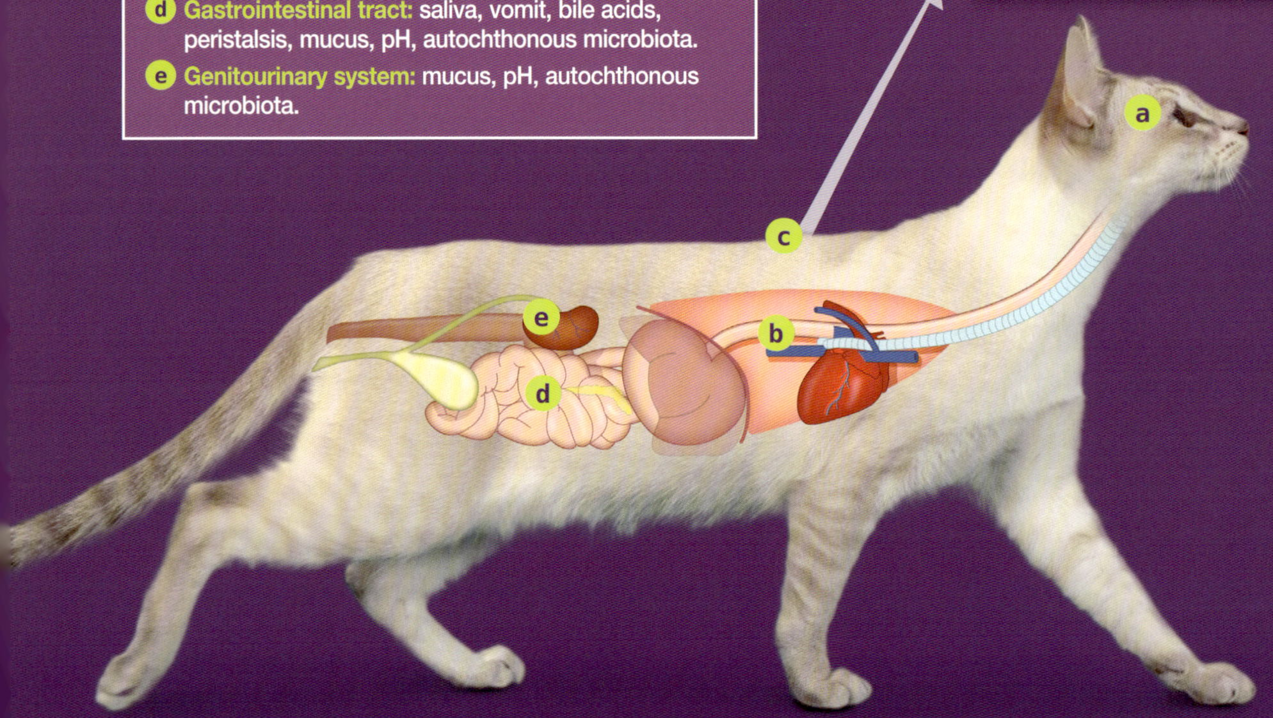

2 When a foreign Ag surpasses the surface barriers, internal innate immunity components and mechanisms are activated.

3 **Internal innate components** are cells (monocytes, macrophages, polymorphonuclear granulocytes, dendritic cells, mast cells, NK cells, intraepithelial $\gamma\delta$ T lymphocytes) and soluble factors (the complement system and certain cytokines such as IFN and TNF).

INNATE IMMUNITY INTERNAL MECHANISMS

4 Internal innate mechanisms include **phagocytosis** (see Chart 9), **complement activation**, the **inflammatory response** (see Chart 7), and the removal of altered cells by **NK cells**.

CYTOTOXICITY MEDIATED BY NK CELLS

5 NK cells are activated by IL-12 produced by the APC. NK cells are innate-surveillance cells with multiple functions; its main function being to destroy abnormal cells much earlier than the acquired immune response is generated.

6 NK cells express **inhibition receptors**, which identify MHC-I, and **activating receptors**, that bind to proteins expressed only on altered cells. The loss of balance between both types of receptors stimulates the secretion of perforins, granulolysins and NK-lysins, which destroy the target cell and activate its apoptosis.

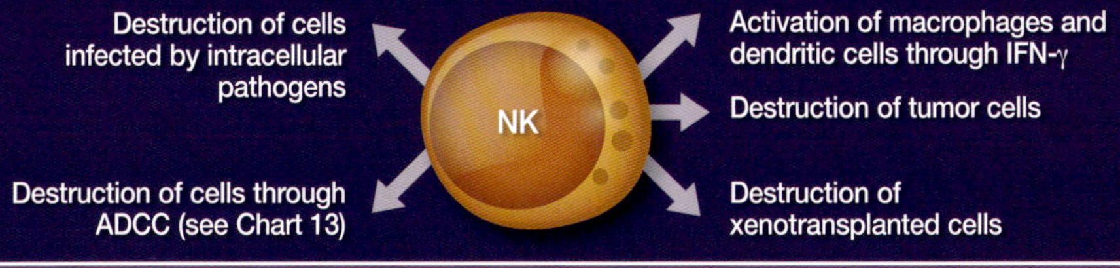

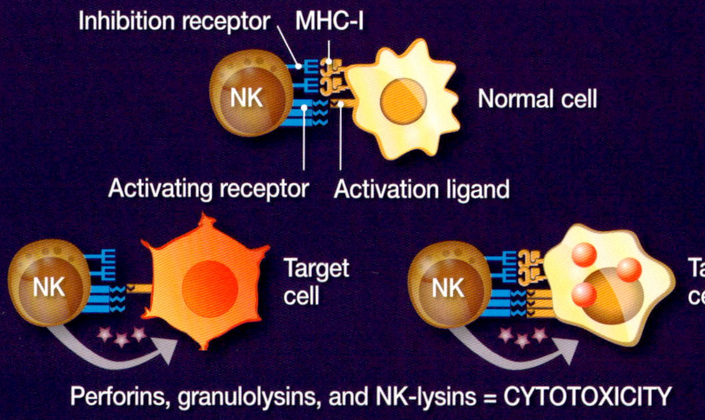

COMPLEMENT SYSTEM

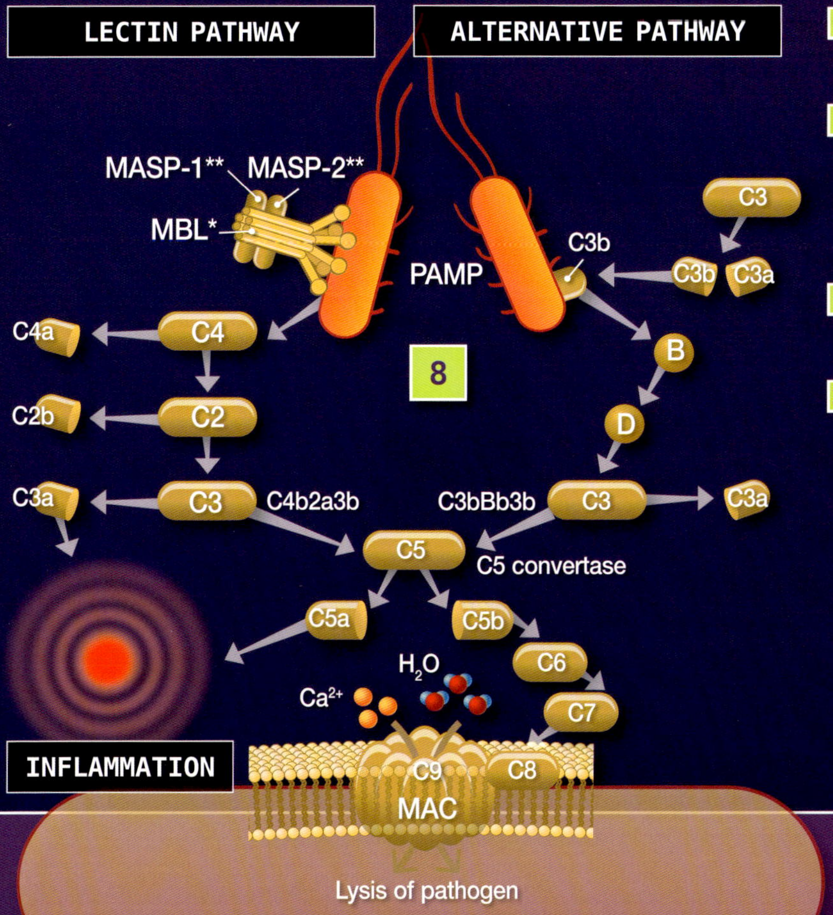

7 The complement system is an essential component of the innate and acquired immune systems. It consists of more than 30 different proteins present in plasma and on the surface of cells, which are designed numerically with the prefix C, or with letters (B, D, P).

8 In the presence of microbial components (PAMP), the complement is activated directly through the **alternative** or through the **lectin pathways**. It is also activated after the formation of immune complexes (through the classical pathway, see Chart 13). Complement activation begins enzymatic cascade routes which culminate in the formation of the **membrane attack complex (MAC)** on the surface of the pathogen, thus, destroying it.

9 Deficiencies in any of the components of the complement system can cause increased susceptibility to infections, such as the recessive autosomal deficiency of C3 described in some dogs of the breed Britanny Spaniel (see Chart 23).

10 Activation of the complement system also plays a fundamental role in inflammation (see Chart 7), in the regulation of the acquired immune system, and in the maintenance of homeostasis.

FUNCTIONS OF THE COMPLEMENT SYSTEM

Innate immunity	Acquired immunity	Homeostasis
• Opsonization. • Lysis of pathogens. • Chemotaxis. • Inflammation. • Cell activation.	• Removal of immune complexes and apoptotic cells.	• Increase of the humoral response. • Activation of T cell responses. • Removal of autoreactive B cells.

* MBL: Mannose-Binding Lectin.

** MASP-1 y MASP-2: Mannose-Associated Serine Protease.

ADAPTIVE IMMUNE RESPONSE

The characteristics of the adaptive immune response (specific or acquired) are specificity, memory (stronger in successive exposures to the Ag), great diversity (it responds to a great variety of Ag), and self-limitation (decreasing after the Ag is no longer present). These responses are dual: HUMORAL, mediated by Ab secreted by B cells after they differentiate into plasma cells; and CELLULAR, mediated by cytotoxic T cells (Tc). Ab are effective against extracellular Ag (extracellular bacteria, viruses, toxins, etc.). Tc destroy cells infected by intracellular pathogens and tumor-like cells.

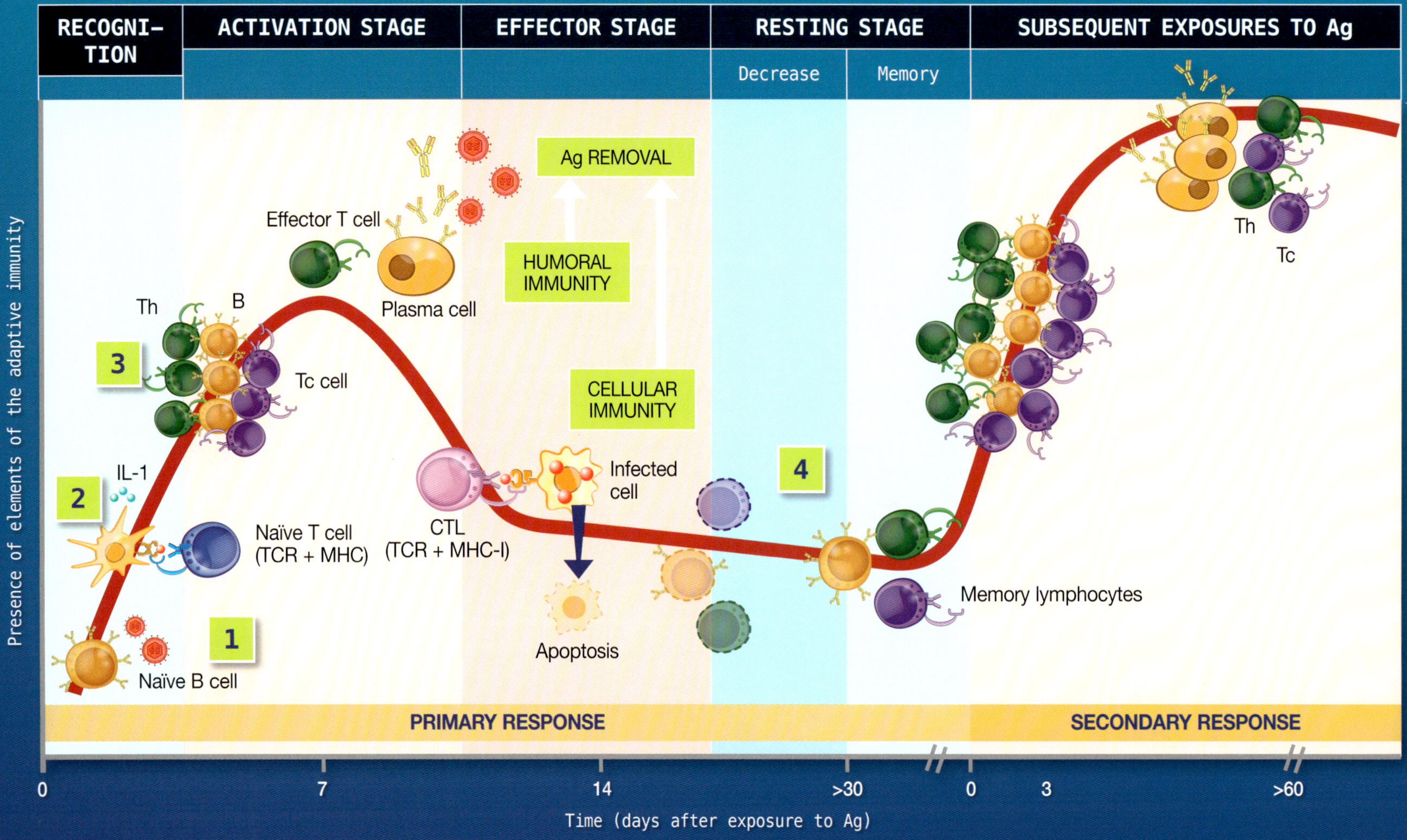

1 The adaptive immune response begins when a naïve lymphocyte (T or B) specifically recognizes an Ag. This recognition induces its **clonal** multiplication (all of its descendants have the same receptors for the Ag as those of the original lymphocyte), and its **differentiation into effector cells**.

2 The antigen presenting cells (APC) present the Ag peptides associated with the molecules of the MHC to the T cells (as T cells do not recognize free peptides): endogenous Ag combine with MHC-I molecules and exogenous Ag with the MHC-II molecules (see Chart 8).

3 T cells differentiate into two major subpopulations: **T helper** (Th, CD4+) and **T cytotoxic** (Tc, CD8+) cells.

4 Once the Ag is eliminated, most of the effector lymphocytes die by apoptosis and the homeostasis (the resting state) is recovered. **Memory lymphocytes** are usually generated. They are responsible for the secondary response raised after subsequent exposures to the same Ag.

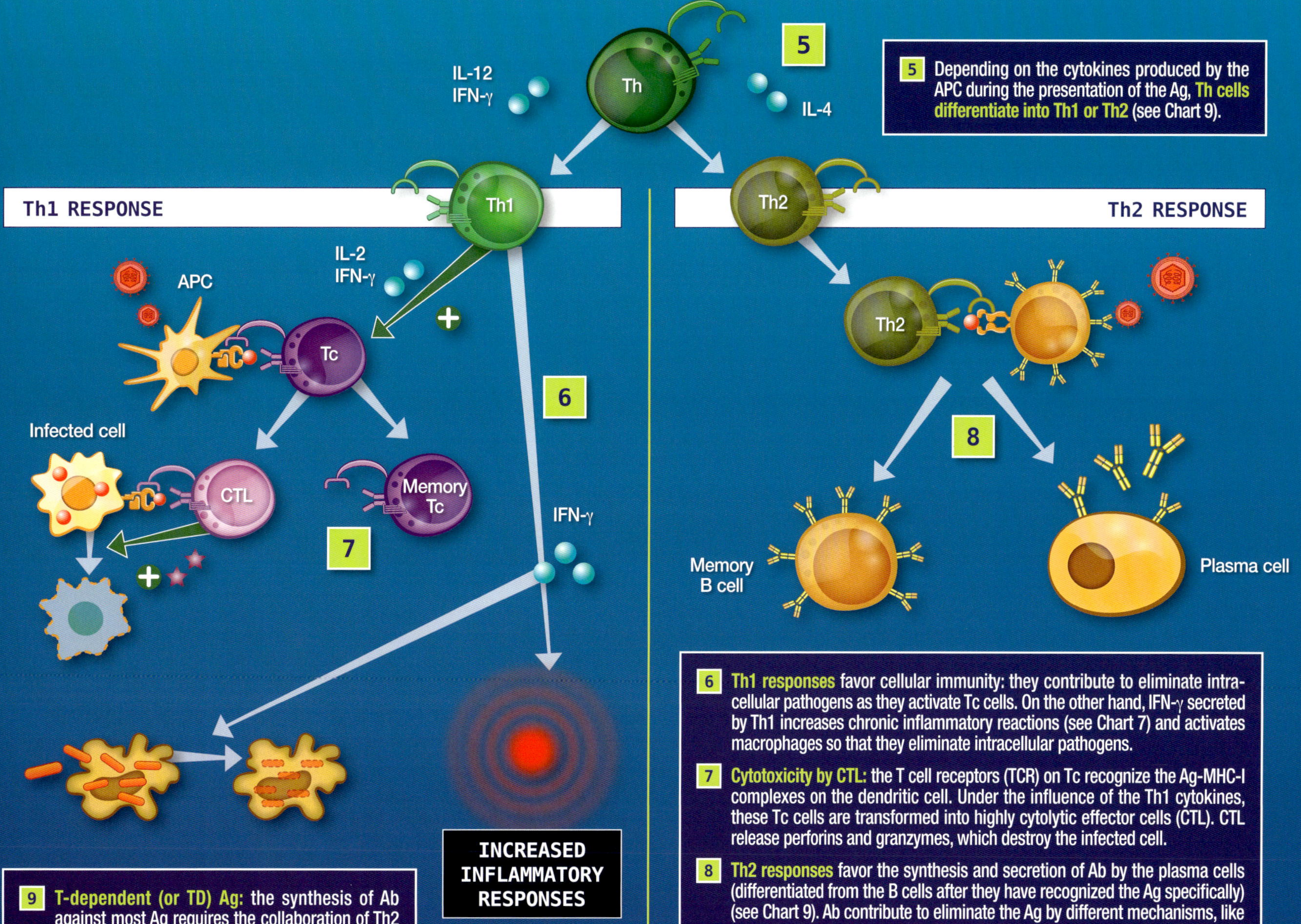

5 Depending on the cytokines produced by the APC during the presentation of the Ag, **Th cells differentiate into Th1 or Th2** (see Chart 9).

6 **Th1 responses** favor cellular immunity: they contribute to eliminate intracellular pathogens as they activate Tc cells. On the other hand, IFN-γ secreted by Th1 increases chronic inflammatory reactions (see Chart 7) and activates macrophages so that they eliminate intracellular pathogens.

7 **Cytotoxicity by CTL:** the T cell receptors (TCR) on Tc recognize the Ag-MHC-I complexes on the dendritic cell. Under the influence of the Th1 cytokines, these Tc cells are transformed into highly cytolytic effector cells (CTL). CTL release perforins and granzymes, which destroy the infected cell.

8 **Th2 responses** favor the synthesis and secretion of Ab by the plasma cells (differentiated from the B cells after they have recognized the Ag specifically) (see Chart 9). Ab contribute to eliminate the Ag by different mechanisms, like neutralization, lysis in combination with the complement, etc. (see Chart 13).

9 **T-dependent (or TD) Ag:** the synthesis of Ab against most Ag requires the collaboration of Th2 cells and B cells, following the scheme shown on the left. The secondary response against these is of greater intensity than the primary one due to the permanence of memory lymphocytes. TD Ag are proteinaceous.

10 **T-independent (or TI) Ag:** other Ag (like lipopolysaccharides) can directly stimulate B cells to produce Ab without the requirement for T cell help. Memory lymphocytes are not produced, and thus, the secondary responses and the primary ones are of equal intensity.

11 In TD Ag, the primary response is characterized by a high relative IgM concentration, whereas in the secondary response, in addition to being of greater intensity, the proportion of IgG is greater.

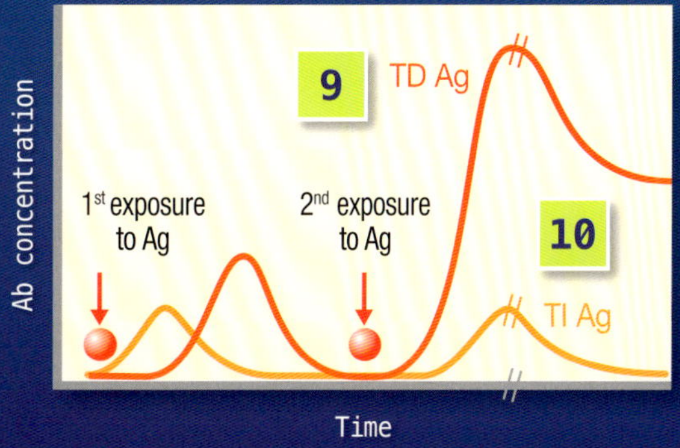

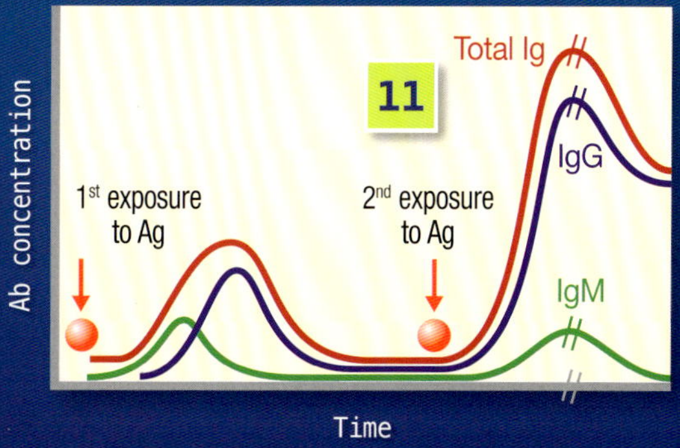

IMMUNOGLOBULINS

Immunoglobulins (Ig) or antibodies (Ab) are glycoproteins that are produced by plasma cells in response to an antigen (Ag), with which they can react specifically. The Ig are the B cell receptors (BCR) once secreted to the extracellular environment (see Chart 3), and are the mediators of the humoral response. They are mainly in the blood, but can also be in other body fluids (milk, saliva), and in the mucosal surfaces.

1 An immunoglobulin has a four chain structure as its basic unit. It is composed of two identical heavy chains (H) and two identical light chains (L). The chains are held together by inter- and intra-chain disulfide bonds. The hinge region confers certain flexibility to the Ig.

2 Each chain consists of a variable (V) and a constant (C) region. The Ag binds with the variable region of the Ig, where specificity resides. Comparisons of the amino acid sequences of V shows three complementarity determining regions (CDR), which form the paratope or site for binding the epitope (sequence of the Ag specifically recognized by the Ig).

3 Immunoglobulins are folded into globular regions (domains): two in the L chains (V_L, C_L) and 4 or 5 in the H chains (V_H, C_H1, C_H2, C_H3 and C_H4), according to the Ig isotype.

STRUCTURE OF THE Ig

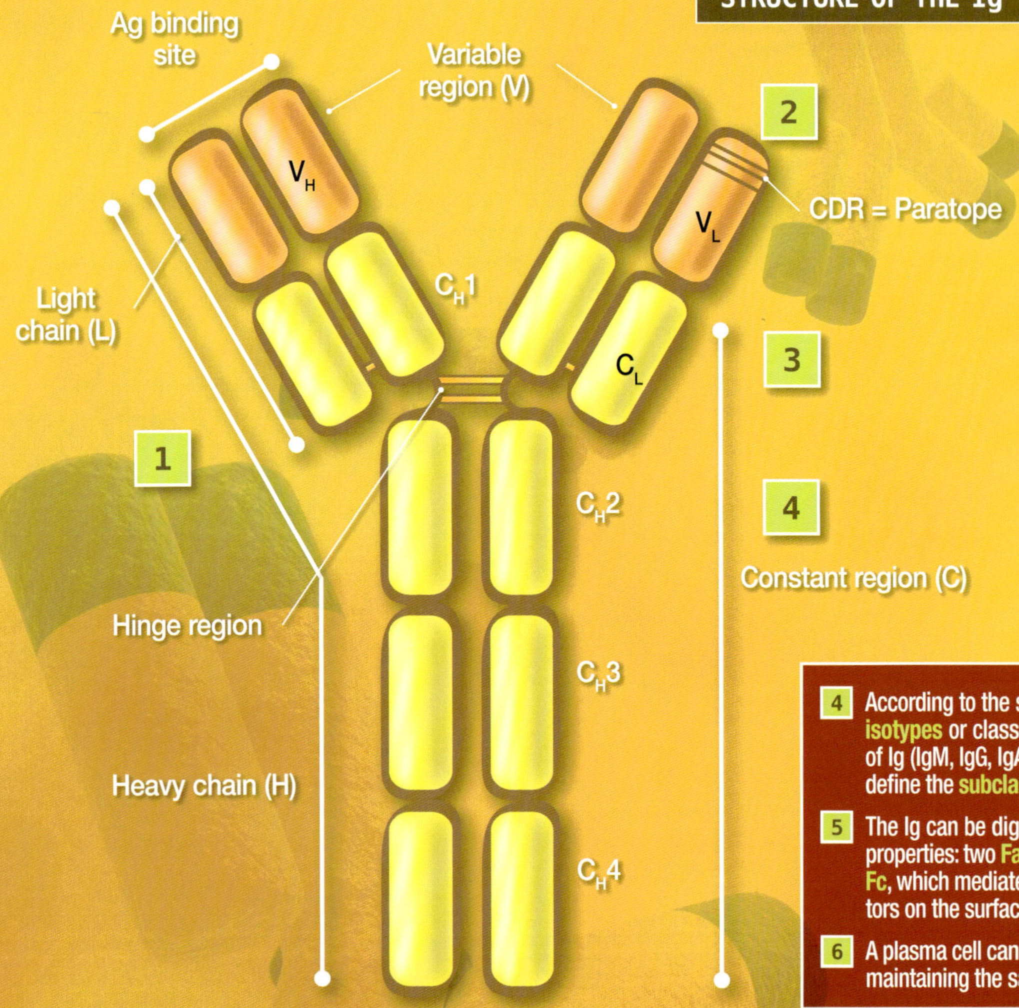

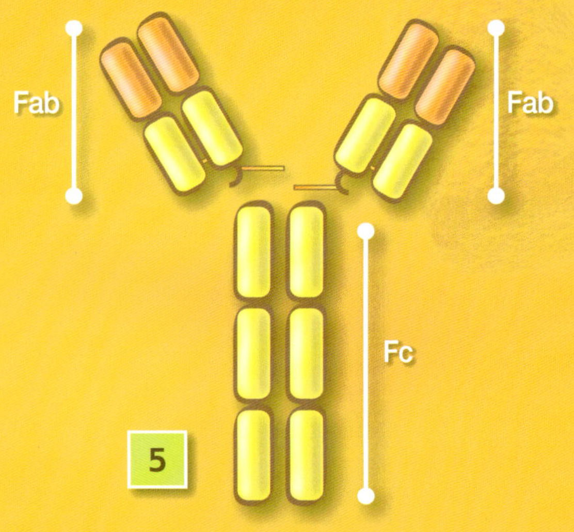

4 According to the sequence of the constant region, heavy chains may be classified into five isotypes or classes, called by Greek letters (μ, γ, α, ε, δ). They form the different classes of Ig (IgM, IgG, IgA, IgE, IgD). Additionally, the small variations of the amino acid sequences define the subclasses, which vary in dogs and cats.

5 The Ig can be digested by proteolytic enzymes in three fragments with different biological properties: two Fab fractions (fragment of Ag binding site) and an easily crystallized fraction, Fc, which mediates the biological functions of the Ig. The Fc is recognized by the FcR receptors on the surface of different cells of the immune system (see Charts 3 and 5).

6 A plasma cell can secrete different Ig isotypes throughout the immune response, but always maintaining the same idiotype (specificity for the Ag).

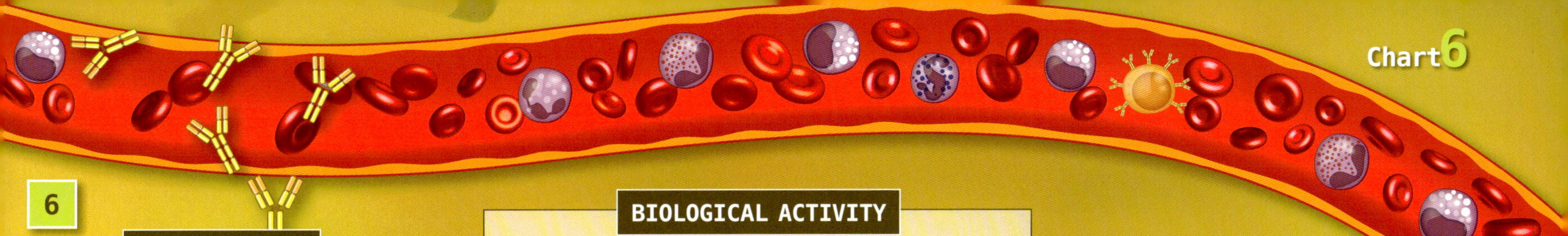

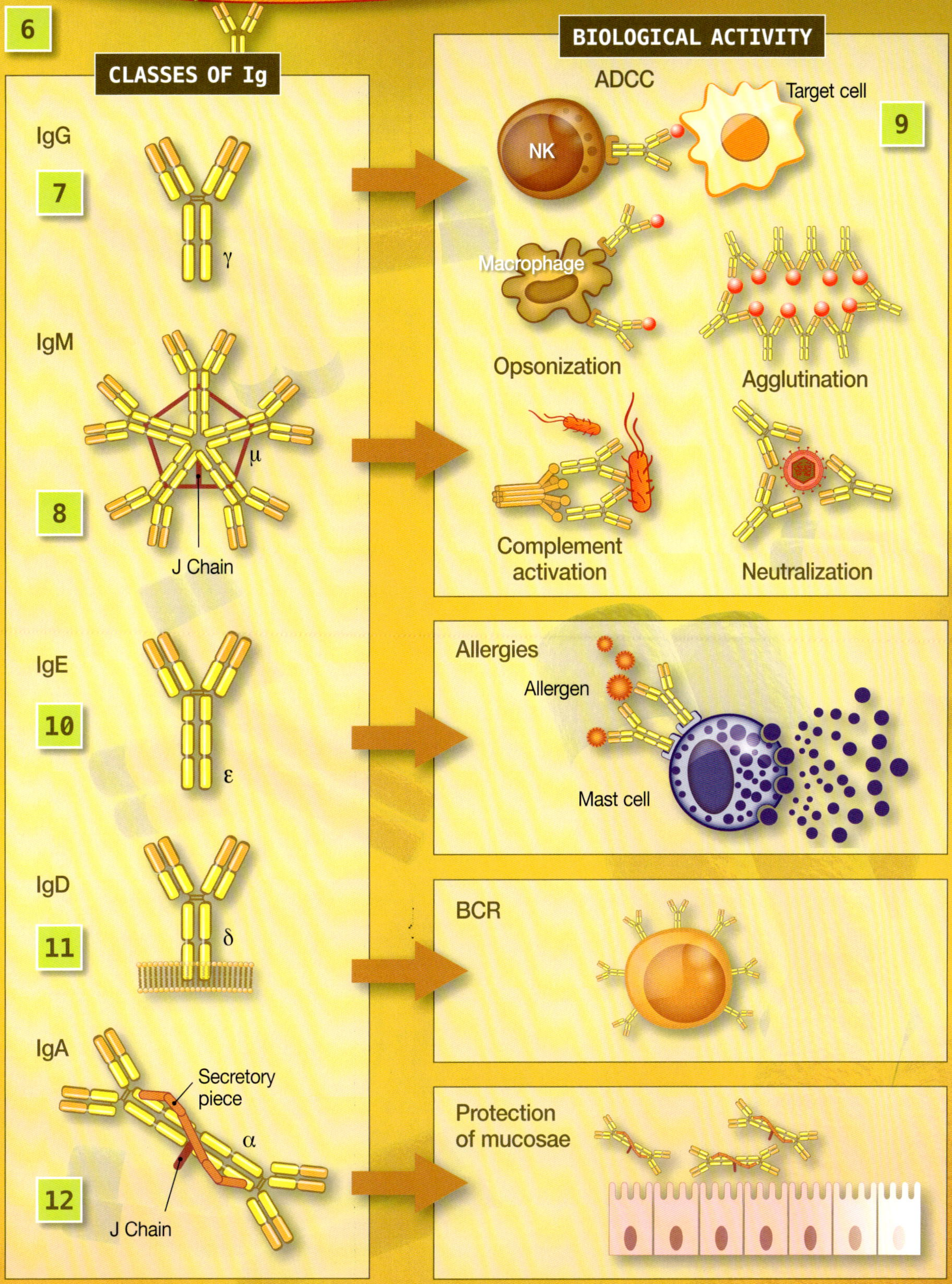

7 **IgG.** Major isotype in the blood and characteristic of the secondary responses (see Chart 5). They are monomers and can cross blood vessels. Four subclasses have been identified in dogs and cats (IgG1-IgG4), and only a small percentage may cross the placenta (see Chart 12).

8 **IgM.** Characteristic isotype of the primary responses (see Chart 5). They are pentamers stabilized by disulfide bonds and with a small peptide (J chain). Its great size prevents them from leaving the circulatory system, but they can cross epithelia by the union of J chain to the epithelial cells.

9 IgG and IgM participate in neutralization, agglutination, precipitation and enhancement of phagocytosis (as opsonins) of Ag, as well as in processes of ADCC (Antibody-Dependent Cellular Cytotoxicity). IgM may activate complement by the classical pathway (see Charts 5 and 13).

10 **IgE.** Characteristic isotype of **allergies** (see Chart 21) and of the protection against helminths (see Chart 18). They combine with their specific receptors (FcεR) on the surface of certain cells, like the mast cells. Two subclasses have been identified in dogs and cats (IgE1 and IgE2).

11 **IgD.** Isotype present exclusively as surface Ig (BCR). IgD has not been identified in cats.

12 **IgA.** Usually present in body secretions as a dimer. It is protected from proteolysis by a peptide, called **secretory piece**, which also helps the IgA to be transported across mucosa, where it participates in immunological defense, neutralizing pathogens (see Chart 11).

LOCAL AND GENERAL INFLAMMATION

The aims of inflammation are to destroy pathogens, prevent the spread of an infection or tissue damage, and repair damaged tissue. If the infection is not removed, cells and accumulated fluid drain into local lymph nodes, where acquired immune responses are triggered.

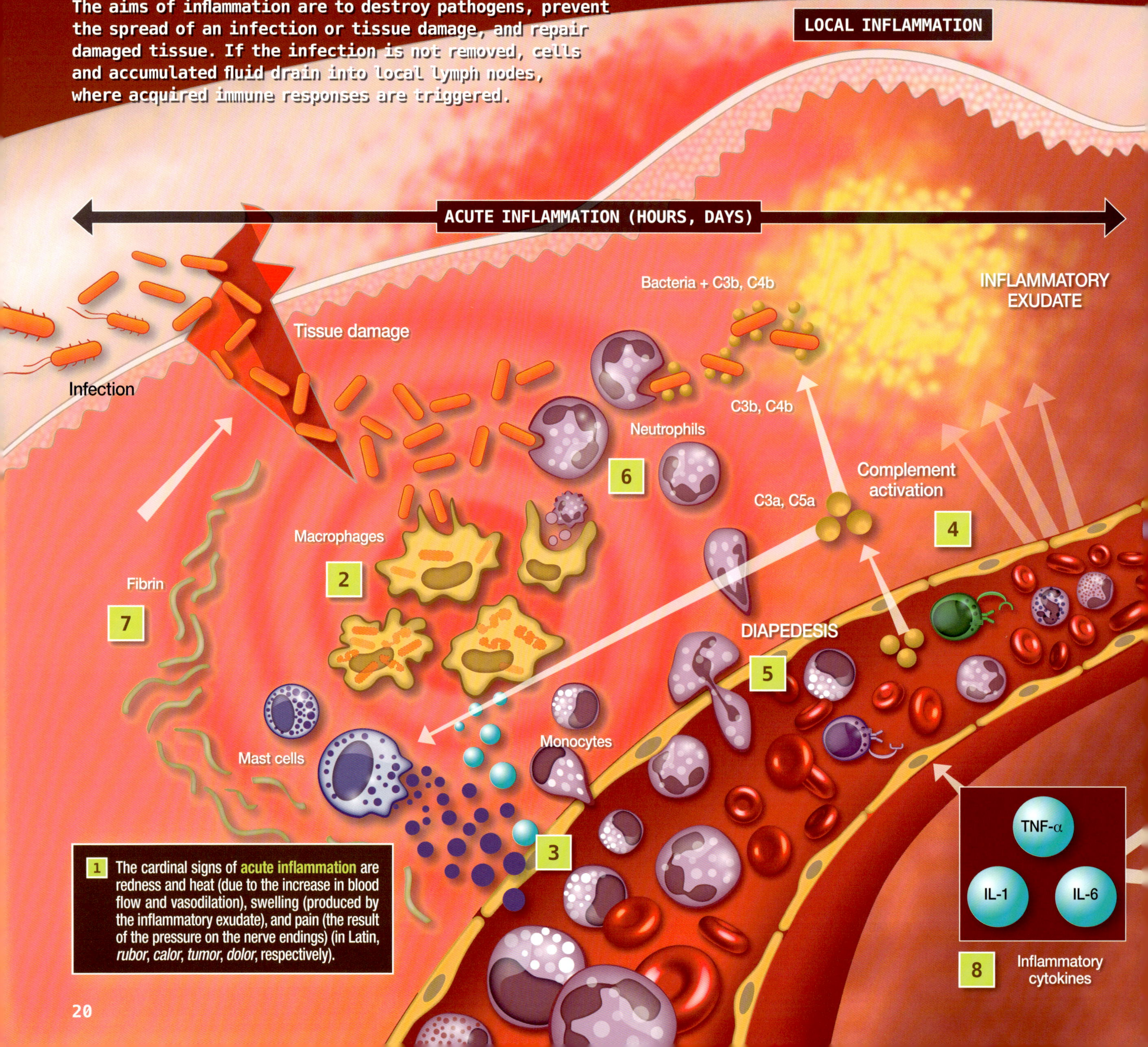

1 The cardinal signs of acute inflammation are redness and heat (due to the increase in blood flow and vasodilation), swelling (produced by the inflammatory exudate), and pain (the result of the pressure on the nerve endings) (in Latin, *rubor*, *calor*, *tumor*, *dolor*, respectively).

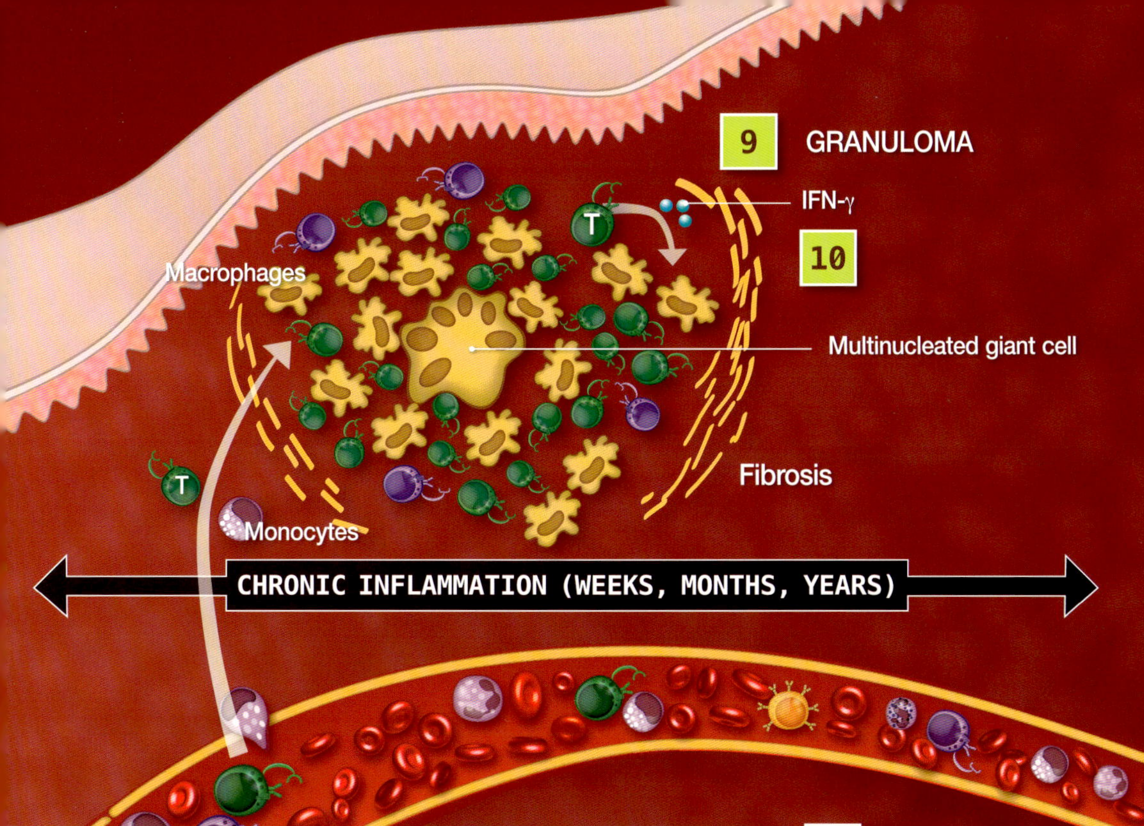

SYSTEMIC INFLAMMATION OR ACUTE-PHASE RESPONSE **11**

Hypothalamus	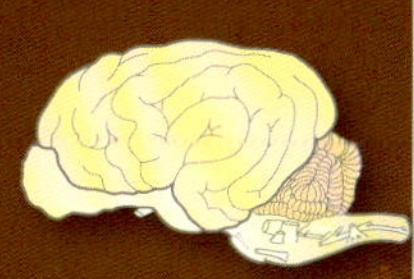	• Fever. • Somnolence. • Loss of appetite.	Body conditions which favor the defense against pathogens.
Bone marrow	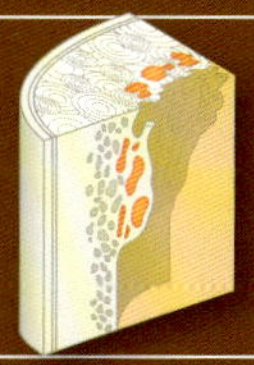	Leukocytosis (neutrophilia).	Phagocytosis and destruction of pathogens.
Liver	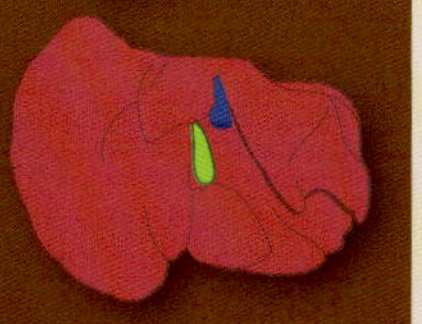	Increased plasma concentration of acute-phase proteins: • C-Reactive Protein (CRP). • Serum amyloid. • Haptoglobin.	• Opsonization and chemotaxis (promoting phagocytosis). • Binding and sequester of plasma iron.

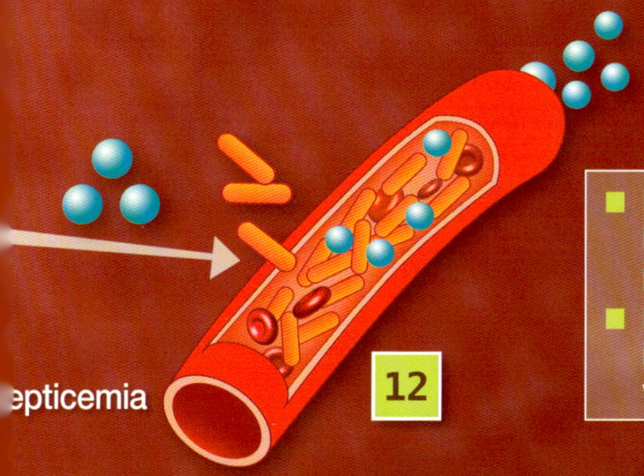

- Increase in vascular permeability
- Increase in general vasodilation

→

- SHOCK
- Disseminated intravascular coagulation (DIC)

→ **DEATH**

2 Tissue macrophages phagocyte and destroy microorganisms, apoptotic neutrophils, and injured tissue debris. In addition, activated macrophages release chemokines and inflammatory cytokines that attract phagocytes to the site of infection by a concentration gradient (**chemotaxis**).

3 Vasoactive molecules (histamines, prostaglandins and leukotrienes) produce vasodilation and increased vascular permeability, allowing plasma leakage (**inflammatory exudate**).

4 The activation of complement releases fractions C3a and C5a (**chemoattractants and anaphylatoxins**), that activate mast cells and endothelial cells promoting the inflammatory response, and C3b and C4b that **opsonize** microorganisms, improving phagocytosis.

5 Phagocytes, attracted by chemotaxis, attach through their integrins (CD11/CD18) to adhesion molecules on endothelial cells (selectins) and migrate between these cells into the tissue (**diapedesis**). Neutrophils migrate first, and 24 hours later monocytes migrate (which differentiate to macrophages).

6 Neutrophils engulf and destroy the microorganisms.

7 Lastly, the coagulation and fibrinolytic systems are activated. This prevents the spread of the focus of infection and facilitates the repair of damaged tissue.

8 IL-1, IL-6 and TNF-α are the **"inflammatory cytokines"** synthesized by the macrophages. Locally, they induce the increase of the vascular permeability and the expression of selectins by endothelial cells. TNF-α activates the formation of clots, preventing the spread of the infection into the bloodstream.

9 **Inflammation becomes chronic** if the microorganisms and particles are difficult to eliminate or degrade. A **granuloma** develops which contains abundant macrophages and T cells. This is the case of immune responses against many pathogens, such as mycobacteria (see Chart 15) and Type IV hypersensitivity against certain particles, such as asbestos (see Chart 21).

10 IFN-γ, released by T cells, induces activated macrophages to phagocyte persistently and to secrete cytokines that attract more cells.

11 Local inflammation is accompanied by a systemic response to protect the whole body. This is termed **"ACUTE-PHASE RESPONSE"** and is coordinated by inflammatory cytokines.

12 In septicemia or after massive tissue damage, very large amounts of inflammatory cytokines, mainly TNF-α, are released into the bloodstream affecting all the small blood vessels of the organism, which may lead to **death**.

PHAGOCYTOSIS AND ANTIGEN PRESENTATION

Phagocytosis is an innate immune mechanism carried out by neutrophils and macrophages, which are able to detect, ingest and destroy antigens.

The presentation of Ag, essential to initiate the activation of the T cells, is performed by macrophages and dendritic cells, and to a lesser extent by B cells. After capturing the Ag, this is processed into small peptides that are expressed together with MHC-II molecules. It is a fundamental process that connects the innate and adaptive immune responses. In addition, any altered cell can present antigens linked to its MHC-I.

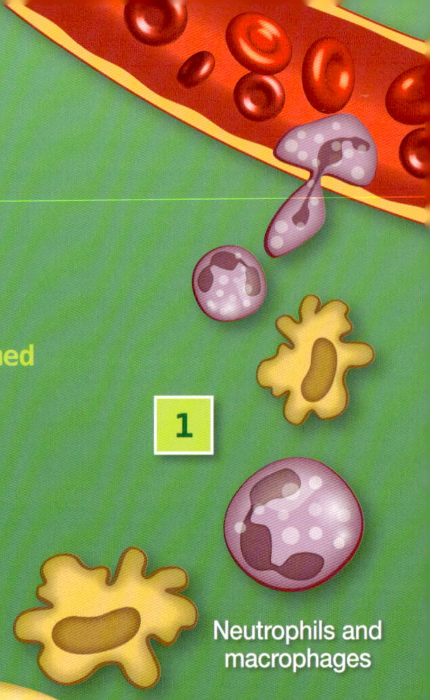

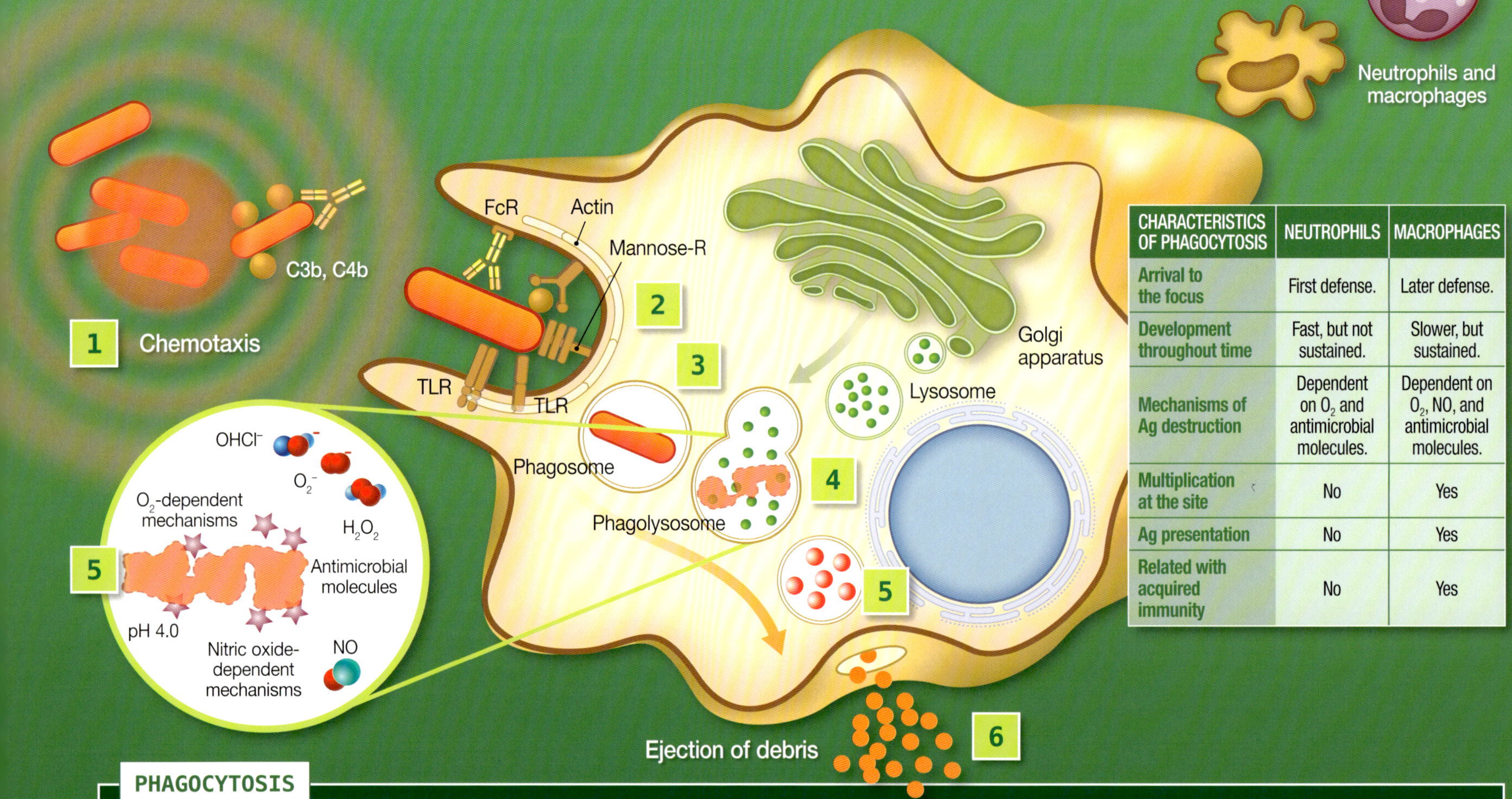

CHARACTERISTICS OF PHAGOCYTOSIS	NEUTROPHILS	MACROPHAGES
Arrival to the focus	First defense.	Later defense.
Development throughout time	Fast, but not sustained.	Slower, but sustained.
Mechanisms of Ag destruction	Dependent on O_2 and antimicrobial molecules.	Dependent on O_2, NO, and antimicrobial molecules.
Multiplication at the site	No	Yes
Ag presentation	No	Yes
Related with acquired immunity	No	Yes

PHAGOCYTOSIS

1 **Chemotaxis.** Attraction of phagocytes by chemotactic factors, such as molecules of the complement systems (C3a, C5a), bacterial products (LPS), derivates of fibrinogen, alarmins, defensins, and chemokines produced by macrophages and other cells (see Chart 7).

2 **Adhesion** of the Ag to receptors present in phagocytes, such as TLR, mannose receptors, opsonin receptors (Ab, factors C3b and C4b of the complement system), fibronectin and collagen receptors.

3 **Ingestion** of the Ag by inclusion in an intracellular vesicle (**phagosome**).

4 **Fusion** of lysosomes with the phagosome resulting in the **phagolysosome**.

5 **Destruction** of the Ag by powerful oxidizing radicals and the action of antimicrobial molecules (lysozyme, hydrolases, cationic proteases, lactoferrin and defensins). Activated macrophages and neutrophils transform the O_2 in microbicidal reactive oxygen species (ROS), a process called "respiratory burst". Only activated macrophages produce the highly toxic nitric oxide (NO) derivates.

6 Non-self material is **ejected** after its degradation. Macrophages can also present processed peptides combined with the MHC-II to specific Th cells.

ANTIGEN PRESENTATION

7 T cells recognize and react with the Ag only if it is processed and associated with MHC-II molecules (Th cells) or MHC-I (Tc cells). There are two routes of Ag-MHC presentation: **exogenous route** for the Th cells, and **endogenous route** for the Tc cells.

EXOGENOUS ROUTE (APC)

ENDOGENOUS ROUTE (APC and nucleated cells)

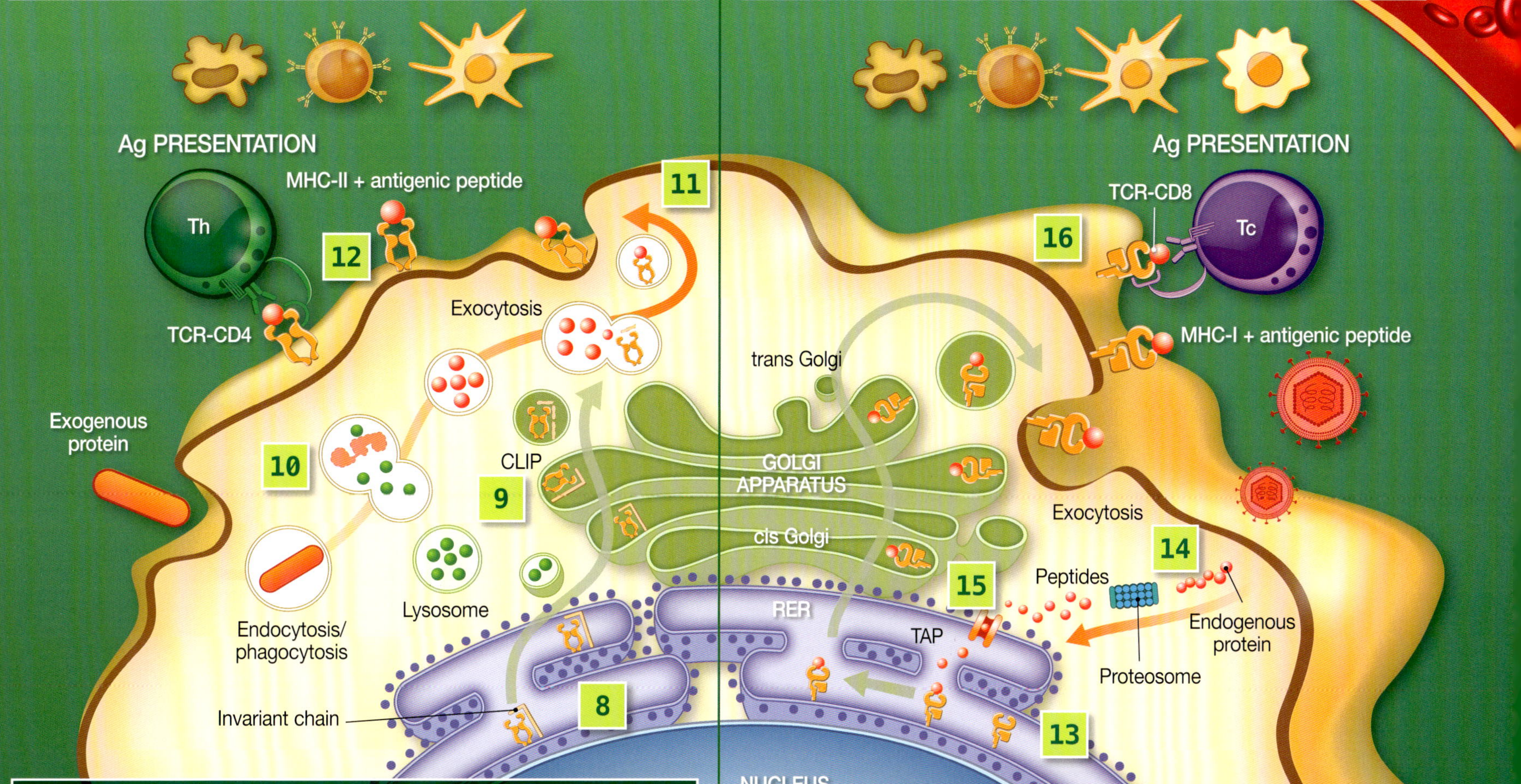

8 Synthesis of the MHC-II molecule in the rough endoplasmic reticulum (RER), associated with a peptide called invariant chain (Ii), which prevents the binding of antigenic peptides to the MHC-II.

9 Transfer of the MHC-II + Ii molecules to the Golgi apparatus and to endosomal vesicles. Digestion of the Ii polypeptide, leaving a residue (CLIP*) associated with the Ag-binding groove.

10 Entry of exogenous Ag (through endocytosis or phagocytosis) and digestion into peptide fragments. Fusion of the endosomes with the vesicles carrying MHC-II + CLIP.

11 Replacement of the CLIP of the MHC-II by an antigenic peptide, and subsequent translocation to the cell surface. Expression (**presentation**) of the peptide-MHC-II complexes on the APC.

12 Recognition of **peptide-MHC-II complex by the TCR-CD4 of the Th cell specific** to each antigenic peptide presented.

13 Synthesis of the MHC-I molecule in the RER.

14 Processing of endogenous Ag (such as molecules of intracellular pathogens in infected cells, or altered-self cellular proteins in the case of tumors) in the proteosome, resulting in peptides.

15 Transport of peptides to the lumen of the RER using the TAP** molecule and binding to the MHC-I. The complex peptide-MHC-I proceeds to the Golgi apparatus and from there to the cell surface.

16 Presentation of endogenous peptides associated with the MHC-I on the cells. Recognition **by the TCR-CD8 of Tc cells specific** to each antigenic peptide presented.

*CLIP: CLass II-associated Invariant chain Peptide.
**TAP: Transporter Associated with antigen Processing.

COOPERATION IN IMMUNE RESPONSES

The innate and acquired immune responses are intimately interconnected, and numerous cooperative actions and signals take place between both. Also, there is a close connection between humoral and cell-mediated acquired responses. Antigen presenting cells (APC), T helper cells (Th) and cytokines are the main protagonists in the cooperation.

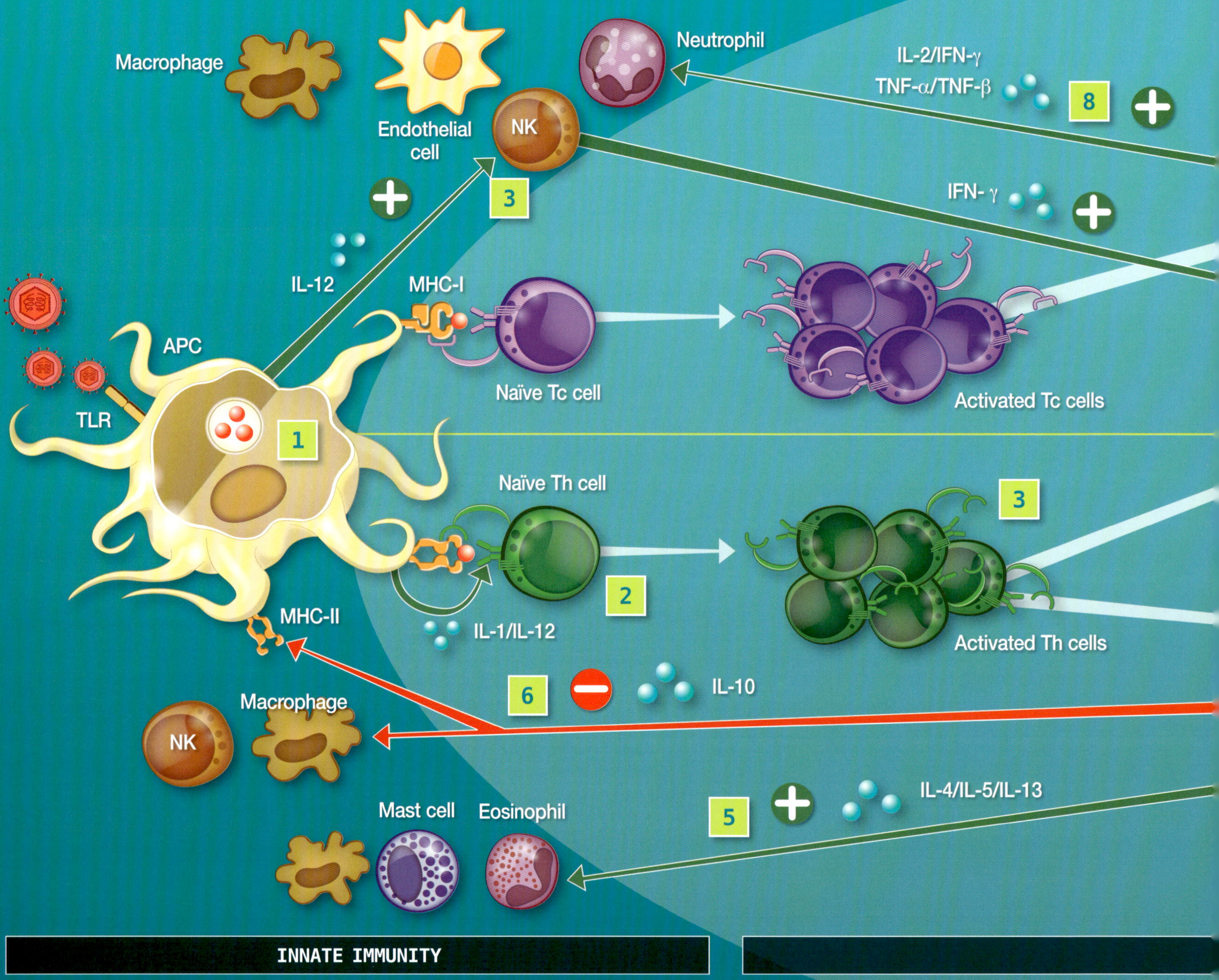

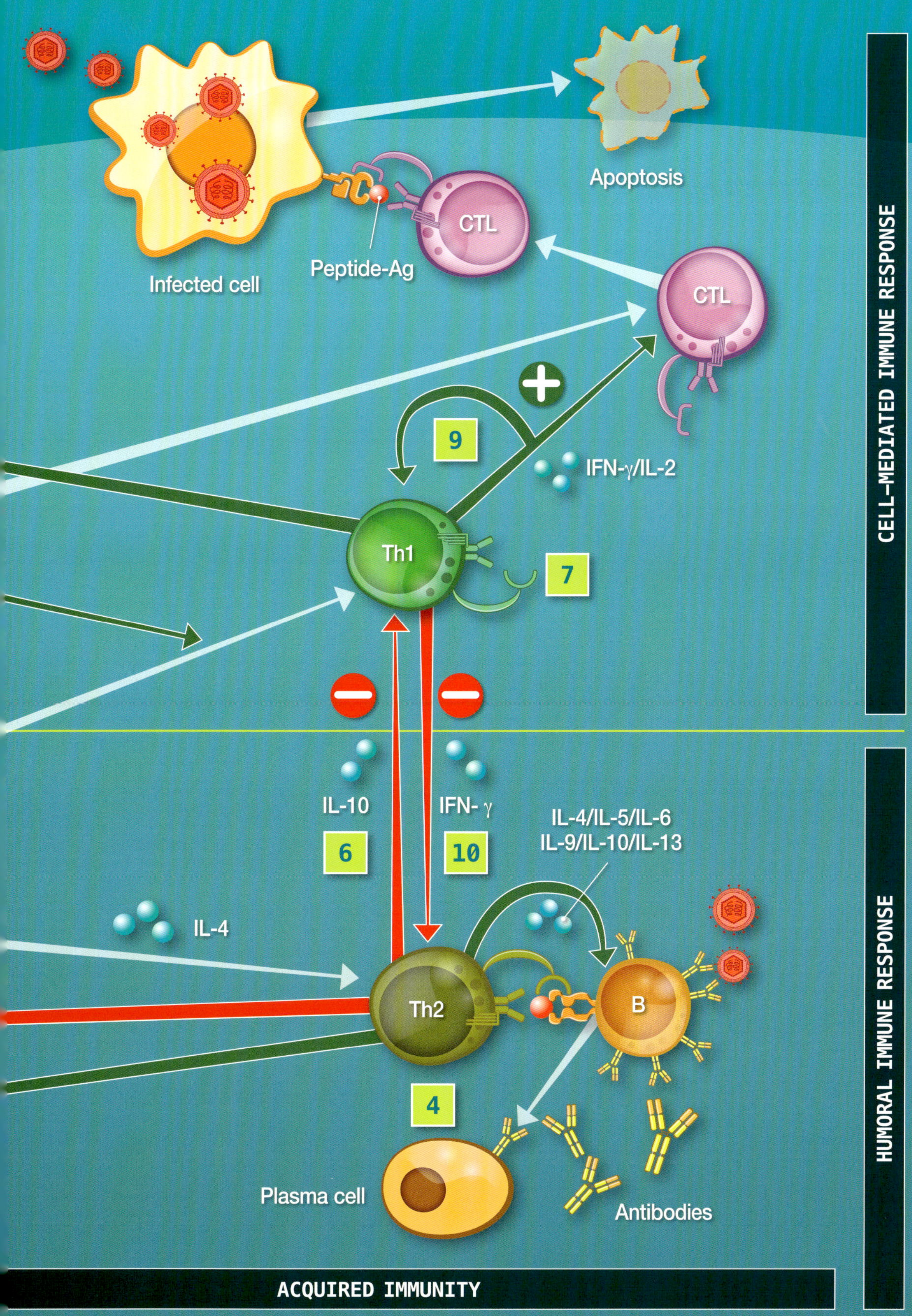

1 APC (especially dendritic cells, DC) process and bind antigenic peptides to their MHC-II for their presentation to the Th cells, and to their MHC-I for their presentation to cytotoxic T cells (Tc).

2 Mature APC secrete polarizing cytokines (IL-1 and IL-12) that act on naïve Th cells, specific to the presented peptide, activating them so that they multiply and differentiate.

3 Activated Th cells differentiate into two subpopulations: Th1 and Th2. IL-1 and IL-2 (secreted by the same Th cells) induce the proliferation of the Th cells. In the presence of IL-4, these Th cells are polarized into the Th2 phenotype. Alternatively, IL-12 (secreted by the APC that has recognized an intracellular antigen) activates naïve Th cells and induces the secretion of IFN-γ by NK cells. Both cytokines are the main polarizing molecules resulting in the Th1 phenotype.

4 Th2 cells establish synapse with the specific B cells and secrete cytokines (IL-4, IL-5, IL-6, IL-9, IL-10 and IL-13) in this synapse, essential for the humoral response (see Chart 5).

5 Several cytokines secreted by Th2 cells activate other cells outside the synapse: IL-5 activates eosinophils; IL-4 activates mast cells, and transforms macrophages into M2 cells with immunosuppressor and antiinflammatory activities; IL-13 and IL-4 stimulate the synthesis of mucus by the Goblet cells and the contraction of the smooth muscle cells.

6 IL-10, synthesized by Th2 cells, inhibits the synthesis of IFN-γ and TNF-α by NK and Th1 cells. Also, IL-10 inhibits the expression of MHC-II and co-stimulatory molecules on dendritic cells and macrophages.

7 Activated Th1 cells participate in cell-mediated immune responses against intracellular Ag by means of the secretion of IFN-γ, TNF-α, TNF-β and IL-2.

8 IFN-γ activates NK cells and macrophages; TNF-β activates neutrophils, macrophages and endothelial cells; TNF-α is a major activator of inflammation; and IL-2 activates NK cells, and stimulates the proliferation of Tc cells and their differentiation to CTL.

9 IFN-γ has an autocrine action on Th1 cells and activates effector Tc cells (CTL), which are in charge of the acquired cell-mediated immune responses.

10 IFN-γ participates in the regulation of the humoral immune response by inhibiting the activity of Th2 cells.

FACTORS THAT AFFECT THE IMMUNE RESPONSES

Self-antigens should not trigger immune reactions. Immunological tolerance is the phenomenon that prevents self-reactivity. The immune response is regulated through both the antigen and the various components of the immune system as well as an individual's factors (age, sex and genetic background). An inadequate regulation can lead to disorders such as immunodeficiency, autoimmunity, hypersensitivity, and other undesirable consequences (abortions, lymphoid tumors).

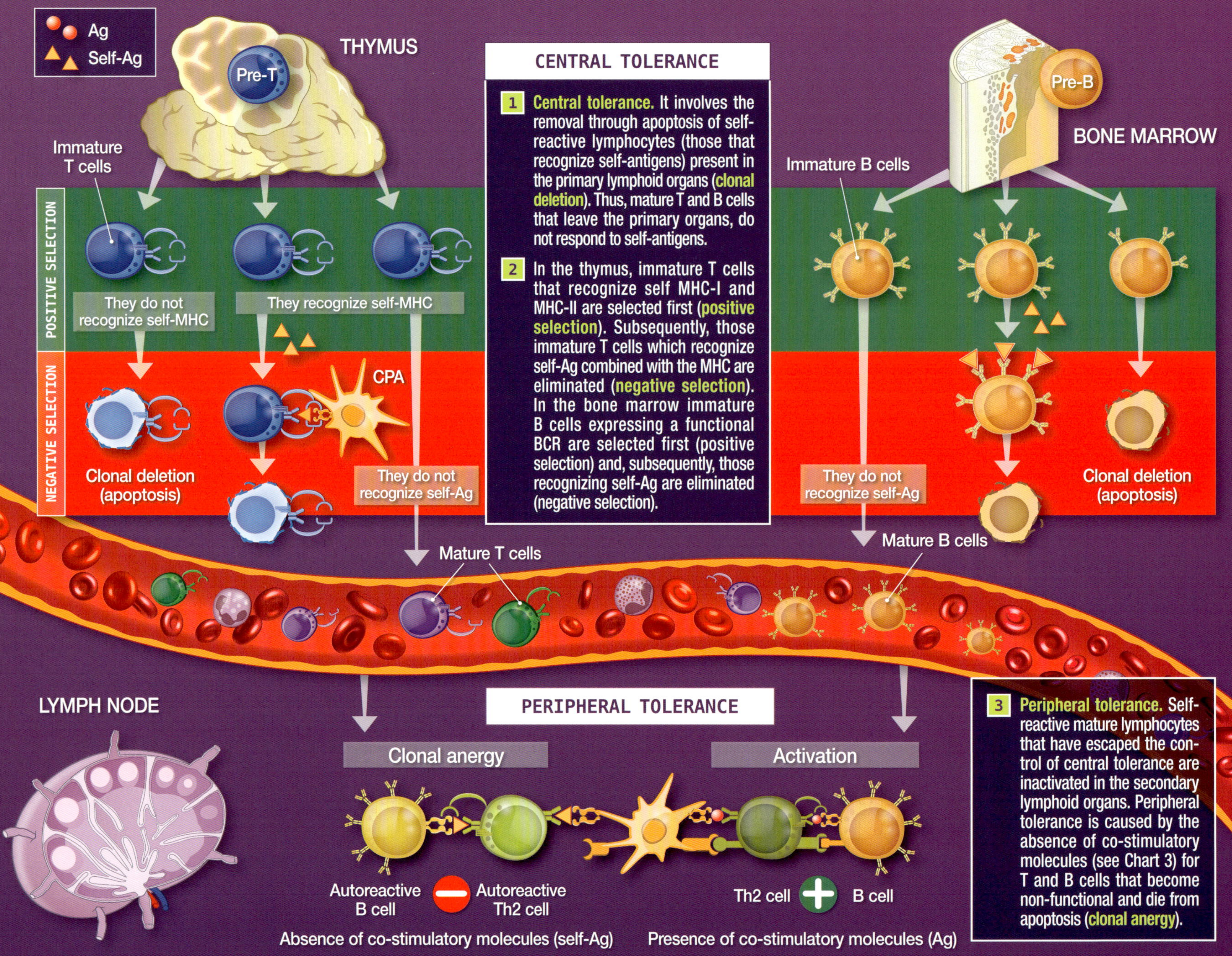

CENTRAL TOLERANCE

1 **Central tolerance.** It involves the removal through apoptosis of self-reactive lymphocytes (those that recognize self-antigens) present in the primary lymphoid organs (**clonal deletion**). Thus, mature T and B cells that leave the primary organs, do not respond to self-antigens.

2 In the thymus, immature T cells that recognize self MHC-I and MHC-II are selected first (**positive selection**). Subsequently, those immature T cells which recognize self-Ag combined with the MHC are eliminated (**negative selection**). In the bone marrow immature B cells expressing a functional BCR are selected first (positive selection) and, subsequently, those recognizing self-Ag are eliminated (negative selection).

PERIPHERAL TOLERANCE

3 **Peripheral tolerance.** Self-reactive mature lymphocytes that have escaped the control of central tolerance are inactivated in the secondary lymphoid organs. Peripheral tolerance is caused by the absence of co-stimulatory molecules (see Chart 3) for T and B cells that become non-functional and die from apoptosis (**clonal anergy**).

REGULATION

4 Antigens. Ag can be immunogenic or tolerogenic (induce tolerance) depending on their quantity (very high or very low doses can induce tolerance), the route of entry (greater immunogenicity by subcutaneous or intramuscular routes) and their persistence.

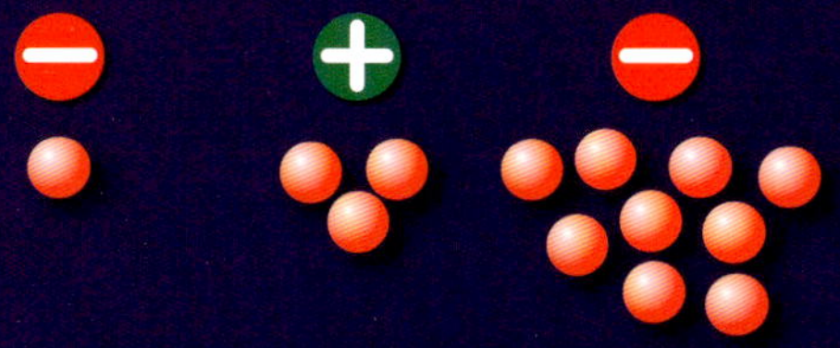

5 Antibodies. Ab can **increase** the immune response by stimulating phagocytosis (see Chart 8). They can also **inhibit** the production of new Ab against an Ag when there are already large amounts of specific Ab against it (negative feedback by Ab). This may prevent successful vaccination in newborn animals due to the presence of maternal Ab (see Chart 41).

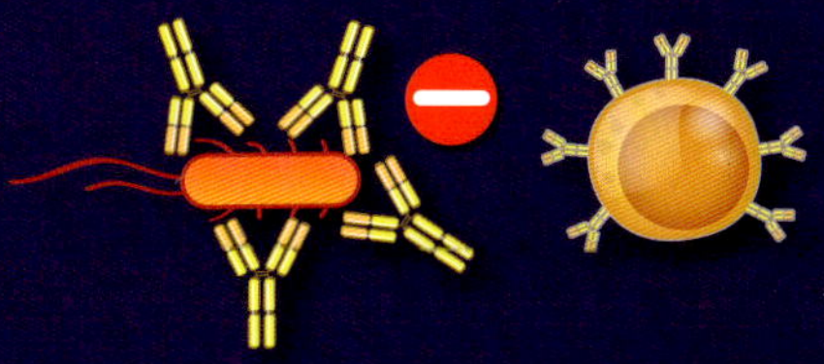

6 Macrophages. When macrophages are activated by IFN-γ they differentiate into proinflammatory M1 cells, whereas when they are activated by IL-4 or IL-13 they differentiate into M2 cells that suppress inflammation and are involved in the induction of tolerance, for instance in the placenta.

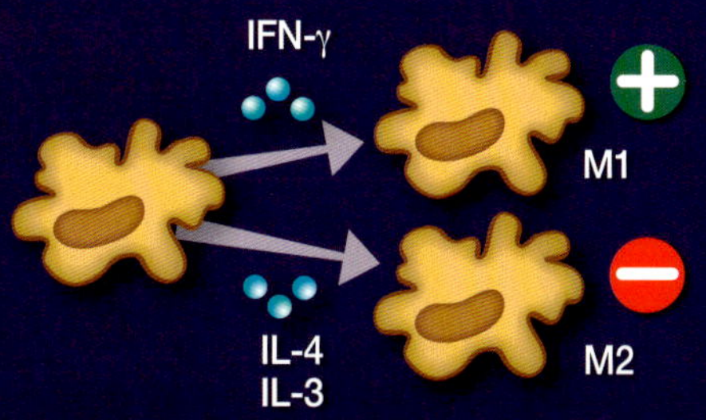

7 T regulatory lymphocytes (Treg). Treg are a subpopulation of T cells (CD4+ CD25+) that control the immune response by suppressing the activation and function of other effector lymphocytes, thus maintaining the homeostasis and self-tolerance. The lack of activity of Treg induces autoimmune diseases (see Chart 22).

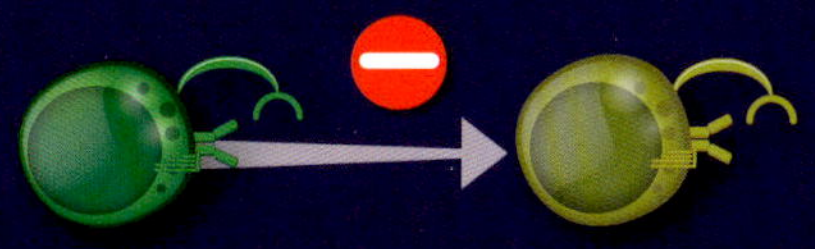

T regulatory cells (CD4+ CD25+)

8 Cytokines. They are the main regulatory molecules of the immune system. The effect of cytokines may be autocrine (on the same secretory cell), paracrine (in neighboring cells), endocrine (on distant cells), synergistic or antagonistic with other cytokines. They are recognized by specific receptors on target cells in which they induce a response. The cytokine environment determines the prevalence of the type of immune response (see Charts 5 and 9).

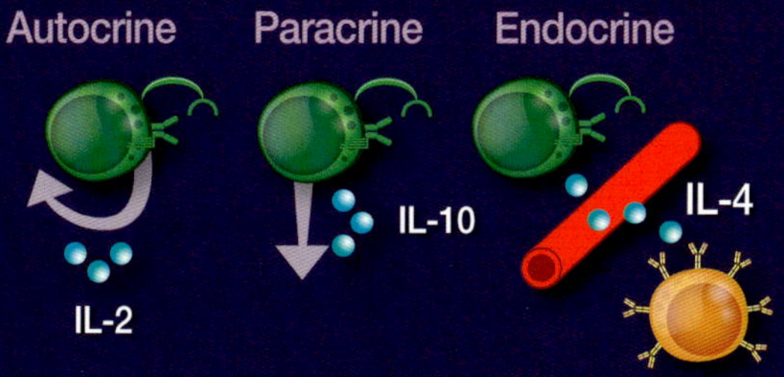

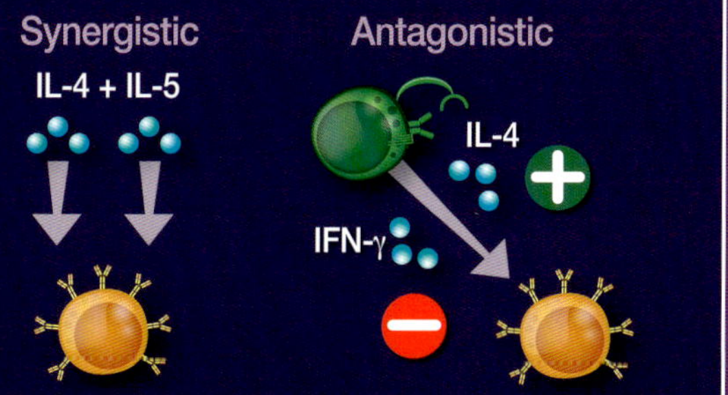

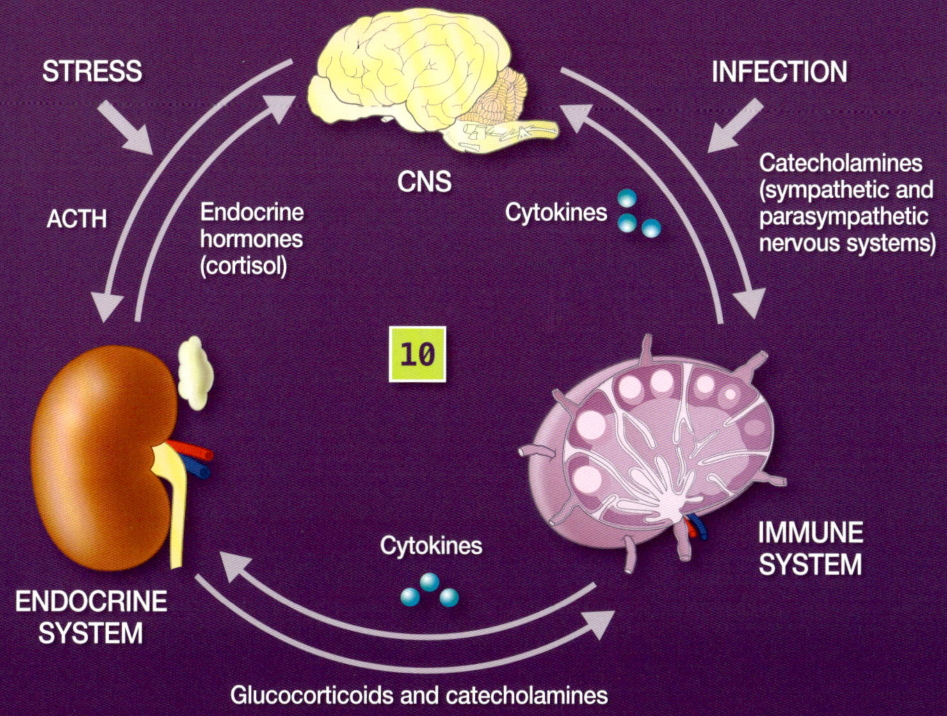

9 Genetic. The immune response depends on the genetic characteristics of the animal. Some relevant genes in immunity are those which encode the MHC, which influence Ag presentation (see Chart 8). Other genes affect the global response, such as B cell proliferation or the ability of macrophages to process Ag.

10 There is a complex network of three-directional communication between the **immune, nervous and endocrine systems.** Stress or an infection can activate and modify the proinflammatory cytokines balance, and stimulate both the hypothalamus-pituitary-adrenal axis (HPA) as well as the sympathetic-adrenal system. This induces the release of ACTH, glucocorticoids and catecholamines (adrenaline and noradrenaline) that affect the immune response.

IMMUNITY AT THE MUCOSA

The mucosa of the gastrointestinal, respiratory and urogenital tracts, as well as the skin and the mammary gland, usually are the sites where invading microorganisms are first encountered. The immune component of these surfaces is located in extensive areas known as mucosa-associated lymphoid tissue (MALT); in MALT the protective immune mechanisms are mediated both by cells and by antibodies.

1

INDUCTIVE SITES	EFFECTOR SITES
NALT Nasal-associated lymphoid tissue.	Lachrymal and nasal areas, tonsils and adenoid, salivary glands.
	Pharynx and ear.
BALT Bronchus-associated lymphoid tissue.	Bronchi.
GALT Gut-associated lymphoid tissue.	Mammary gland.
Peyer's patches.	Small intestine.
Lymphoid tissue associated with solitary lymphoid nodules in the colon, rectum and appendix.	Large intestine.
GENALT Genital-associated lymphoid tissue.	Urinary tract.
	Genital tract.

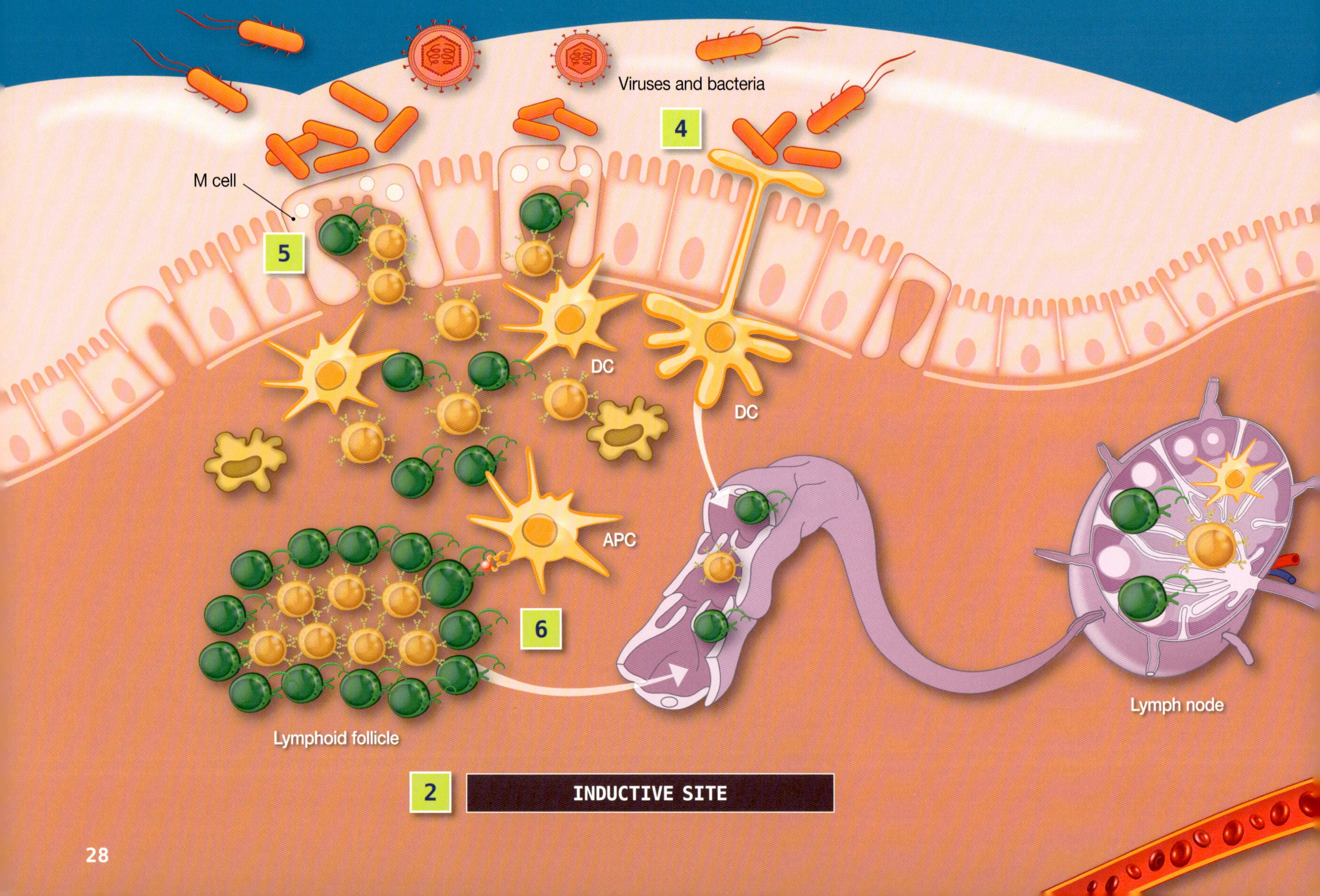

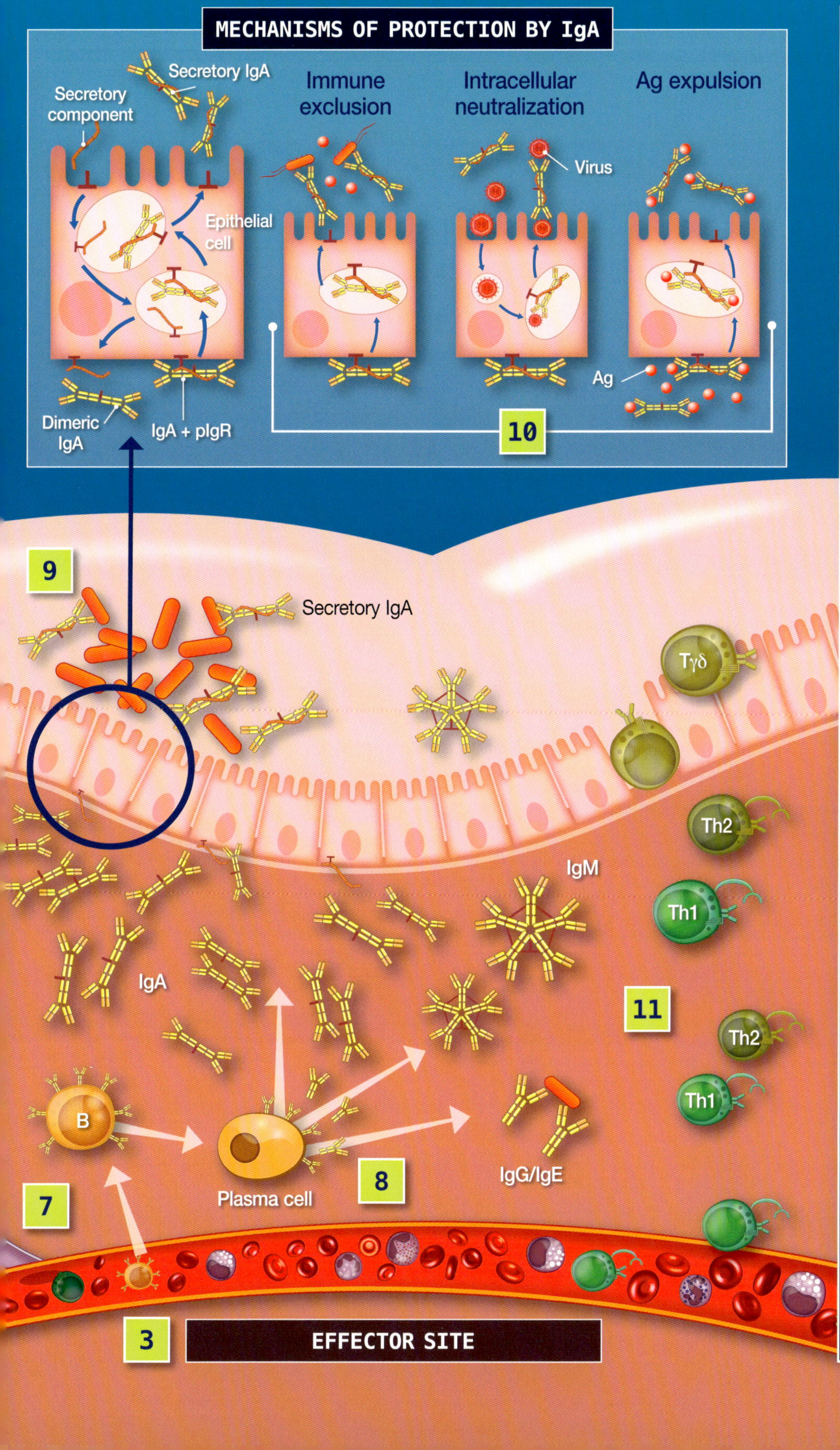

1 Mucosal lymphoid tissues (MALT) fall into two groups: **inductive sites**, where Ag are recognized and processed and immune responses are initiated (NALT, GALT, BALT), and **effector sites**, where Ab and cell-mediated responses are generated.

2 **The MALT of inductive sites** is usually organized and combines several features: it contacts closely with the mucosal surface, it is densely infiltrated with T and B cells and APC, and has cells specialized in the uptake of Ag (M cells) that are situated between epithelial cells.

3 **The MALT of the effector sites** is usually diffuse and contains B cells and plasma cells, which primarily secrete IgA, $\alpha\beta$ T cells (Th and Tc lymphocytes), and **$\gamma\delta$ T cells** (**intraepithelial lymphocytes, IEL**, particularly abundant in the intestine).

4 Ag can penetrate the intact epithelium and reach the MALT by two routes which involve either M cells or dendritic cells in the submucosa, which extend their cytoplasmic processes between the epithelial cells into the lumen.

5 **M cells** (present in NALT and GALT) take up Ag from the lumen of the mucosa and deliver it via transcytosis to the APC and intraepithelial lymphocytes located in a large pocket-like structure on their basolateral side.

6 APC process and present the Ag to the naïve Th and Tc cells, activating them in the lymphoid follicle of the MALT. Activated T and B cells leave the inductive site through the lymphoid vessels to adjacent lymph nodes (see Chart 1). There, the Th cells interact with the specific B cells, inducing the Ab class switch to IgA.

7 Subsequently, activated lymphocytes migrate via the bloodstream to different effector sites. This transfer of antibody-producing cells from the induction sites ensures that a secretory immune response protects at a systemic level.

8 Plasma cells secrete primarily **IgA**, and, to a lesser degree, IgM, IgE and IgG. Protection mechanisms include: **exclusion**, which consists of blocking Ag penetration (by IgA, and to a lesser extent, IgM), and **elimination**, which is the neutralization of the Ag that has penetrated the mucosa (by IgE and IgG).

9 To make the immune exclusion possible it is necessary for the IgA to be transported to the outside of the mucosal surface. Immature epithelial cells present in their basolateral membrane a specific receptor (pIgR) with affinity for the J chain of IgA (see Chart 6). Once the IgA binds to the receptor, it is transferred by transcytosis towards the lumen, retaining part of pIgR and becoming **secretory IgA**.

10 IgA confers protection at three different levels: on the surface of the mucosa (exclusion), within epithelial cells (neutralization), and within the submucosa (expulsion).

11 T cells are the most important effector cells in the intestinal mucosa and they are situated both below and within the epithelium. The IEL are $\gamma\delta$ T cells which can recognize the Ag without having been processed by the APC. These cells can act as APC, some work as NK cells and others act as Tc cells against parasites. They also secrete cytokines, such as IFN-γ, that stimulate macrophages and enterocytes to produce nitric oxide, important in the defense of the intestinal mucosa.

IMMUNITY IN THE FETUS AND IN THE NEWBORN

The immune system of mammals develops and matures during pregnancy. At birth, both dogs and cats are able to respond to potentially infectious agents. However, this immune response is not very effective, so it is essential that they acquire maternal antibodies through the colostrum.

STRUCTURE OF THE PLACENTA

2

1

3

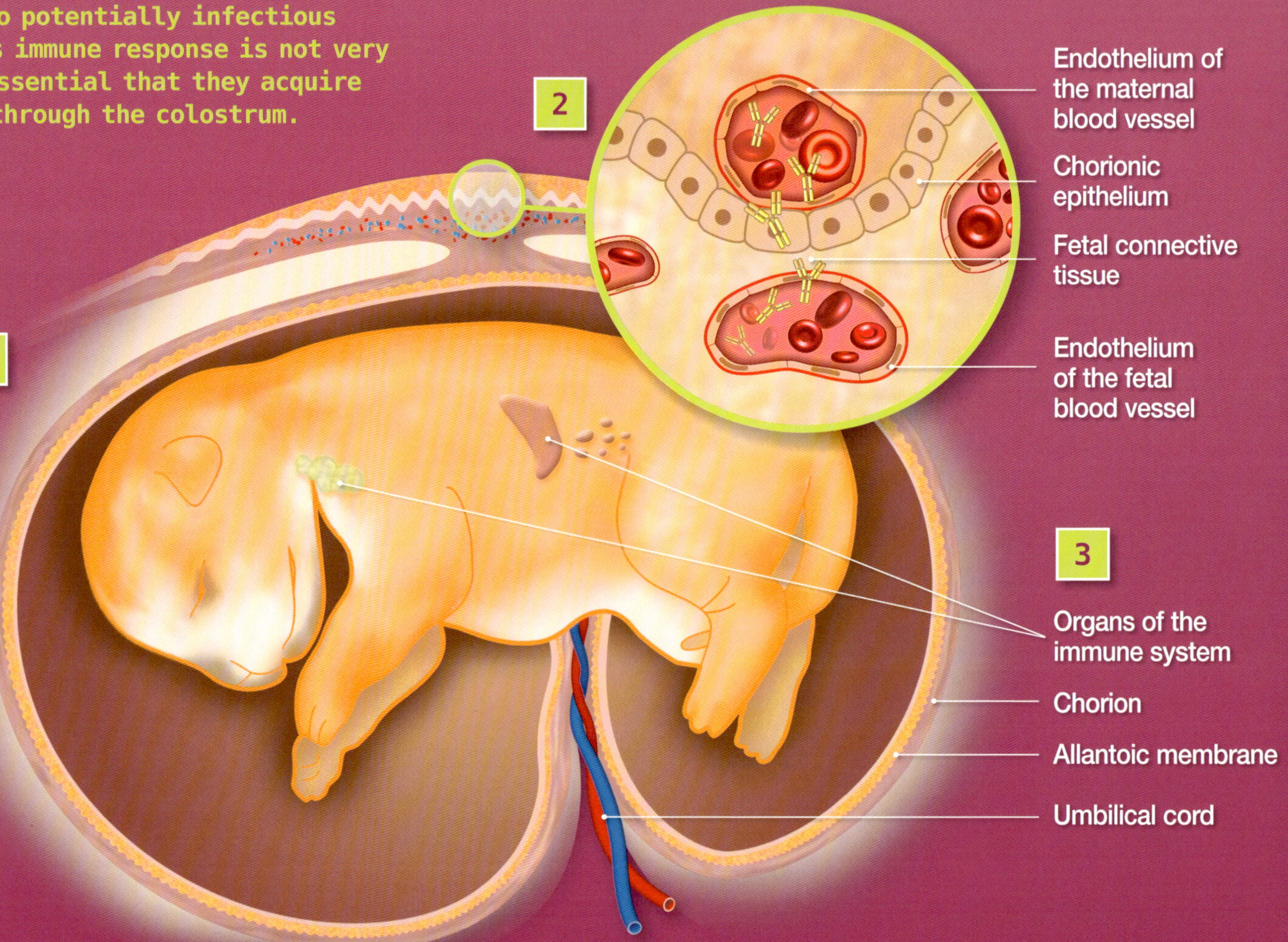

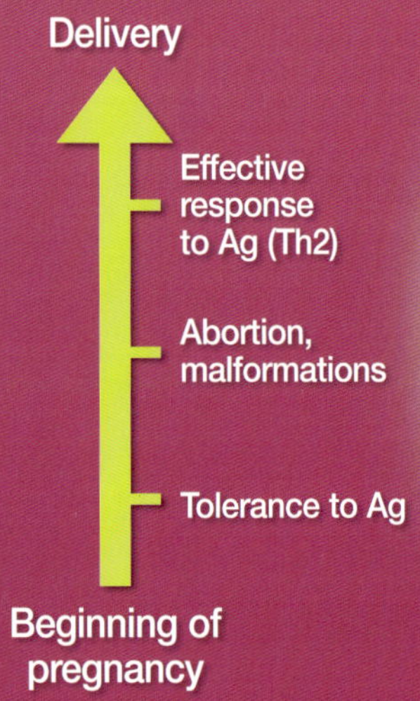

4

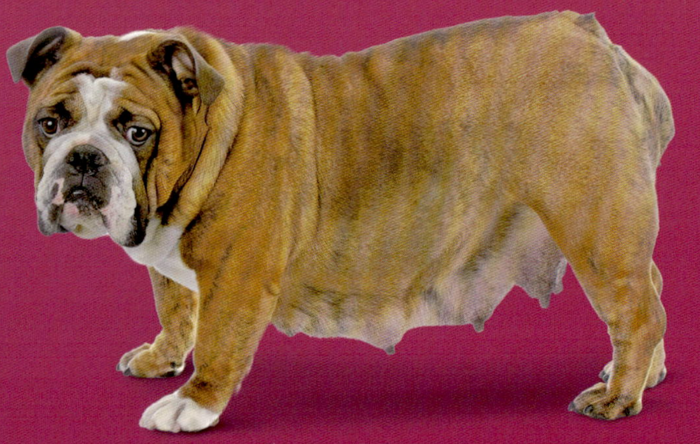

1 The hormonal and immune mechanisms responsible for maintaining pregnancy foster a **maternal Th2 immune response**, both at the peripheral level and at the placenta, which contributes to protect the fetus against the rejection by the immune system of the mother.

2 Carnivores have an **endotheliochorial placenta**: the fetal chorionic epithelium is in contact with the endothelium of the maternal blood vessels. This only allows the passage of 5-10 % of IgG from the mother's circulation to the fetus.

3 The immune system develops gradually in the fetus: the thymus appears between 23-33 days of gestation and culminates its development at 45 days; a rudimentary spleen may be detected at 28 days; lymph nodes arise later, and the Peyer's patches at an even more advanced stage of gestation.

4 As the fetus has not been exposed to any foreign Ag, its immune system is considered naïve. The response to a potential infection in the uterus depends on the pathogen, the immune status of the mother and, mainly, the **gestational age of the fetus**.

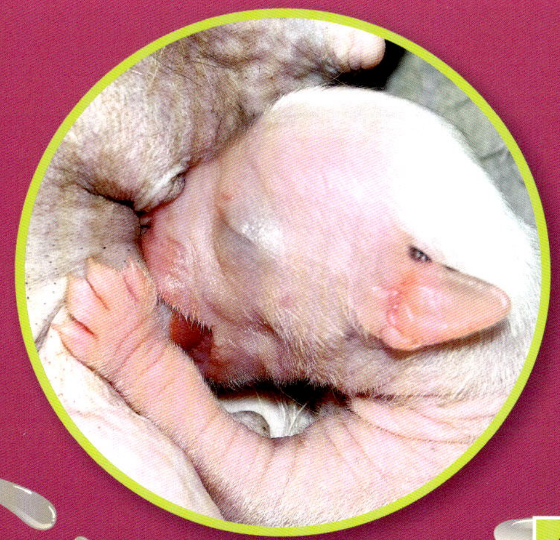

5 **Maternal passive immunity** is transferred to the newborn through the colostrum during the first hours of life. Intestinal absorption of Ig in this period allows concentration values of IgG in the serum of newborns to be similar to the IgG concentration in the serum of their mothers.

6 **Colostrum** contains secretions from maternal blood, accumulated in the mammary gland during the final period of gestation. It contains mainly **IgG (in the queen)**, **IgA (in the bitch)** and small amounts of IgM.

7 Part of the IgA in the colostrum remains in the intestine of the newborn, thus protecting it against enteric infections.

8 The **failure of passive transfer of immunity (FPT)** is caused by no or insufficient ingestion of colostrums. It can happen due to agalactia or mastitis in the mother, a very numerous litter, low weight or very weak puppies or kittens and newborns rejected by their mothers. It may also be due to defects in the absorption of the Ig in the intestine of the newborn.

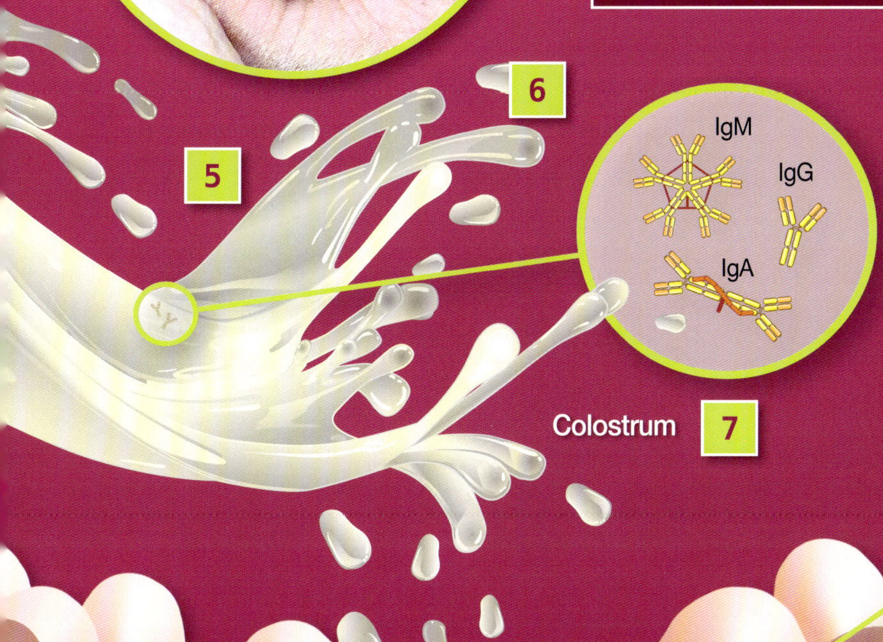

IMMUNOGLOBULIN ABSORPTION IN THE NEWBORN INTESTINE

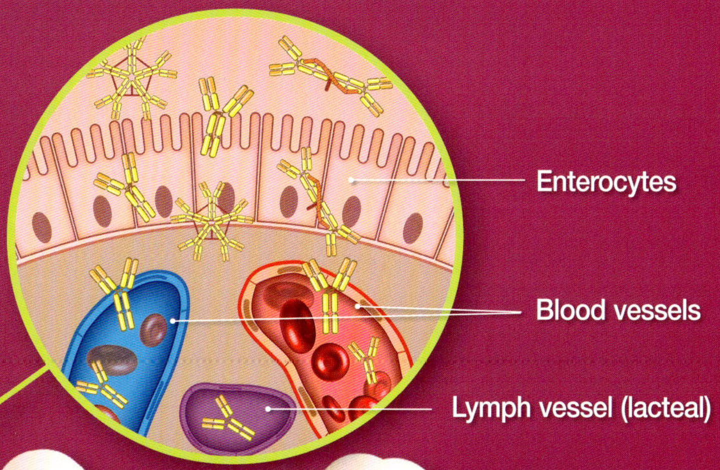

Ig absorption in the intestine of the newborn is possible due to:

- Presence of trypsin inhibitors in the colostrum.
- Low activity of proteases.
- Transient expression of Ig receptors (FcRn) on enterocytes.

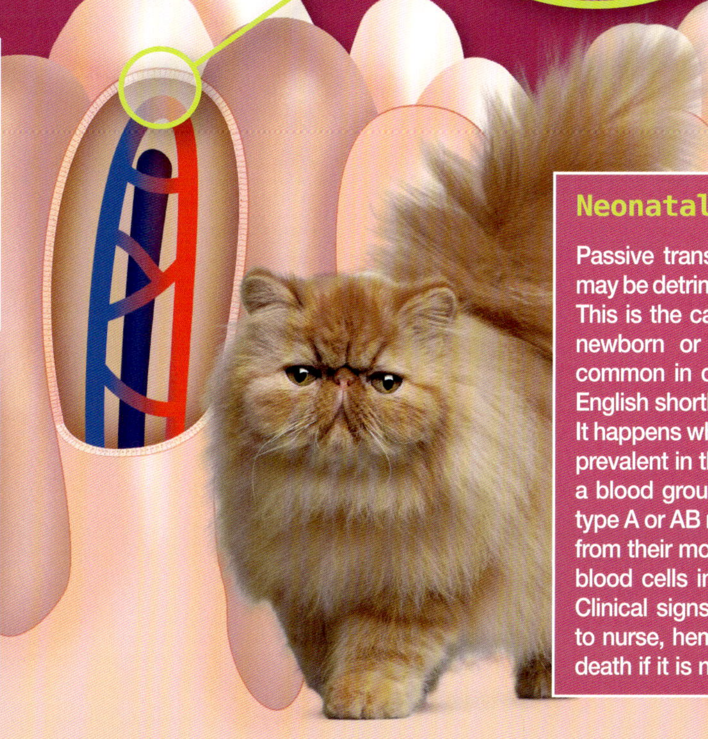

9 Maternal Ig inhibit the synthesis of Ab in the newborn; thus, **very young animals which still maintain maternal immunity should not be vaccinated** (see Chart 41).

10 Newborns have the ability of responding against numerous Ag, both through the innate and adaptive immunities. Specific reactions are primary responses, with a prolonged latency phase. This response is less effective than in adults and is mainly of the **Th2-type (humoral)**.

Neonatal isoerithrolysis

Passive transfer of Ig by colostrum sometimes may be detrimental to the newborn (see Chart 21). This is the case of the hemolytic disease of the newborn or neonatal isoerithrolysis, relatively common in cats of the Persian, Burmese, Rex, English shorthair, Abyssinian and Somali breeds. It happens when a queen of blood group B (more prevalent in these breeds) has been mounted by a blood group A male, and the kittens of either type A or AB receive colostrum with Ab anti-A Ag from their mother. These Ab produce lysis of red blood cells in the kittens and originate anemia. Clinical signs in kittens include lethargy, refusal to nurse, hemoglobinuria, jaundice, and sudden death if it is not treated in time.

GENERAL MECHANISMS OF THE IMMUNE RESPONSE AGAINST PATHOGENS

EVOLUTION

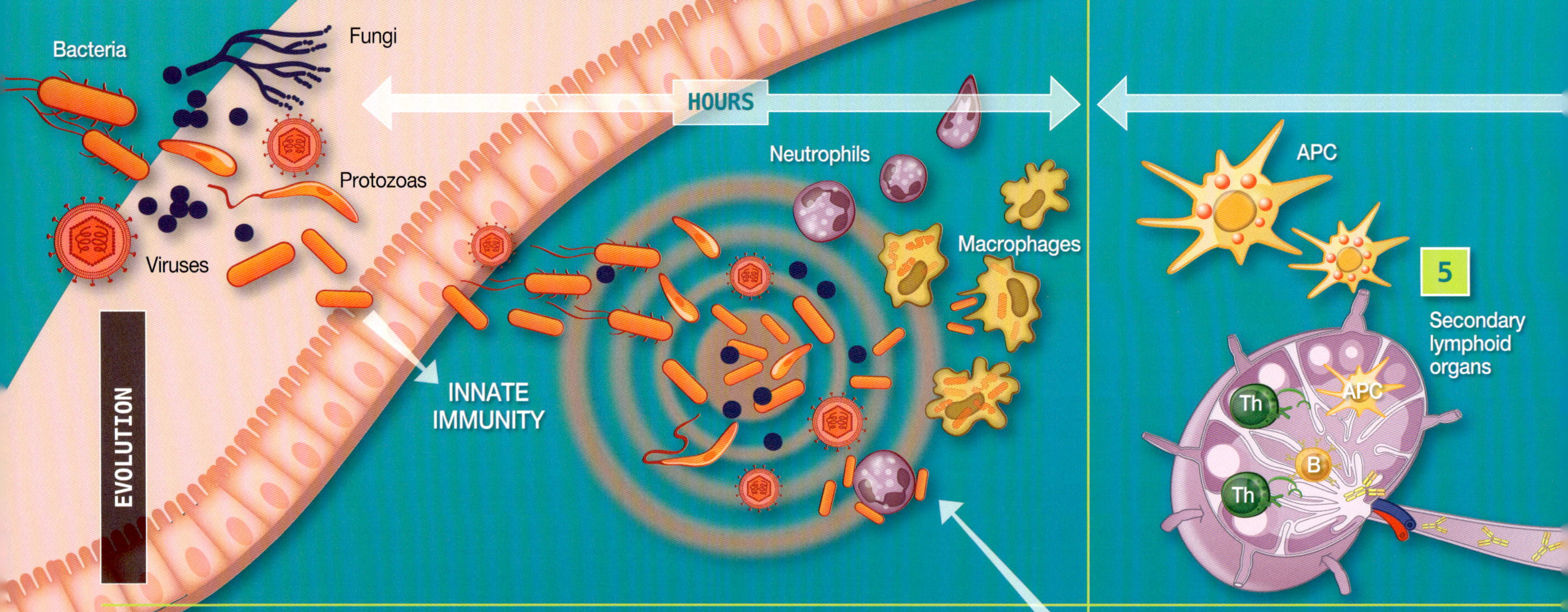

MECHANISMS

1 Extracellular pathogens can directly activate the complement through the **alternative pathway or the lectin pathway** (see Chart 4). Complement activation consists of an enzymatic cascade in which, after recruiting a component, it is cleaved. One of the fragments is released and has biological activity, while the other binds covalently to the surface of the pathogen and recruits the next protein to continue the process.

FUNCTIONS OF THE COMPLEMENT SYSTEMS

2 Fragments C3a and C5a of complement act as **anaphylotoxins**: they attract inflammatory cells to the focus of infection (see Chart 7).

3 Fragments C3b and C4b bind covalently to the surface of the pathogen, serving as **opsonins**. When they are recognized by their receptors on phagocytes the efficiency of phagocytosis is improved.

4 The last stage of the complement activation is the aggregation of the "membrane attack complex" (MAC), which forms pores on the surface of the pathogen, inducing its osmotic **lysis**.

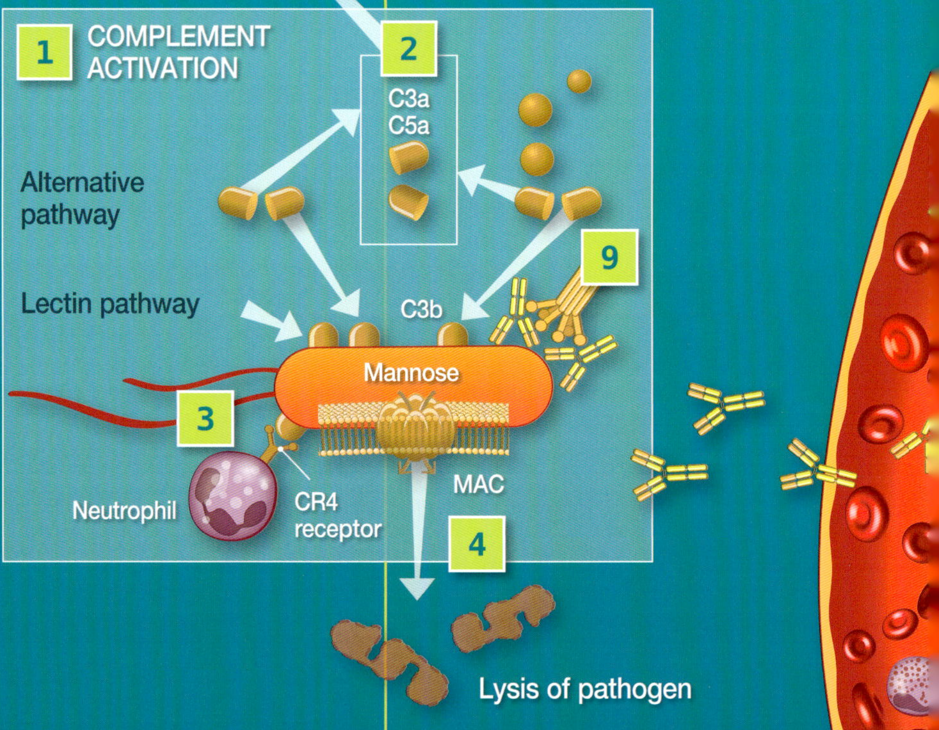

INNATE MECHANISMS

Invading pathogens have to deal first with the ever present innate defenses of the animal, which offer immediate protection. If the pathogen is not eliminated, it is captured by the APC and transported to the regional lymph nodes. This starts the acquired immune response, which requires more time to develop when it is first exposed to the Ag. Depending on several factors, the predominant immune response is either HUMORAL (usually against extracellular pathogens) or CELL-MEDIATED (against intracellular pathogens).

DAYS – WEEKS → MEMORY

5 The APC trap the Ag and present it to Th cells in the secondary lymphoid organs (lymph nodes, spleen, or MALT). The Th cells are activated following the specific recognition of the Ag-MHC-II by their TCR and they secrete "polarizing" cytokines that promote cellular or humoral responses upon leaving the secondary lymphoid organs (see Charts 5 and 9).

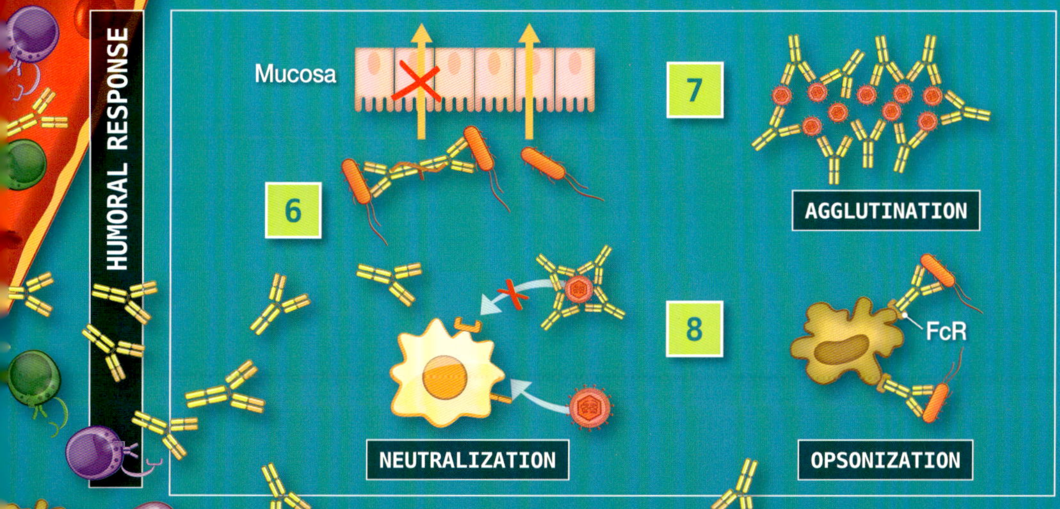

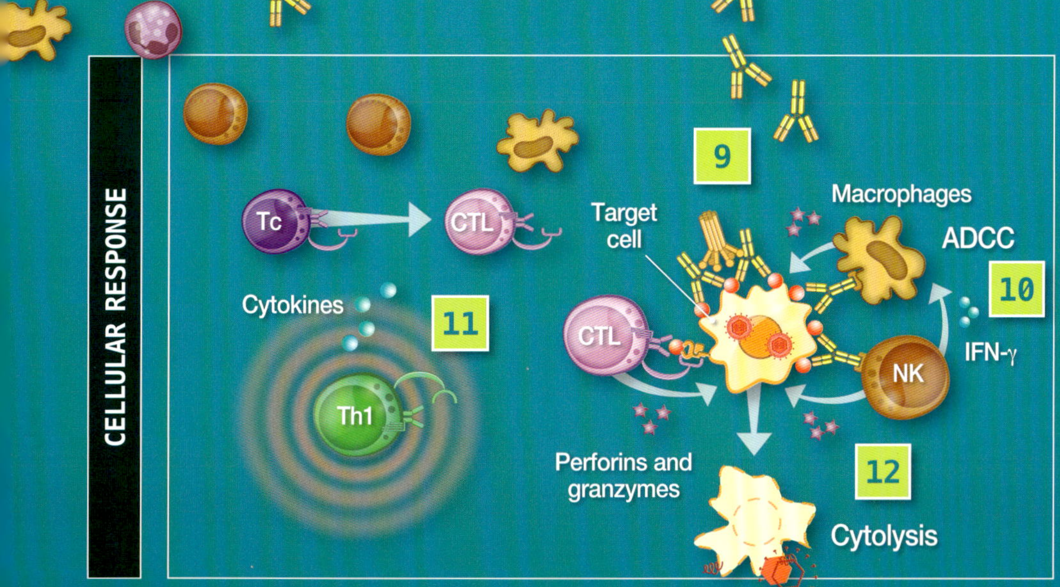

FUNCTIONS OF THE SECRETED Ig

6 **Neutralization:** blocking of the recognition of pathogens and toxins by the receptor on target cells, preventing their penetration into the cell. Ab also block adhesion and penetration of pathogens through the mucosa (see Chart 11).

7 **Agglutination:** clumping of extracellular pathogens, which prevents their spread and facilitates their detection by the immune cells.

8 **Opsonization:** phagocytic cells possess receptors for Fc of the Ig (FcR). They recognize Ig-coated Ag, which are endocytosed, processed, and disposed of or presented to the Th cells.

9 **Complement activation by the classical pathway:** the formation of Ag-Ab complex initiates the classical complement cascade.

10 **Antibody dependent cellular cytotoxicity (ADCC):** the Ag of the pathogen that are expressed on the **surface of infected cells** react with specific Ab. These are recognized by the FcR of monocytes and macrophages, NK cells, neutrophils, and eosinophis. Subsequently, these cells produce enzymes that destroy the infected cell.

11 **Th1 cells enhance the cellular response.** They secrete cytokines that activate and recruit macrophages and NK cells so that they act on the infected cell and activate the CD8+ T cells, which become CTL.

12 **CTL** and **NK** cells identify target cells (cells infected by viruses, tumor or transplanted cells) and release **lytic enzymes** (perforins, granzymes) which destroy the target cell. They also elicit the mechanism of programmed cell death or **apoptosis** through the recognition of the cell receptor CD95 (also called FasR) on the target cell by the ligand CD95L (FasL) located on the surface of CTL and NK cells.

13 **Memory and protection.** Following the elimination of the Ag, the effector mechanisms of adaptive immunity wane, although memory lymphocytes persist. This makes subsequent responses to the same Ag more intense and rapid (see Chart 5).

ADAPTIVE MECHANISMS

IMMUNITY AGAINST VIRUSES

Viruses are very simple infecting particles that need live cells to replicate. The innate immunity comprises the physical defenses (the skin, the mucus, etc.), molecules like the interferons, and cells like the NK and the macrophages. The specific immunity is created by the antibodies and, mainly, by cytotoxic T lymphocytes (CTL).

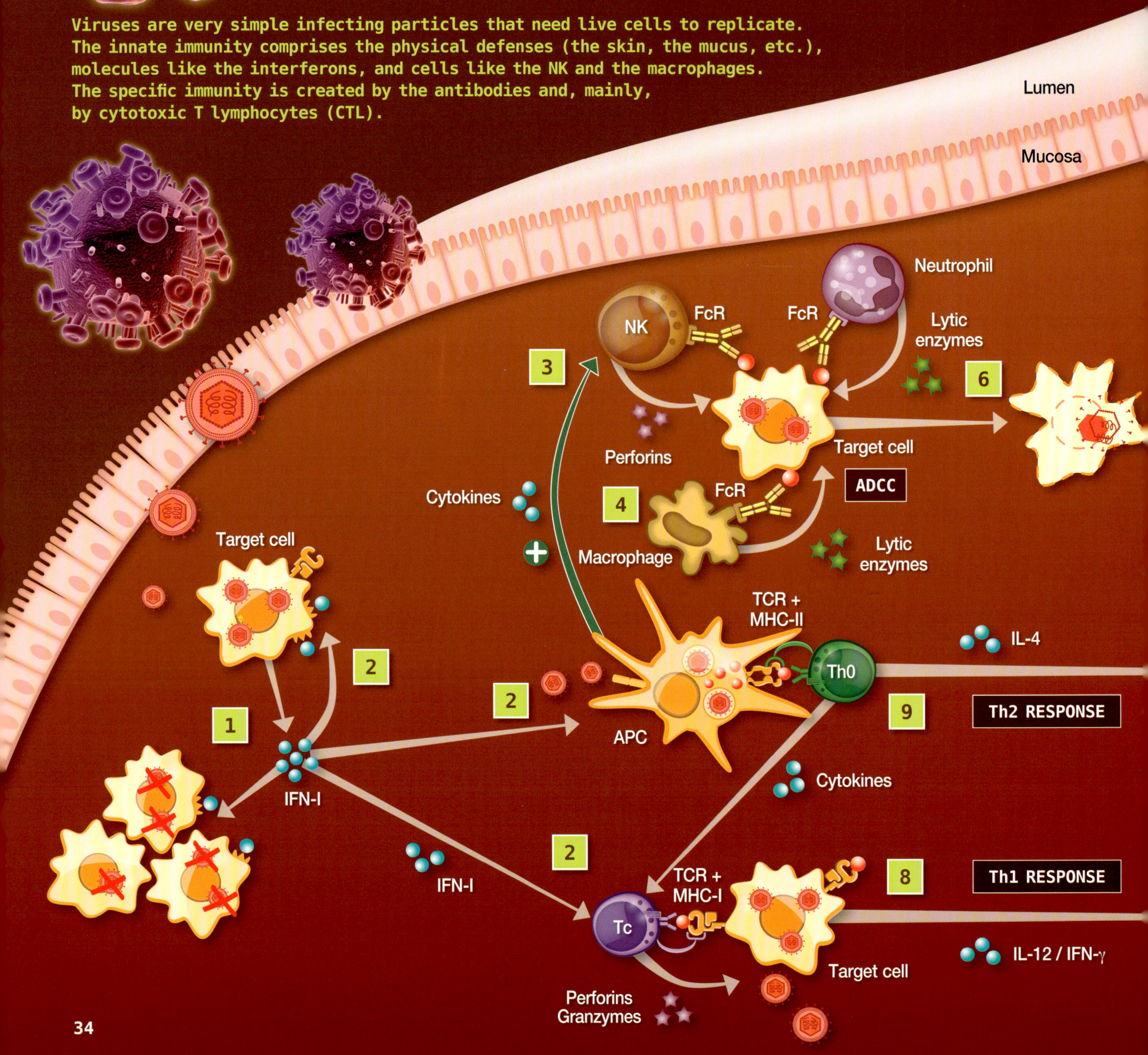

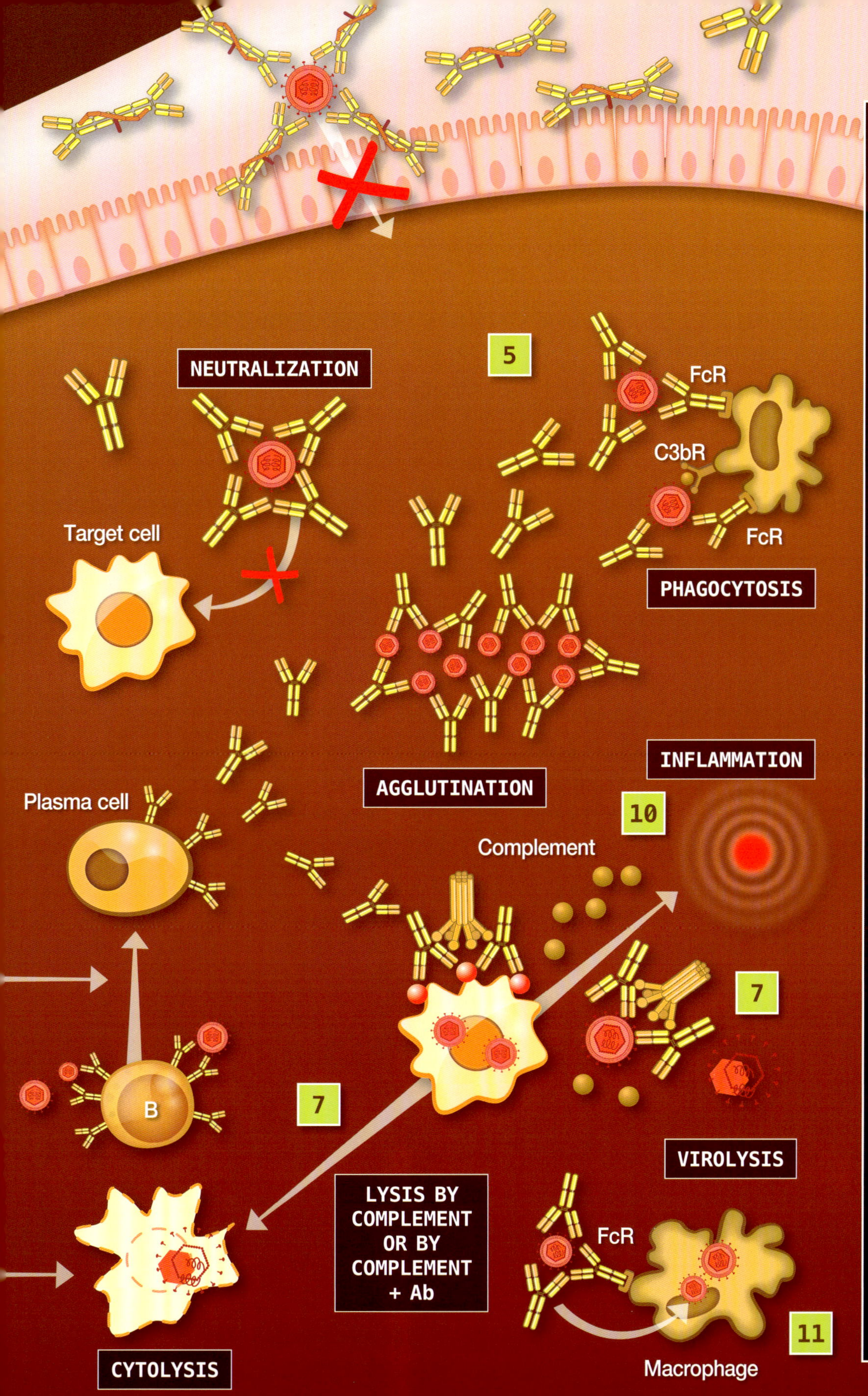

1 The infection of cells by viruses stimulates the production of **type I interferons** (IFN-I) that promote the synthesis of new proteins, some of which have antiviral activity. IFN-I (IFN-α, IFN-β) specifically bind to their receptors on the cells, to which they induce an antiviral state, preventing the formation of new viral particles. IFN-I take several days to degrade.

2 IFN-I increase the expression of the MHC-I in the infected cells (favoring CTL activity) and of the MHC-II in the APC (favoring Ag presentation), and has antiproliferative activity.

3 Frequently, the expression of MHC-I on virus-infected cells is decreased or abolished. This is detected by the **NK cells**, which respond immediately. In addition, NK cells can destroy infected cells through ADCC (antibody dependent cellular cytotoxicity).

4 The **macrophages** also act very early in infection. Their antiviral action is both intrinsic (degrading phagocytosed viruses) and extrinsic (cytotoxic action, destroying cells by ADCC).

5 **Antibodies** are essential for fighting extracellular viruses. They **neutralize** viruses by blocking their entry to the cell. In addition, they can **opsonize** (enhancing phagocytosis), and **agglutinate**.

6 Antibodies also can coat infected cells so that they are eliminated by **ADCC** mediated by NK cells, macrophages and neutrophils (see Chart 13).

7 **Complement** can be activated directly through the alternative pathway, or triggered by immune complexes through the classical pathway. The result of both activation pathways is the **lysis** of **viruses** and of **infected cells**.

8 **CD8+ T cells** (Tc and CTL) recognize viral Ag synthesized in the cytoplasm of infected cells associated with the MHC-I. This promotes the lysis of the infected cell.

9 **CD4+ T cells** (helper or Th) recognize exogenous Ag processed by the APC and presented by these cells associated with the MHC-II. Thus, they collaborate with the CTL response and with the maturation of B cells.

10 The immune response to viruses can have undesirable consequences, such as the formation of large amounts of circulating immune complexes that obstruct the capillaries and excessively activate complement (type III hypersensitivity, see Chart 21). This entails the release of vasoactive amines, the recruitment of inflammatory cells and tissue damage (*e.g.*, glomerulonephritis in feline infectious peritonitis).

11 Viruses coated by antibodies can penetrate in cells that have the FcR receptor but that are incapable of eliminating them; this is a mechanism of cell entry of some viruses.

IMMUNITY AGAINST BACTERIA

Immune responses against extracellular and intracellular bacteria are different: humoral defenses predominate in responses against the former, while cellular defenses predominate in responses against the latter.

EXTRACELLULAR BACTERIA

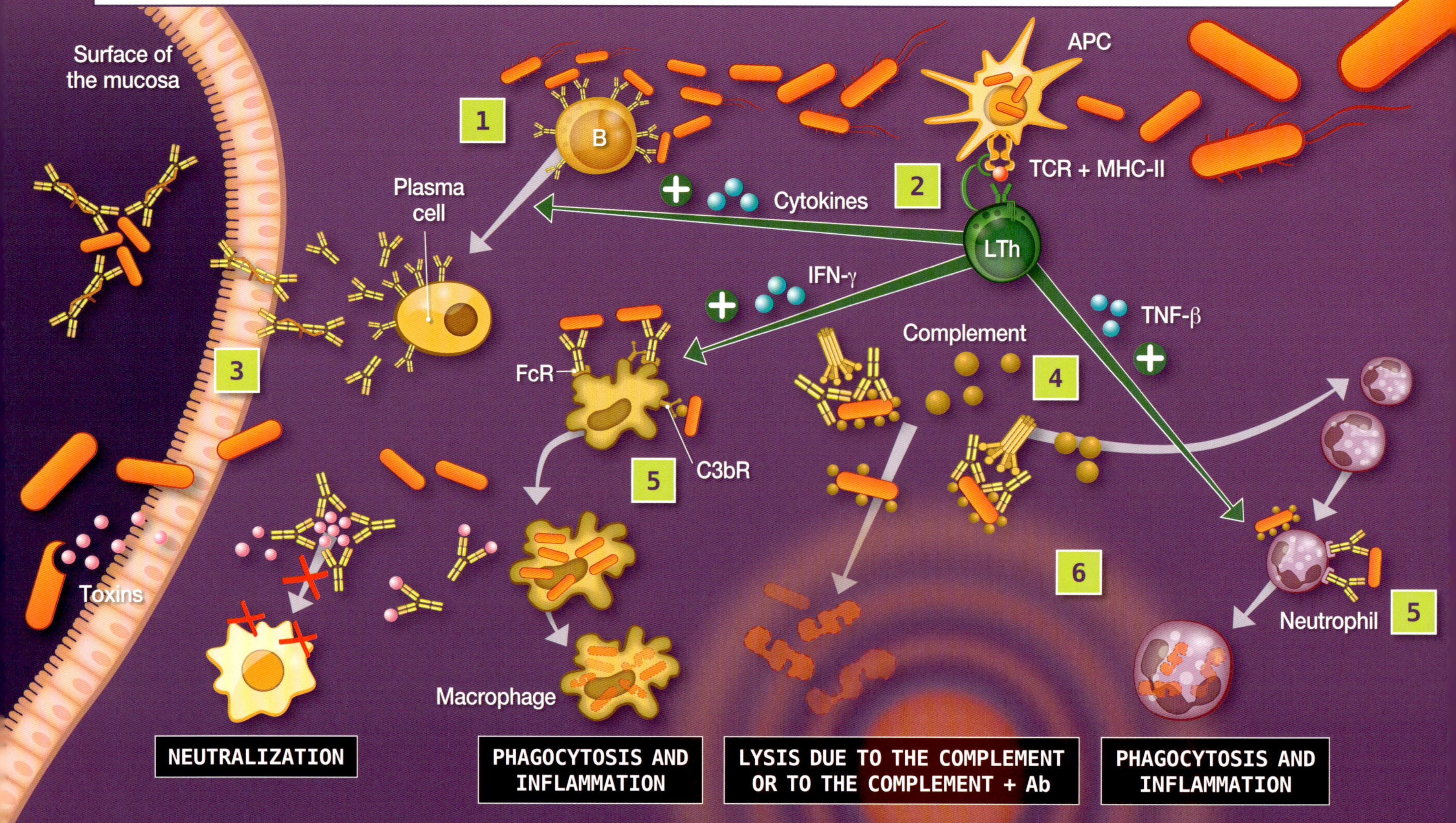

1 Ag of extracellular bacteria partially activate B cells.

2 APC (primarily dendritic cells) that have endocytosed or phagocytosed extracellular bacteria present the Ag combined with the MHC-II to Th cells (CD4+). These cells secrete cytokines that induce B cells to differentiate into Ab-producing plasma cells (see Charts 5 and 9).

3 Secreted Ab **inhibit the adhesion** of bacteria to mucosal surfaces or **neutralize** bacterial toxins.

4 The complement can be activated by bacteria (through the alternative pathway or through the lectin pathway) or after the formation of antigen-antibody complexes (by the classical pathway; see Chart 13). The direct consequence of the **activation of complement is bacterial lysis.**

5 Bacteria coated by Ab and/or by C3b complement fraction (**opsonized**) are phagocytosed more effectively, since macrophages and neutrophils possess receptors that bind to Ig (FcR) and to the C3b fraction (C3bR).

6 The activation of complement generates **chemotactic molecules** (C3a, C5a) that attract neutrophils and other cells of the immune system to the site where the bacteria are multiplying. These cells are then activated by TNF-β secreted by the Th cells causing local inflammation (see Chart 7). Phagocytes secrete cytokines that also promote inflammation.

INTRACELLULAR BACTERIA

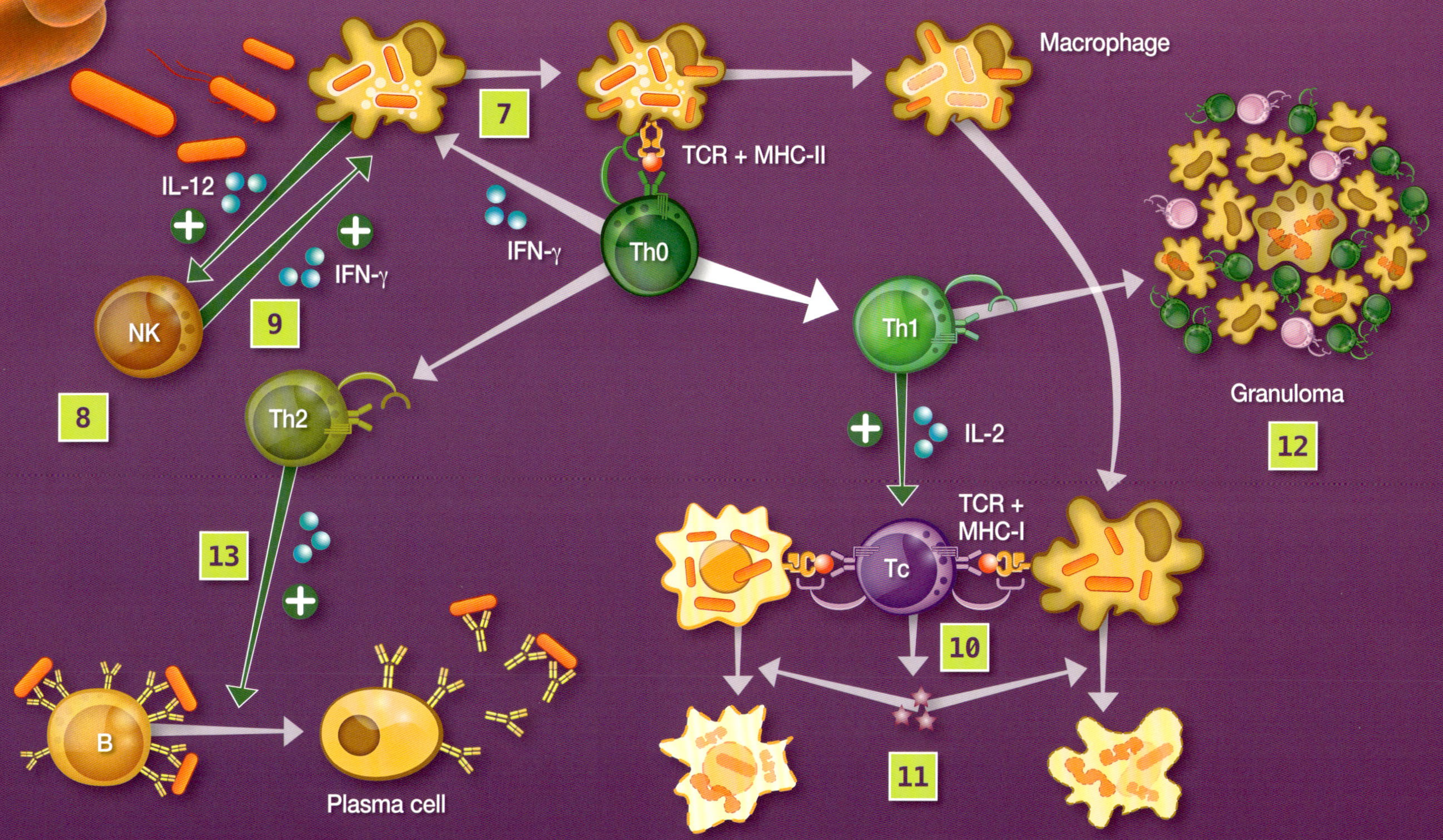

7 Some intracellular bacteria infecting macrophages **can resist** the destruction mechanisms in the phagolysosome.

8 NK cells are activated by intracellular bacteria and/or IL-12, secreted by macrophages that have phagocytosed bacteria. These activated NK cells secrete IFN-γ (see Chart 9).

9 IFN-γ activates macrophages to effectively destroy bacteria in the phagolysosomes. After processing the Ag, the macrophages present them associated with the MHC-II to Th cells (CD4+). These cells secrete more IFN-γ that amplifies the process.

10 Some bacteria, such as mycobacteria, escape the phagolysosomes and multiply in the cytoplasm. Under these circumstances, or in any other infected cell, bacterial Ag are presented to Tc cells (CD8+) associated with the MHC-I (see Chart 8).

11 The Tc cells are activated by cytokines (IL-2), secreted by the Th1 cells, and are transformed into CTL that synthesize perforins and granzymes that destroy the infected cell (see Chart 5).

12 If the bacteria are difficult to destroy, the infection becomes chronic and granulomas can develop; these are full of T cells and macrophages (see Chart 7), as occurs in tuberculosis.

13 If the humoral responses prevail over the cellular responses, intracellular bacteria are not effectively removed (only in their extracellular phase), making the prognosis worse.

IMMUNITY AGAINST PROTOZOA

Acquired immunity plays an essential role in the defense against protozoa. Th1 mechanisms are associated with an effective immune response to protozoa and Th2 with the spread of the protozoan invasion. Nevertheless, given how well parasites are adapted to the host, they are seldom eliminated, and many protozoa induce chronic infections.

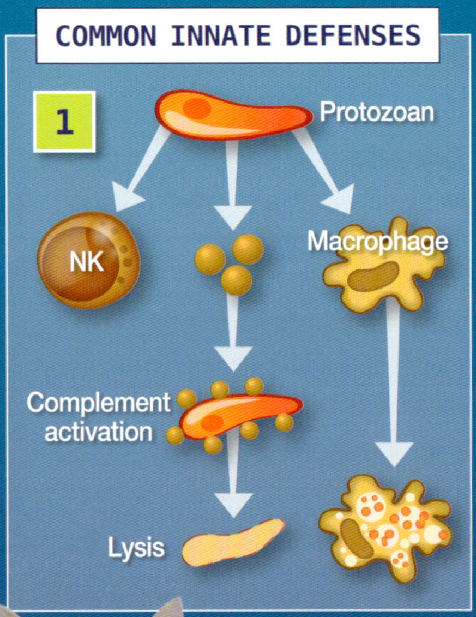

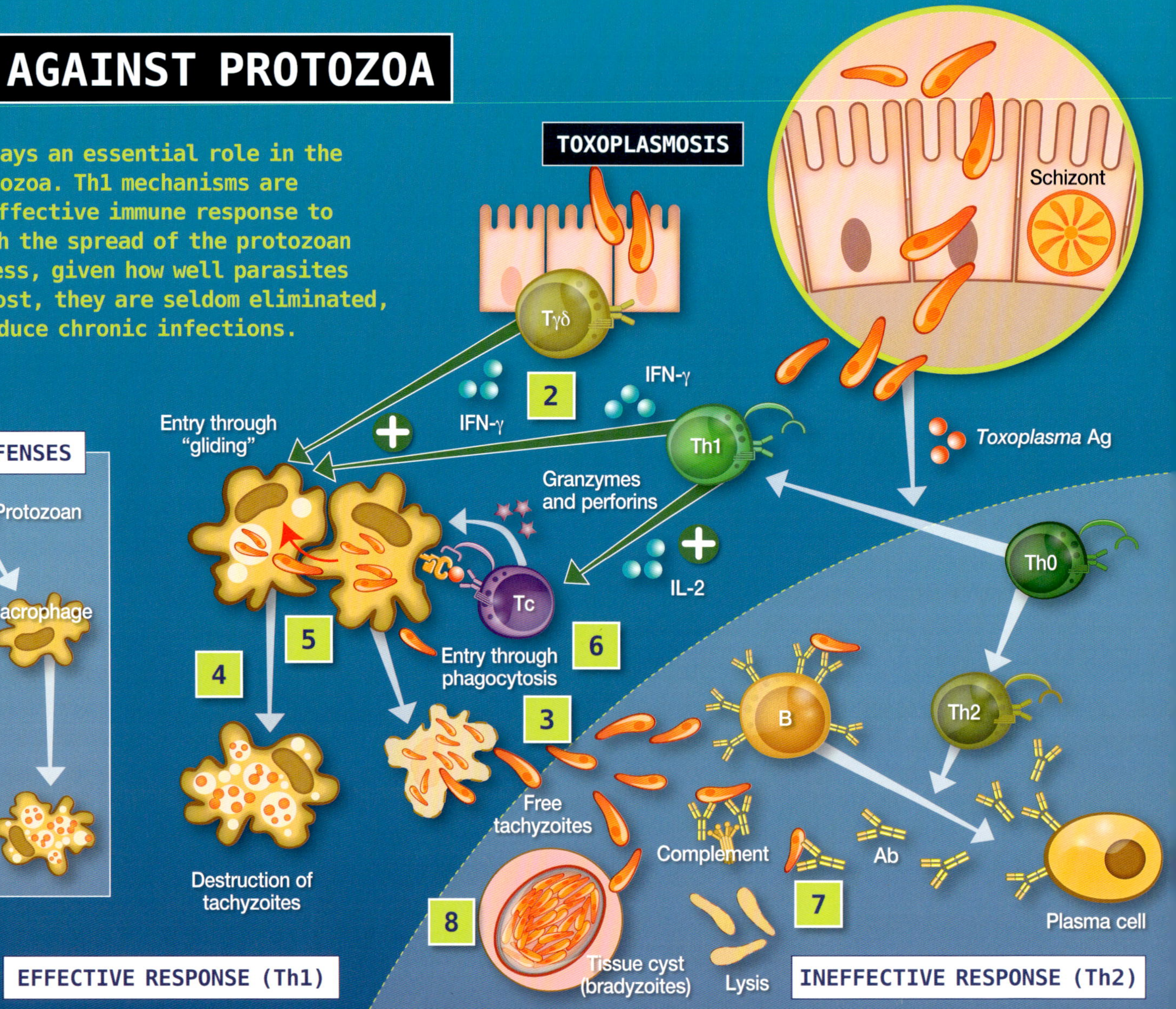

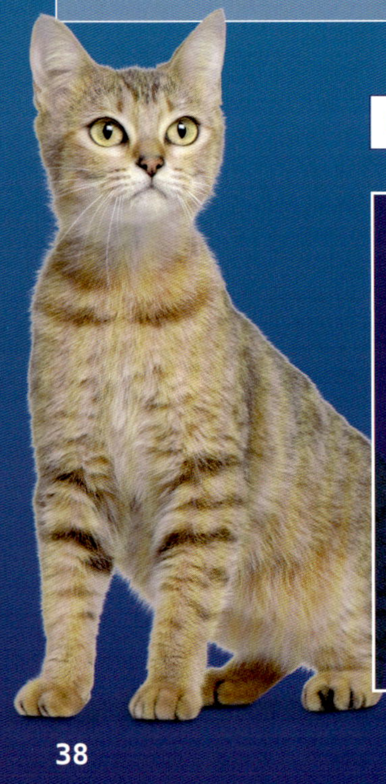

1. The innate defenses against protozoa include the activation of the complement by the alternative pathway (that causes protozoal lysis or opsonization), the lytic activity of NK cells, and the intracellular destruction of protozoa in activated macrophages. *Leishmania* and *Toxoplasma* are able to evade these mechanisms.
2. **Intraepithelial γδ T cells** (IEL) of the mucosa respond to the heat shock protein (HSP), released by the cells infected by *Toxoplasma*, producing early IFN-γ and the lysis of the infected cell.
3. In the macrophages, *Toxoplasma* reside in modified vacuoles. These do not fuse with lysosomes. As a result, macrophages are unable to eliminate the protozoa, which grow within these cells until the macrophages rupture, releasing tachyzoites.
4. Only macrophages activated by IFN-γ, produced by NK cells, γδ T lymphocytes and Th1 cells specific for *Toxoplasma* Ag, can fuse their lysosomes with the vacuoles that contain toxoplasma parasites, destroying them.
5. Tachyzoites can infect other macrophages by "gliding" through molecular junctions. By this mechanism they **evade the immune system**.
6. Th1 lymphocytes secrete IL-2 that activates CD8+ T cells (Tc and CTL) that destroy the infected cells (see Chart 5).
7. Th2 response generates antibodies that, together with complement or through ADCC, destroy free tachyzoites. Nevertheless, this mechanism does not eliminate intracellular tachyzoites.
8. *Toxoplasma* tachyzoites can develop to bradyzoites that get encased in cysts. By this mechanism they may also evade the immune response.

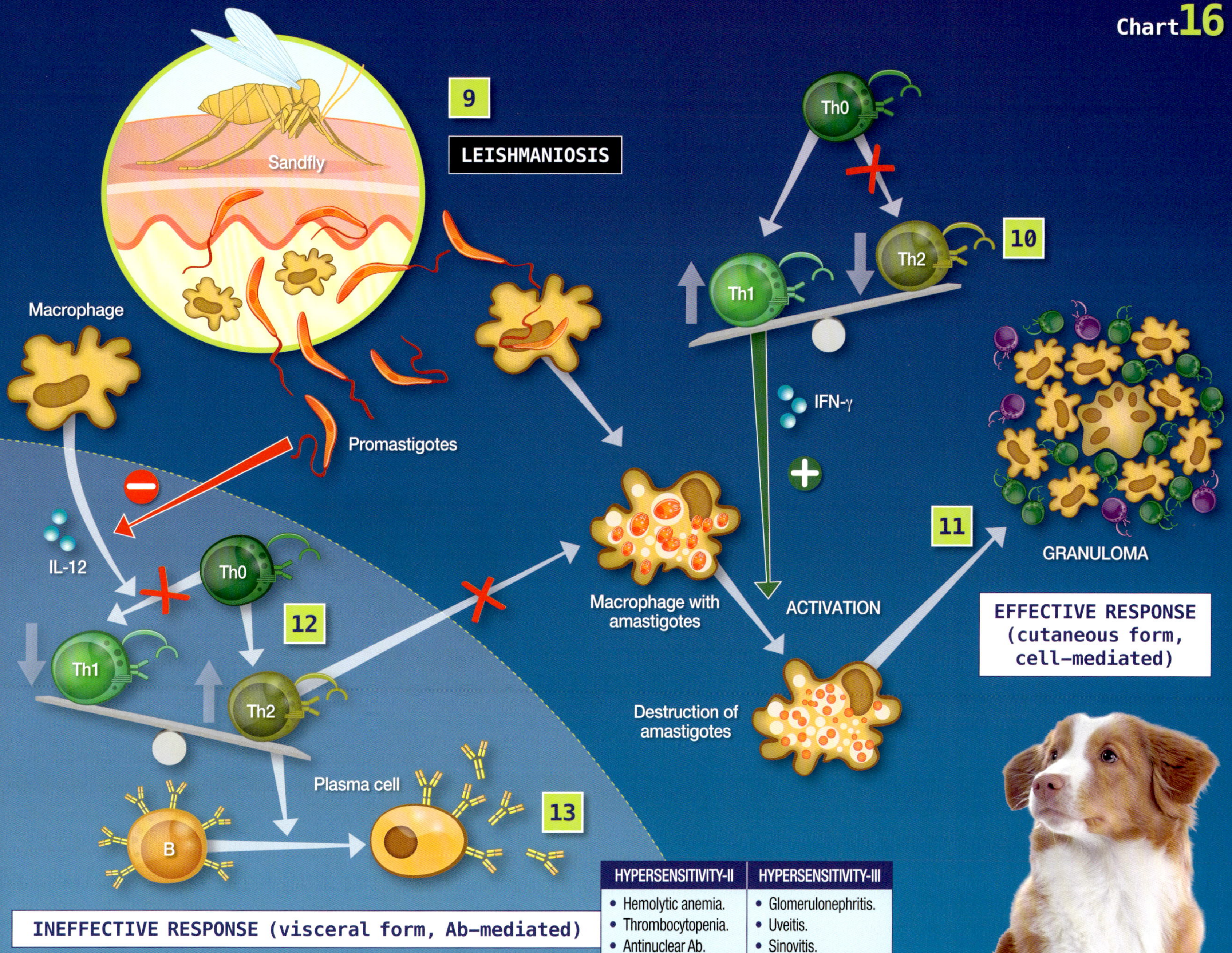

HYPERSENSITIVITY-II	HYPERSENSITIVITY-III
• Hemolytic anemia.	• Glomerulonephritis.
• Thrombocytopenia.	• Uveitis.
• Antinuclear Ab.	• Sinovitis.

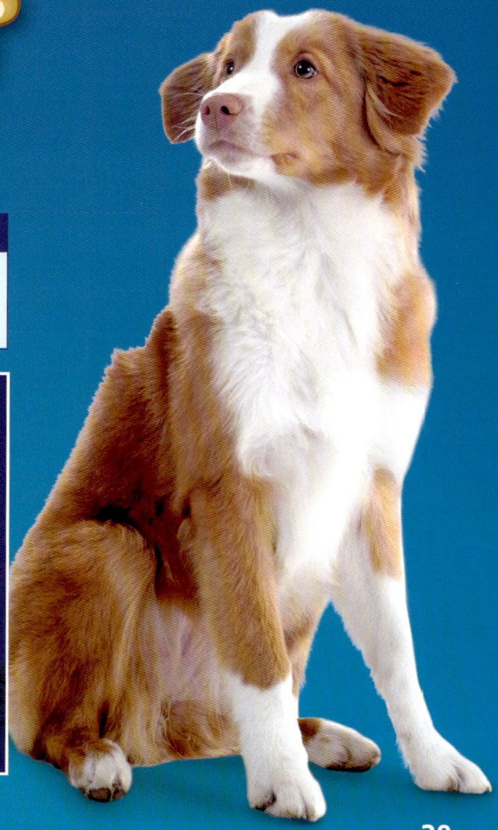

9 *Leishmania* promastigotes penetrate the dog through sandfly bites and are rapidly phagocytosed by subdermic macrophages, where they divide and become amastigotes (see Chart 34). The evolution of the disease depends on whether the animal develops an effective or ineffective immune response.

10 In the effective immune responses, Th1 mechanisms predominate over the Th2 and the infection is restricted to the skin (**cutaneous form**). IFN-γ is secreted; it activates the infected macrophages, partially destroying intracellular *Leishmania*.

11 Cutaneous leishmaniosis is characterized by chronic inflammation and formation of granulomas rich in T cells and macrophages (Type IV hypersensitivity, see Chart 21).

12 Ineffective immune responses result from the suppression of IL-12 by *Leishmania*, ensuring Th2 responses. The parasites **invade the organs**, resulting in a progressive, chronic infection in which there are numerous infected macrophages that spread the parasites.

13 *Leishmania* induce polyclonal B cell activation, which is manifested as the classic hypergammaglobulinemia that accompanies leishmaniosis. The excess of Ab produces Type II and Type III hypersensitivity (see Chart 21).

IMMUNITY AGAINST FUNGI

The immune reaction against fungi usually develops in the entry tissue (*e.g.*, nasal sinuses for *Aspergillus* or *Histoplasma*, skin for dermatophytes) or in those tissues where they reside (digestive and urogenital mucosa for *Candida*, ear for *Malassezia*). The most effective defense mechanisms against fungi are innate, which in immune competent individuals are able to eliminate them. Neutropenia hampers the control of fungal infections.

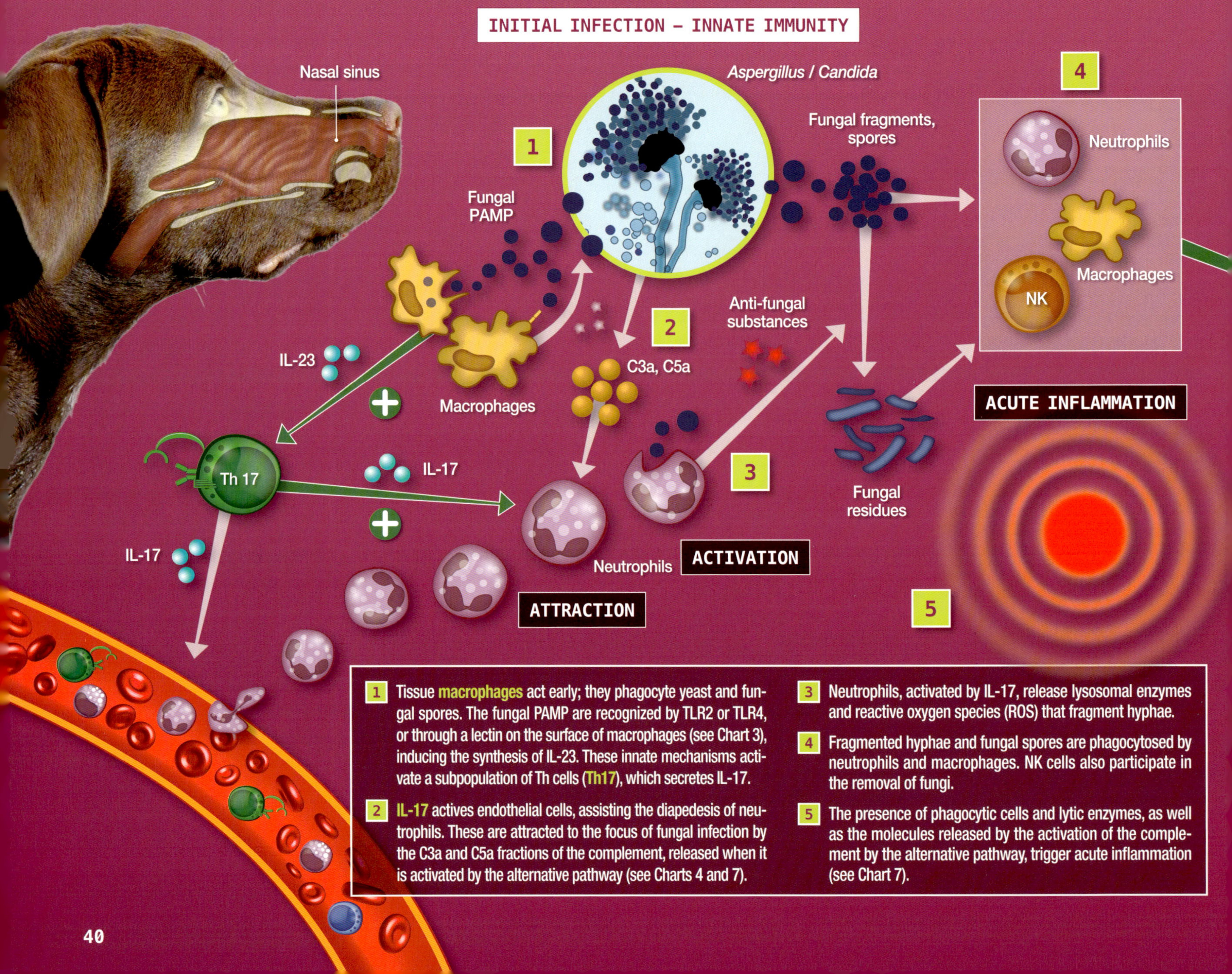

1 Tissue **macrophages** act early; they phagocyte yeast and fungal spores. The fungal PAMP are recognized by TLR2 or TLR4, or through a lectin on the surface of macrophages (see Chart 3), inducing the synthesis of IL-23. These innate mechanisms activate a subpopulation of Th cells (**Th17**), which secretes IL-17.

2 **IL-17** actives endothelial cells, assisting the diapedesis of neutrophils. These are attracted to the focus of fungal infection by the C3a and C5a fractions of the complement, released when it is activated by the alternative pathway (see Charts 4 and 7).

3 Neutrophils, activated by IL-17, release lysosomal enzymes and reactive oxygen species (ROS) that fragment hyphae.

4 Fragmented hyphae and fungal spores are phagocytosed by neutrophils and macrophages. NK cells also participate in the removal of fungi.

5 The presence of phagocytic cells and lytic enzymes, as well as the molecules released by the activation of the complement by the alternative pathway, trigger acute inflammation (see Chart 7).

ESTABLISHED INFECTION – ACQUIRED IMMUNITY

6 In established fungal infections, acquired defenses enter in action.

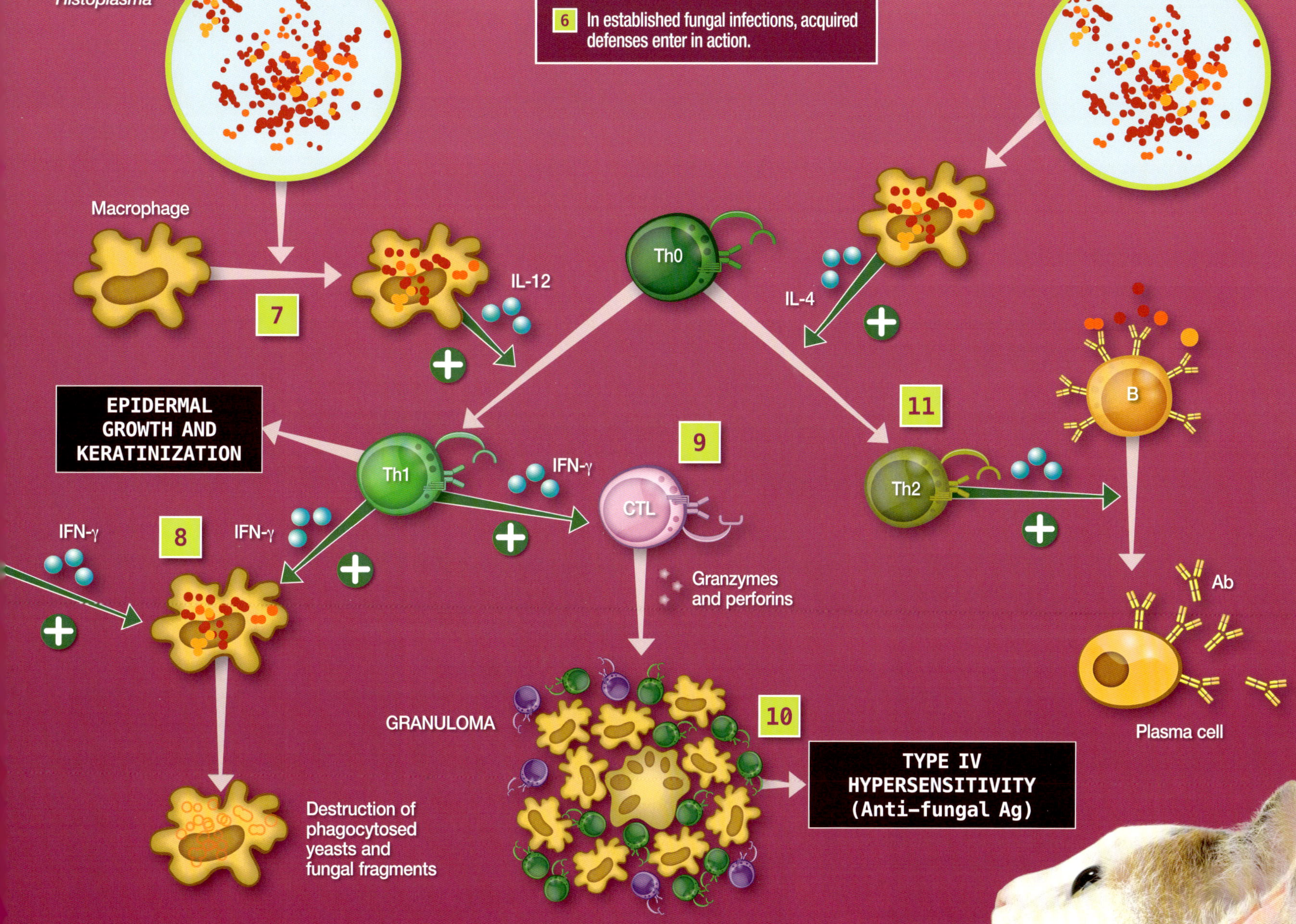

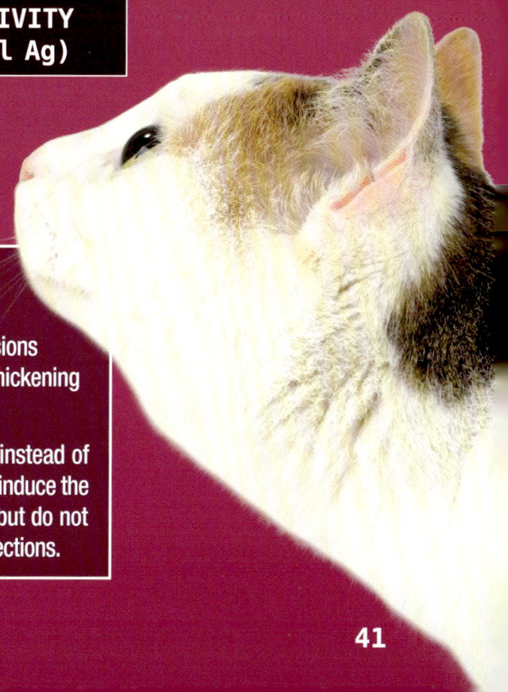

7 Some yeasts can survive inside macrophages. These infected macrophages secrete **IL-12**, which induces Th0 to differentiate into **Th1** cells, responsible for the solely effective responses to intracellular fungi.

8 Macrophages with phagocytosed fungal fragments or with intracellular yeasts are activated by IFN-γ synthesized by the Th1 or NK cells. Once activated, they destroy the foreign elements.

9 CD8+ T cells are activated by cytokines secreted by the Th1 cells and become **CTL** which synthesize granzymes and perforins.

10 Continuous secretion of cytokines by Th1 cells attracts macrophages, Th and Tc cells, triggering an exacerbated cellular immune response that causes granulomatous lesions (Type IV hypersensitivity, see Chart 21). It also produces thickening of the skin by epidermal growth and keratinization.

11 Occasionally, macrophages and other APC secrete **IL-4** instead of IL-12. In this case the **Th2** responses are activated. These induce the synthesis of antibodies, which are useful for diagnosis, but do not have a clear protective nature in the majority of fungal infections.

IMMUNITY AGAINST HELMINTHS

The eosinophils and the IgE are the main protagonists in the immune response against helminths. Helminths penetrate the body most frequently through the mucous membranes, where the immune responses are triggered. The phenomenon of premunition, characteristic of parasitic infections, is a state in which the immune defenses of a host infested by helminths are enough to protect it from the superinfestation, but insufficient to kill the worm.

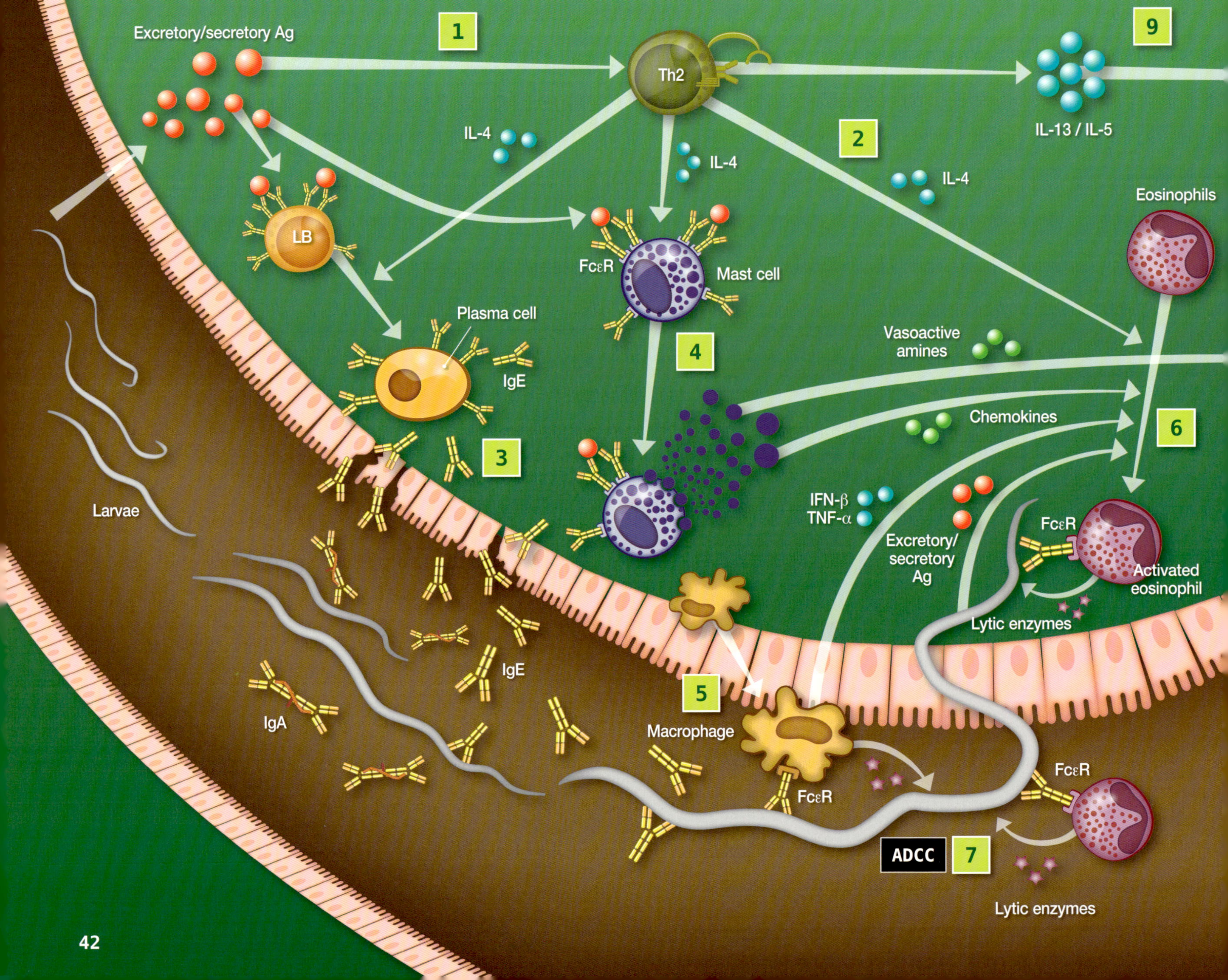

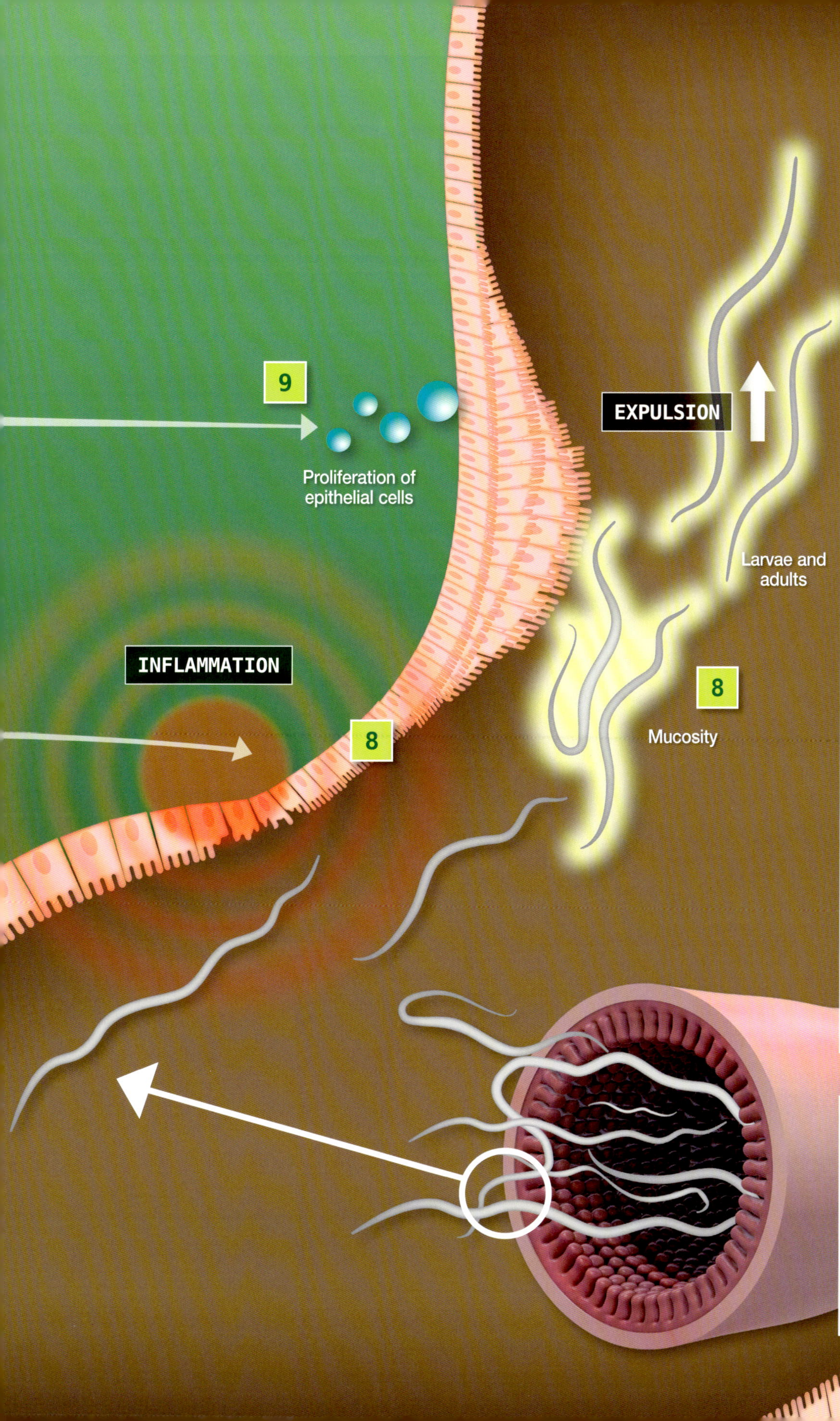

1 Excretory/secretory antigens produced by helminths promote **Th2 responses** (distinctive of the response to these parasites), characterized by the secretion of IL-4.

2 **IL-4** produces the accumulation of mast cells in the submucosa, the mobilization of eosinophils, and the differentiation of B cells to plasma cells which secrete IgE, specific against the parasitic Ag. IgG and IgA can also be synthesized.

3 Due to the high concentration of **IgE**, helminth infestations are often accompanied by Type I hypersensitivity reactions, with eosinophilia, edema, pruritus and asthma (see Chart 20).

4 **Mast cells** bind IgE thanks to their receptors for this immunoglobulin (FcεR). The recognition of Ag by the specific IgE produces the degranulation of these sensitized mast cells, releasing vasoactive amines (which induce local inflammation) and chemotactic substances (see Chart 20).

5 **Macrophages** also have FcεR, through which they bind the Ab attached to the parasite. When this happens, they become activated, increasing their lysosomal activity and releasing lytic enzymes on the parasite.

6 **Eosinophils**, attracted by chemokines to the site where the parasite is located, are activated by different factors (IL-4, TNF-α, etc.).

7 Because they have FcεR, eosinophils can bind to antibody-coated helminths, degranulate, and release their granule contents directly on the parasite. These contents include lytic enzymes, radicals of oxygen, etc., which are very effective in destroying helminths.

8 **Vasoactive amines** increase vascular permeability and muscle contraction, and stimulate the Goblet cells to produce **mucus**, which coats the parasites facilitating their expulsion. In the intestine, the absorption of sodium is also inhibited, causing **diarrhea**.

9 Helminths are also eliminated by the action of IL-13, which stimulates the **proliferation of epithelial cells**. This forces the parasites to detach from the mucosa.

Evasion strategies

Helminths may evade the immune system by any of the following mechanisms:

a resisting complement and lytic enzymes due to their thick cuticle;

b shedding their loose-fitting coat;

c changing the expression of surface antigens at each molt.

IMMUNITY AGAINST TUMORS

The immune system plays an important role in the prevention and elimination of tumors, but its effectiveness depends on the type of tumor and its growth rate. In addition, many tumors go unnoticed to the immune system, either due to their location or because they can evade the immune response. Cells of the innate immunity, and especially the NK cells, are critical for controlling the onset of the tumor focus, and the CTL are decisive in preventing its progression.

UNCONTROLLED MULTIPLICATION OF THE TRANSFORMED CELL

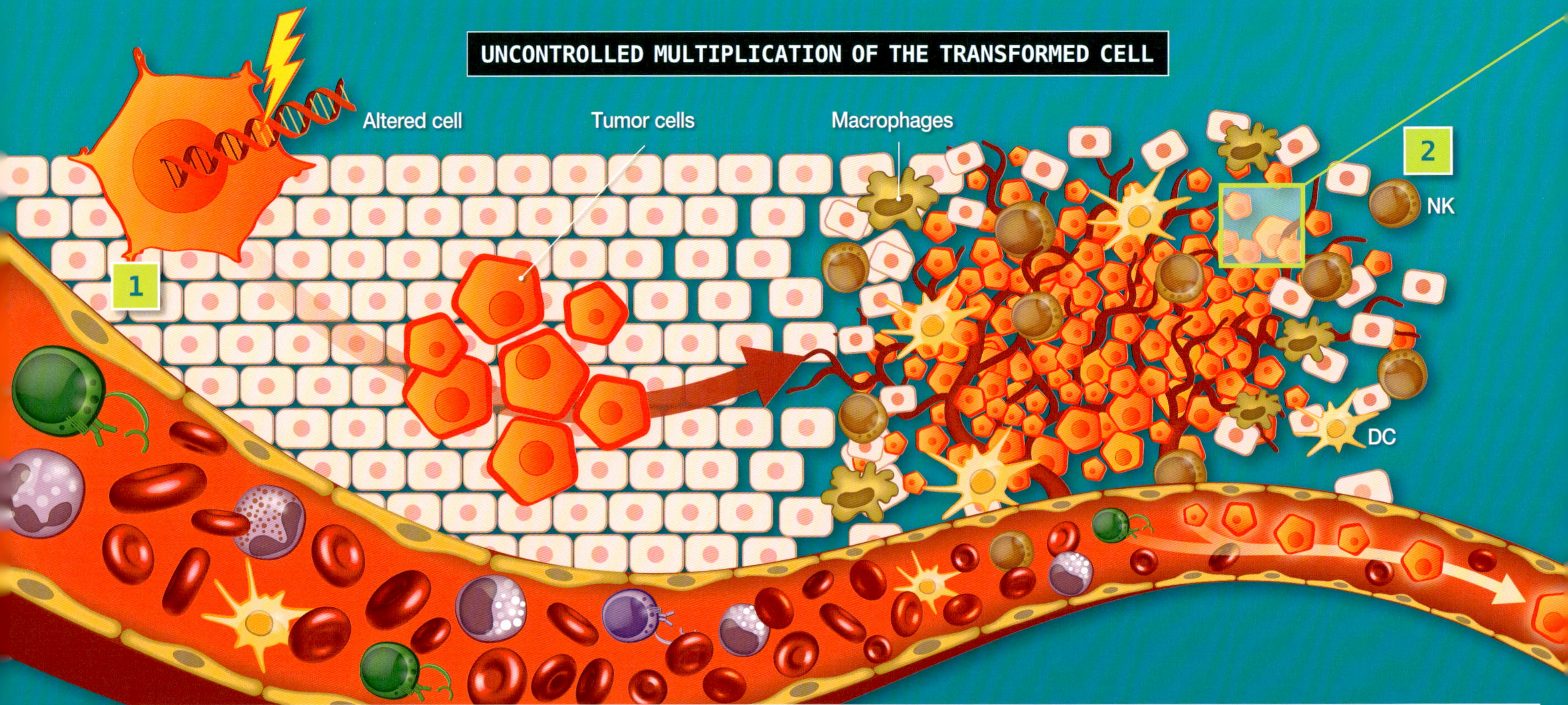

1 The genetic alteration of the tumor cell may be inherited or caused by physical (UV radiation), or chemical agents (certain pesticides), or oncogenic viruses (*e.g.*, feline leukemia virus, canine oral papilloma). The risk of developing tumors increases with age.

2 The chemokines produced by altered tissue attract NK cells and activate infiltrating macrophages and dendritic cells. In addition, enzymes that destroy the extracellular matrix and the basal cell layer of the tissue are released in malignant tumors. This favors the spread of tumor cells through the bloodstream and lymph to other tissues.

3 The **NK cells** in the blood and tissues recognize tumor cells with **altered or few MHC-I molecules** (see Chart 4) and destroy them through the perforins, granzymes and NK-lysins, and through the activation of apoptosis of tumor cells by FasL (see Chart 13). The activated NK cells produce antitumor cytokines (such as **IFN-γ**), which activate macrophages and other cells of the immune system.

4 Depending on the type of tumor and the cytokines produced, macrophages are differentiated into two populations: **M1**, with tumoricidal and Ag presentation abilities; and **M2**, associated with the progression of the tumor (see point 10). The tumoricidal activity of macrophages activated by IFN-γ is applied either directly, through TNF-α, proteases, reactive oxygen species (ROS), and nitric oxide; or indirectly, as a result of the destruction of the tumor vessels by TNF-α.

5 M1 macrophages, in turn, secrete cytokines (TNF-α and IL-12), which stimulate the proliferation and activity of the Tc cells and again, of macrophages and NK cells.

6 Some tumor Ag are recognized by the dendritic cells and presented to Th1 cells that release cytokines (IFN-γ and IL-2), which activate NK and Tc cells and M1 macrophages.

7 **The CTL recognize tumor Ag bound to MHC-I** and destroy tumor cells through the release of granzymes and perforins and through the activation of their apoptosis by FasL (see Chart 13).

8 When the tumor cells are destroyed by the M1 macrophages infiltrating the tumor, tumor peptides are bound to MHC-II and are presented to Th2 cells, promoting humoral response and the production of Ab specific for tumor Ag. **NK cells, neutrophils and macrophages are able to destroy tumor cells by ADCC** (see Chart 13). This antitumor mechanism does not seem to be very effective *in vivo*.

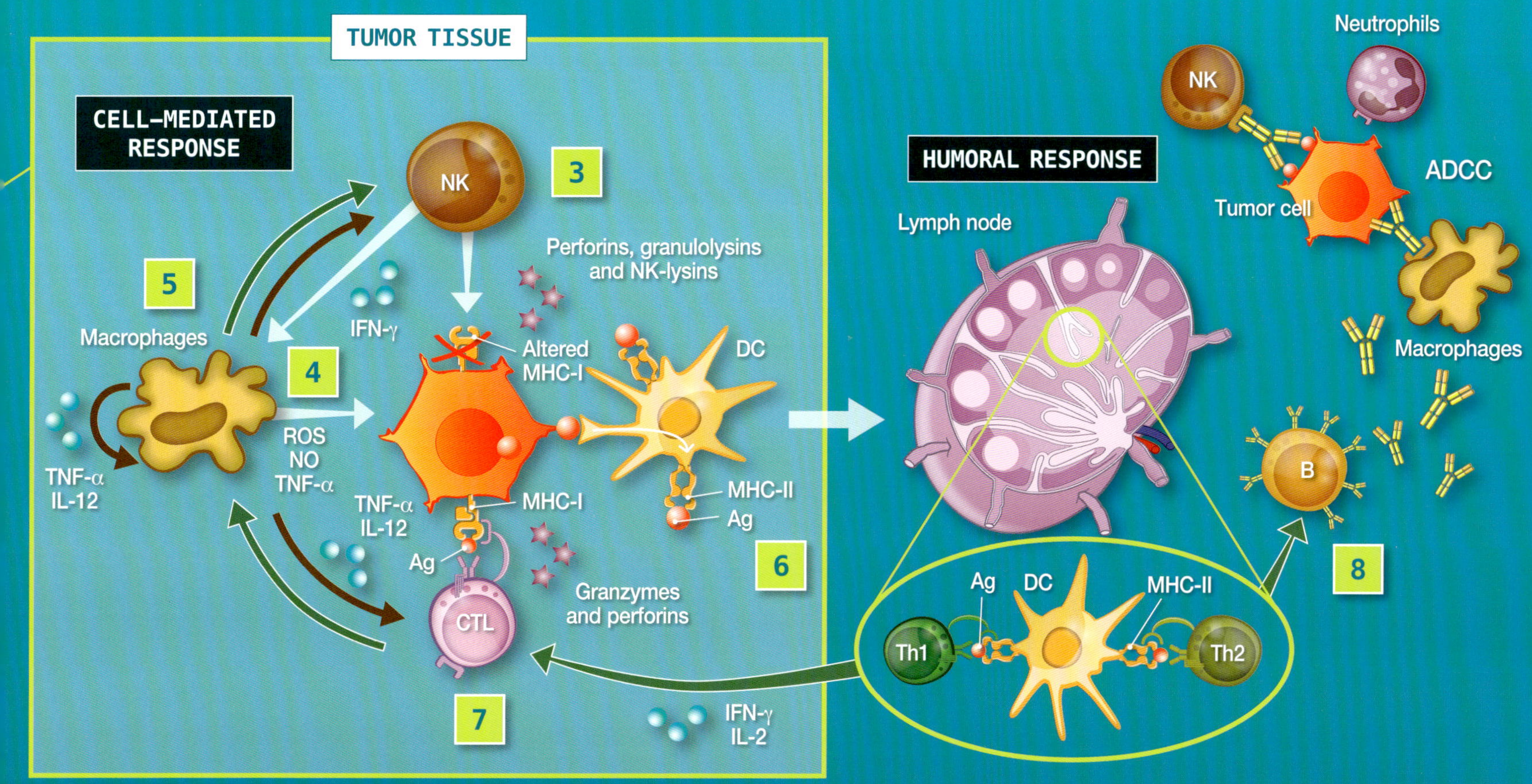

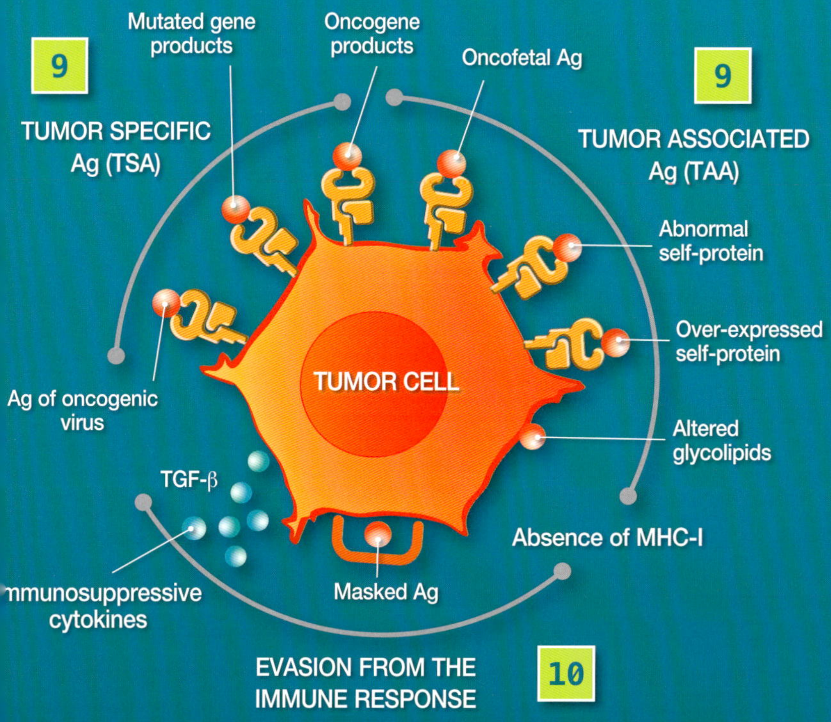

9 The most immunogenic **tumor Ag** are products of oncogenes, viruses and mutated genes. Oncofetal Ag and Ag that are expressed on normal cells but are over-expressed in tumor cells can induce immune response or tolerance.

10 **Tumors can evade the immune response** through different mechanisms. For example, the MHC-I molecules may be altered or absent, tumor cells can produce mucopolysaccharides which mask Ag, or cytokines (TGF-β) that induce immunosuppression or determine the differentiation of M2 macrophages.

11 The use of immunohistochemical techniques and the presence of certain markers (*e.g.*, telomerase activity) or tumor Ag (*e.g.*, carcinoembryonic Ag), allow for rating the prognosis and treatment of the tumor.

TREATMENT

12 **Immunotherapy with cytokines** (TNF-α, IFN-α, IL-2) may be applied to complement the radio- or chemotherapy following removal of some malignant tumors of dogs and cats, such as the feline squamous cell carcinoma and mammary carcinoma.

13 Other immunological treatments may include the administration of **therapeutic vaccines**, such as the DNA vaccine (see Chart 42), developed against oral melanoma. Other vaccines, still in their experimental stage, use extracts of tumor cells and recombinant cytokines.

ALLERGY

Hypersensitivity is an excessive and inappropriate immune response against usually harmless antigens, resulting in tissue damage and systemic alterations. An allergy is an immediate hypersensitivity reaction (Type I) mediated by high levels of IgE. It develops in genetically predisposed individuals (atopic), who are sensitized to a particular allergen. Clinical signs are the result of a sudden and massive release of inflammatory mediators from mast cells.

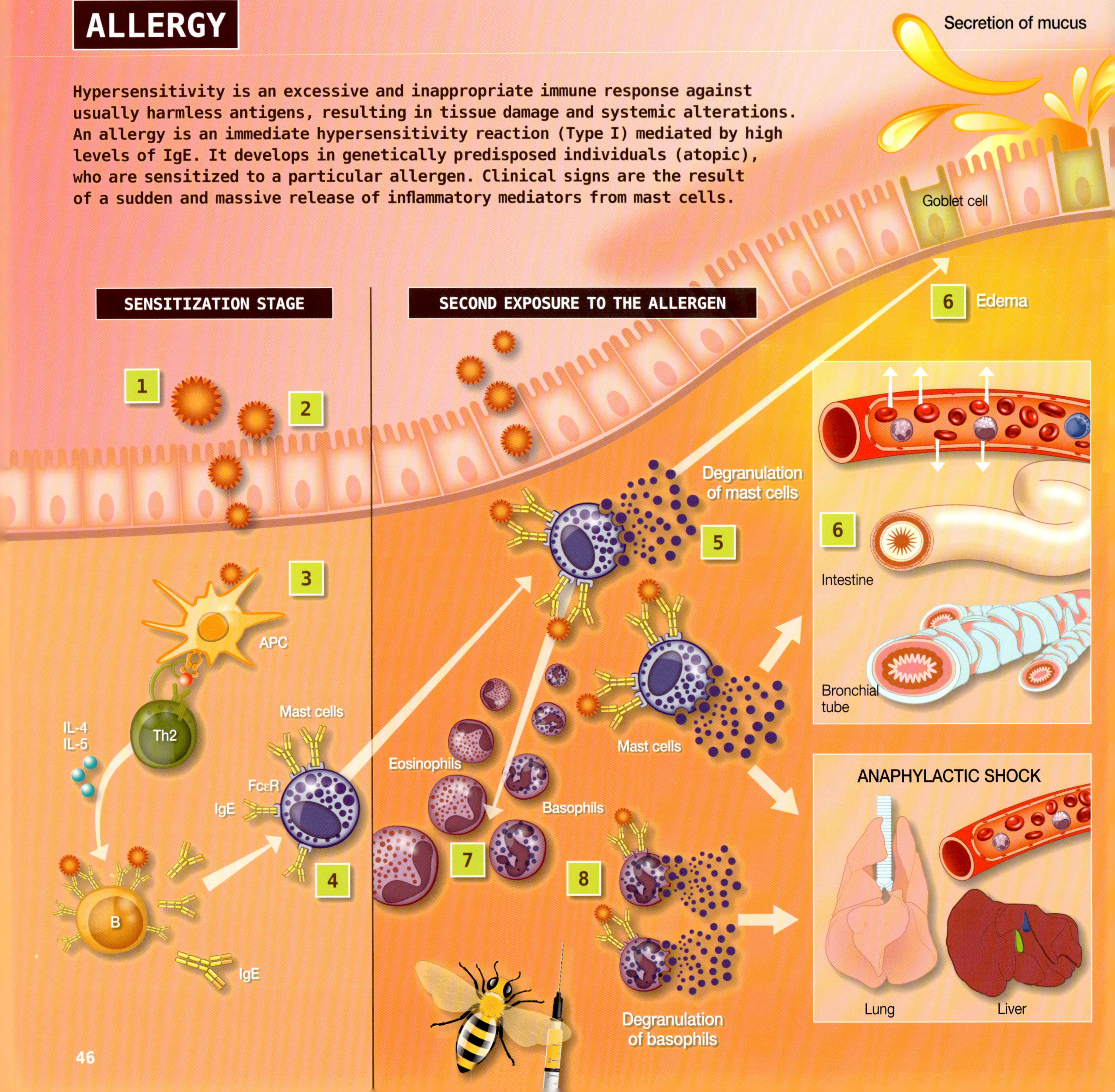

1 An **allergen** is a normally ubiquitous environmental Ag which induces an allergic response. Most allergic reactions are localized, affecting the mucosal and cutaneous surfaces (eye, respiratory, digestive) through which the allergen enters.

2 The first phase of the allergic reaction is the **sensitization** of the immune system by a first contact with the allergen. The second exposure to the same allergen gives rise to a hypersensitivity reaction and clinical alterations, which appear 15-30 minutes later.

3 Allergens are captured by the APC which present them to the Th cells, which differentiate to Th2 cells. In atopic individuals, these Th2 cells promote B cells to secrete high levels of **IgE**.

4 IgE bind their specific receptors on the surface of **mast cells** and sensitize them. They also bind to a lesser extent to basophils and eosinophils.

5 In a second exposure to the allergen, it cross-links two IgE attached to the mast cell, causing its **degranulation** and the release of **inflammatory mediators**, whose effect is immediate (histamine, serotonin, heparin, proteases) or more delayed (leukotrienes, prostaglandins, platelet-activating factor and certain cytokines).

6 At the local level, the inflammatory mediators originate vasodilatation and edema, smooth muscle contraction in the bronchi and gastrointestinal tract, increased secretion of mucus, and pruritus.

7 A **late-phase reaction** sometimes occurs 6 to 12 hours later in cutaneous reactions, involving basophils and eosinophils, attracted to the tissues by the chemotactic factors released by mast cells.

8 The parenteral administration of an allergen causes a generalized degranulation of basophils and mast cells, with massive release of inflammatory mediators. This leads to an **anaphylactic reaction** or **anaphylaxis**, with collapse and death of the animal in a short time. Dogs tend to suffer liver and heart failures, whereas in cats lung and intestine are more affected.

9 The most common allergies are to flea-bites, some proteins in the diet, vaccines and drugs, inhaled Ag such as pollen, and contact with some allergens. Clinical signs depend on the route of entry of the allergen, although food allergies are accompanied by skin reactions as well as by digestive signs.

10 The majority of the animals develop allergies to several allergens. Certain breeds, such as French Bulldog or Yorkshire Terrier, are more predisposed to suffer from allergies.

Main allergies in the dog and cat

Skin allergic reactions usually are seen on ears, face, axillae, feet, abdomen and perianal area.

RESPIRATORY AND OCULAR ALLERGIES

- Rhinitis and conjunctivitis
- Asthma
- Nasal exudates and lachrymal discharge

FOOD ALLERGIES

- Diarrhea
- Vomiting
- Highly pruritic skin reactions

SKIN ALLERGIES

- Dermatitis
- Erythema
- Pruritus
- Edema
- Scabbing
- Pyoderma
- Hyperpigmentation

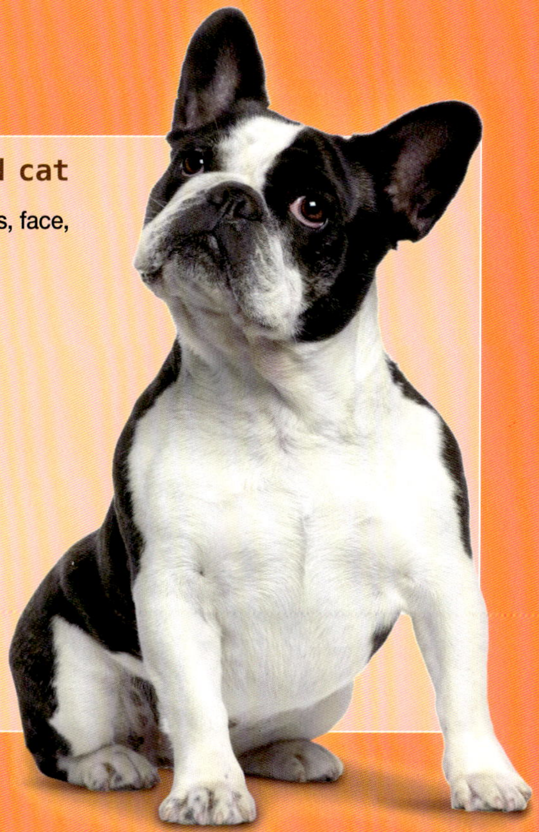

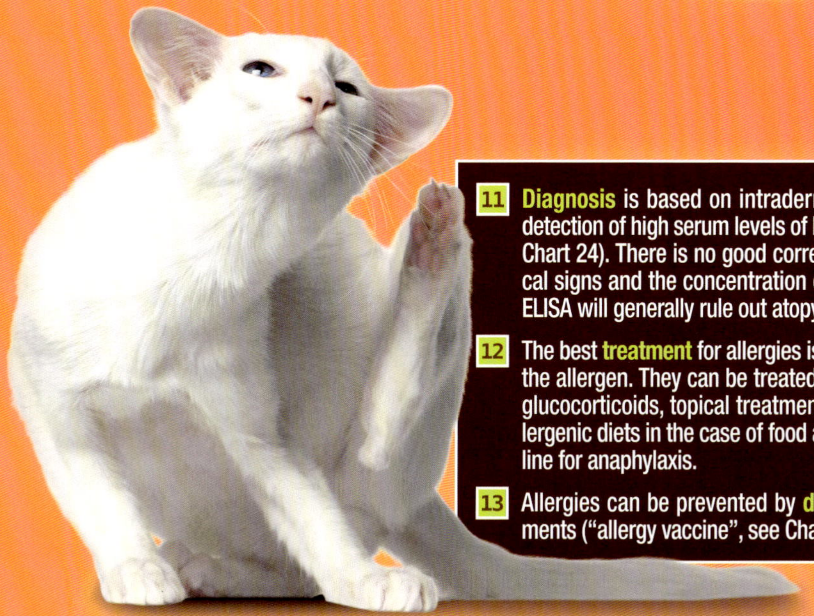

11 **Diagnosis** is based on intradermal skin testing and detection of high serum levels of IgE (by ELISA test, see Chart 24). There is no good correlation between clinical signs and the concentration of IgE, but a negative ELISA will generally rule out atopy.

12 The best **treatment** for allergies is to avoid exposure to the allergen. They can be treated with antihistamines, glucocorticoids, topical treatment of pruritus, hypoallergenic diets in the case of food allergies, and adrenaline for anaphylaxis.

13 Allergies can be prevented by **desensitization** treatments ("allergy vaccine", see Chart 25).

NON-ALLERGIC HYPERSENSITIVITY REACTIONS

ANTIBODY-MEDIATED

TYPE II HYPERSENSITIVITY

1 **Type II hypersensitivity** is an antibody-mediated cytotoxicity that develops within a few hours. Ab (IgG or IgM) bind to the Ag on the cell surface, mediating its destruction by various mechanisms of cytotoxicity (ADCC, lysis by complement activation, and release of lytic enzymes when unable to engulf the cell).

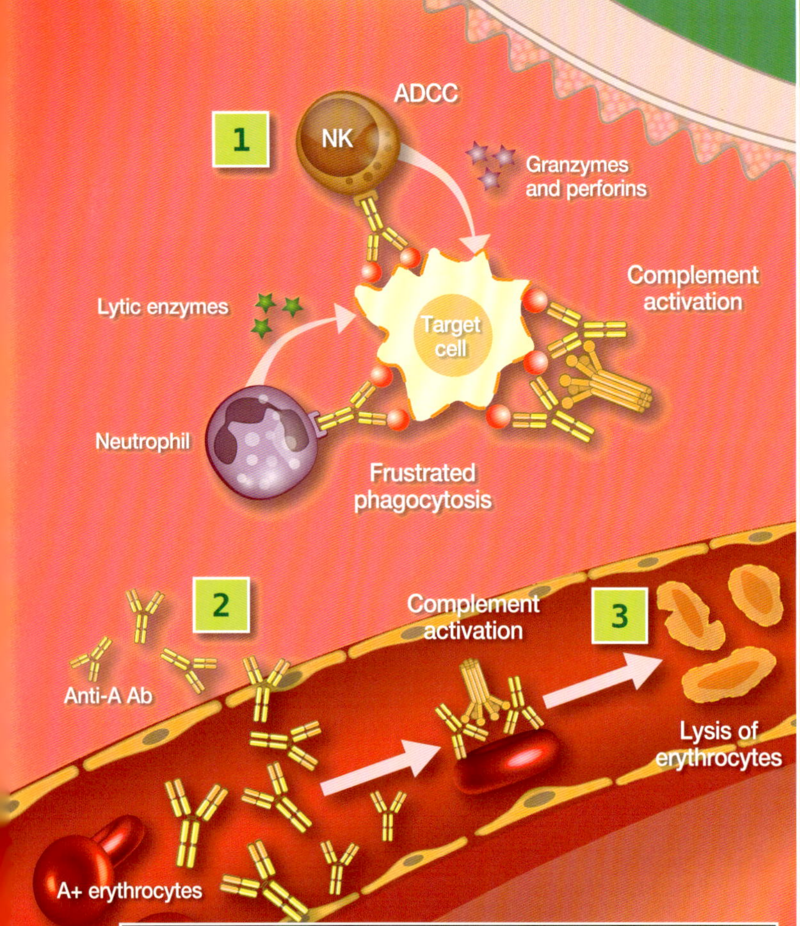

2 In the **hemolytic disease of the newborn**, erythrocytes of the puppy or kitten are lysed by Ab anti-erythrocytes present in maternal colostrums (see Chart 12).

3 Type II hypersensitivity is also involved in the lysis of erythrocytes in transfused incompatible blood, in the hemolytic anemia due to the reaction to certain drugs such as antibiotics, in the hyperacute rejection of transplants, and in some autoimmune diseases such as pemphigus.

TYPE III HYPERSENSITIVITY

4 **Type III hypersensitivity** occurs 3 to 10 hours after the entry of a soluble Ag in the presence of high levels of circulating Ab (IgG or IgM). Large quantities of immune complexes are formed, which accumulate and are deposited in capillaries and tissues. This activates the complement, which attracts neutrophils (that release their lytic enzymes directly on the tissue) and mast cells, promoting an acute inflammatory reaction (see Chart 7).

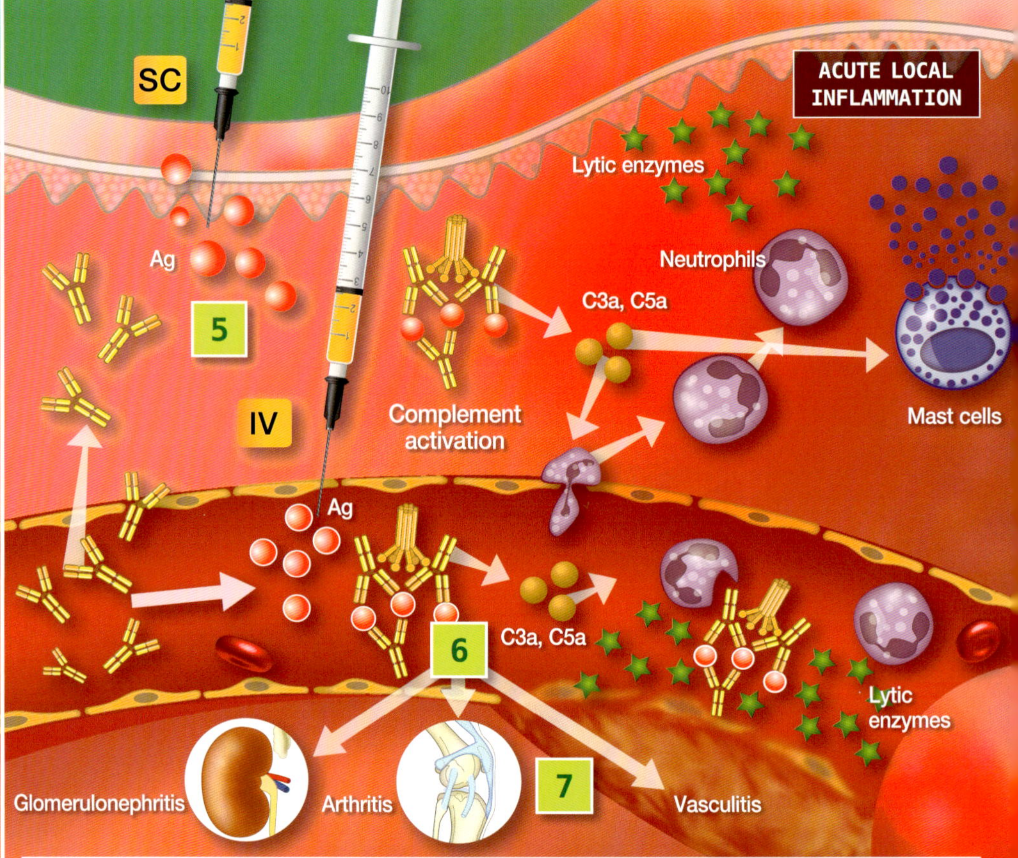

5 If the Ag penetrates through the subcutaneous route, the immune complexes accumulate at the site of entry, leading to a local inflammation (**"Arthus reaction"**). The "blue eye" is an edema and corneal opacity that can occur in dogs vaccinated or infected with infectious canine hepatitis virus, caused by the deposit of immune complexes (see Chart 41).

6 After the intravenous administration of a high dose of Ag, the immune complexes may be deposited on the walls of the capillaries (**vasculitis**), in the renal glomerulus (**glomerulonephritis**) and in the synovial capsule of joints (**arthritis**).

7 Type III hypersensitivity is involved in the pathogenesis of certain infectious and parasitic diseases, such as feline infectious peritonitis, visceral leishmaniosis, etc.; in some autoimmune diseases, such as rheumatoid arthritis; and in reactions to specific antibiotics.

Non-allergic hypersensitivity reactions may be mediated by Ab (Types II and III) or cells (Type IV), and are characterized because they take longer to develop than allergies, from hours to days or weeks.

CELL-MEDIATED

TYPE IV HYPERSENSITIVITY

8 **Type IV hypersensitivity** (or delayed hypersensitivity, since it takes more than 24 hours to occur) is a chronic local inflammatory reaction mediated by sensitized Th1 cells, following a second contact with the Ag.

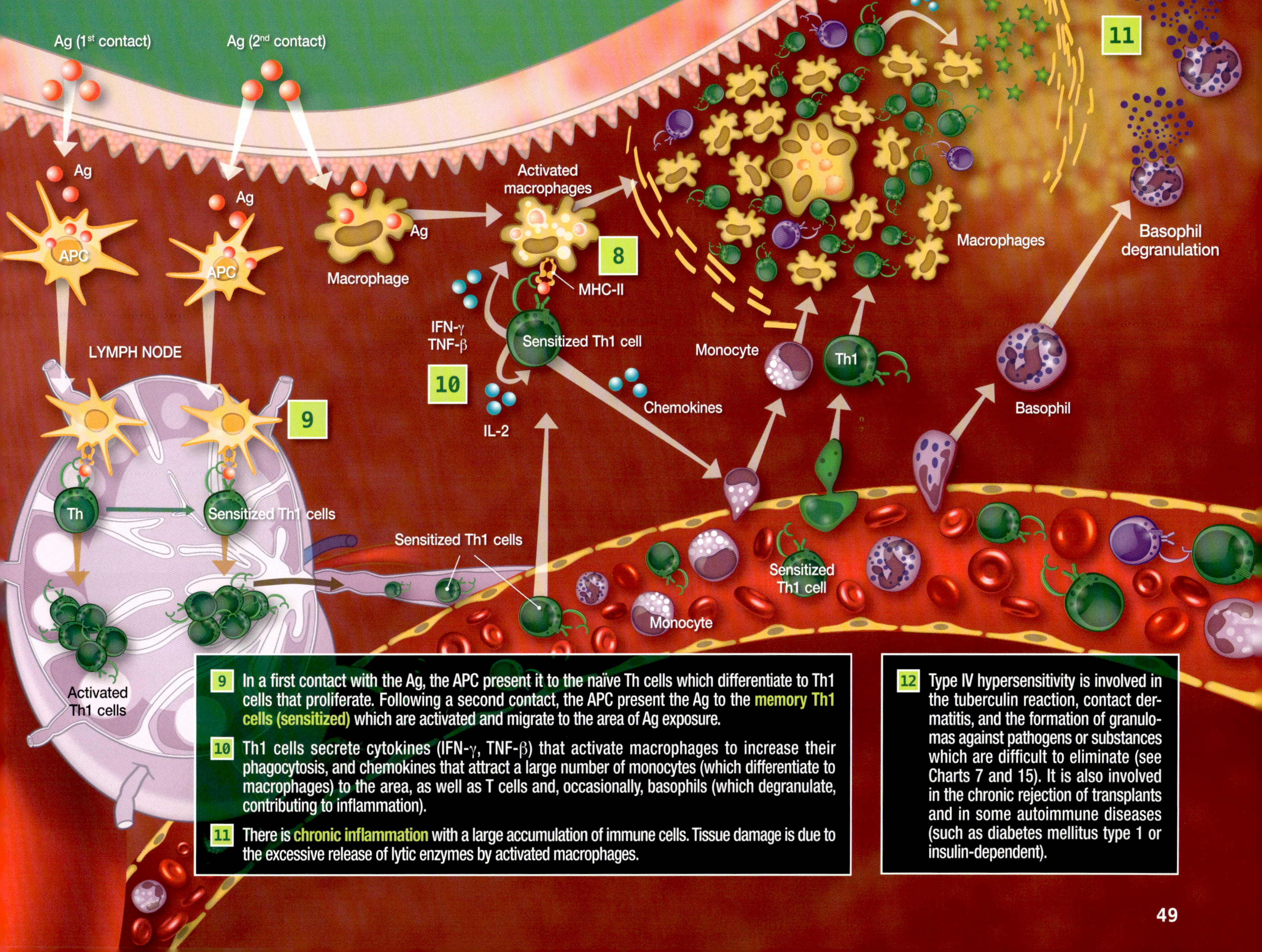

9 In a first contact with the Ag, the APC present it to the naïve Th cells which differentiate to Th1 cells that proliferate. Following a second contact, the APC present the Ag to the **memory Th1 cells (sensitized)** which are activated and migrate to the area of Ag exposure.

10 Th1 cells secrete cytokines (IFN-γ, TNF-β) that activate macrophages to increase their phagocytosis, and chemokines that attract a large number of monocytes (which differentiate to macrophages) to the area, as well as T cells and, occasionally, basophils (which degranulate, contributing to inflammation).

11 There is **chronic inflammation** with a large accumulation of immune cells. Tissue damage is due to the excessive release of lytic enzymes by activated macrophages.

12 Type IV hypersensitivity is involved in the tuberculin reaction, contact dermatitis, and the formation of granulomas against pathogens or substances which are difficult to eliminate (see Charts 7 and 15). It is also involved in the chronic rejection of transplants and in some autoimmune diseases (such as diabetes mellitus type 1 or insulin-dependent).

AUTOIMMUNITY

Autoimmunity is the process by which the immune system reacts against self-antigens (autoantigens). It is associated with a failure of the self-tolerance mechanisms which gives rise to autoreactive lymphocytes and autoantibodies that attack the cells, causing an autoimmune disease. Multiple predisposing and triggering factors are involved in its emergence, and as a consequence, it's difficult to prevent and control.

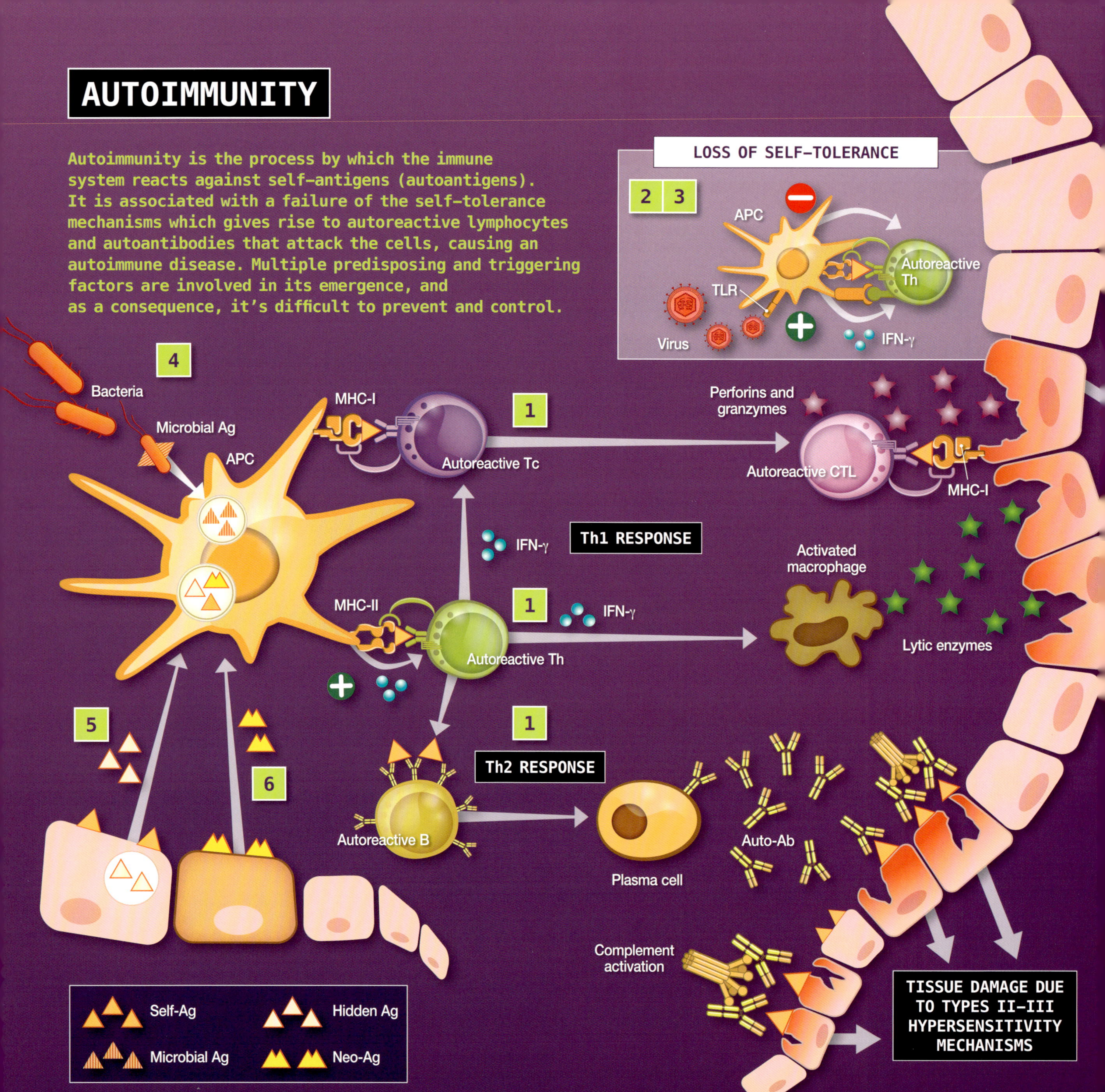

1 The autoimmune response is initiated when an APC presents an autoantigen to an autoreactive Th cell. If the self-tolerance mechanisms fail (see Chart 10), this Th cell is activated and can induce the production of **auto-Ab** (Th2 response) or the activation of **autoreactive Tc cells** and macrophages through the production of cytokines, such as IFN-γ (Th1 response). One or several mechanisms of hypersensitivity (II, III, IV) may be involved in the cell damage (see Chart 21).

2 The **loss of self-tolerance** can occur due to a failure in the negative selection of autoreactive T cells in the thymus, the failure of the anergy of the T and B cells, and the insufficient suppressor activity of T regulatory cells (see Chart 10).

3 **Failure of anergy:** an infectious agent may bind the TLR of an APC which is presenting self-antigens, and activate it. This triggers co-stimulatory signals which terminate anergy and allow the synthesis of cytokines, resulting in the activation of the autoreactive T cell.

4 One of the mechanisms by which autoimmunity is developed is the **molecular mimicry**, whereby a microbial Ag which shares epitopes with a self-Ag gives rise to Ab that react to both (*e.g.*, Ab produced against *Streptococcus* recognize epitopes of myocardial cells).

5 An autoimmune response can be induced against cellular Ag with which the immune system has had no prior contact, and therefore has not developed self-tolerance. This is the case of **hidden Ag** inside cells or tissues, which are exposed because of an infection or injury (*e.g.*, antinuclear Ab or ANA, typical of systemic lupus erythematosus).

6 An infectious agent or a chemical compound (some antibiotics), among others, can **modify the self-Ag** originating **neo-antigens** (neo-Ag) that activate the immune response.

7 There is a **genetic predisposition** to autoimmunity, since it is associated with certain MHC haplotypes (variants).

8 Autoimmunity affects **adult or senior animals** more frequently, possibly associated with immunosenescence (decreased immune response at older age, mainly affecting the suppressor activity of regulatory T cells).

9 Autoimmune diseases tend to appear after a **triggering factor**, such as an infection (the most frequent cause), ultraviolet light, stress, cancer, antibiotic treatment, vaccination, etc.

TISSUE DAMAGE DUE TO TYPE IV HYPERSENSITIVITY MECHANISM

10 Autoimmune diseases are more prevalent in dogs than in cats. In addition, they are more common in certain dog breeds and pedigrees (Cocker Spaniel, Golden Retriever, Doberman, etc.). There is no sex predisposition.

11 In dogs, autoimmunity may be associated with an IgA deficiency, which causes weakening of the mucosal immunity and increased susceptibility to infections (see Chart 23).

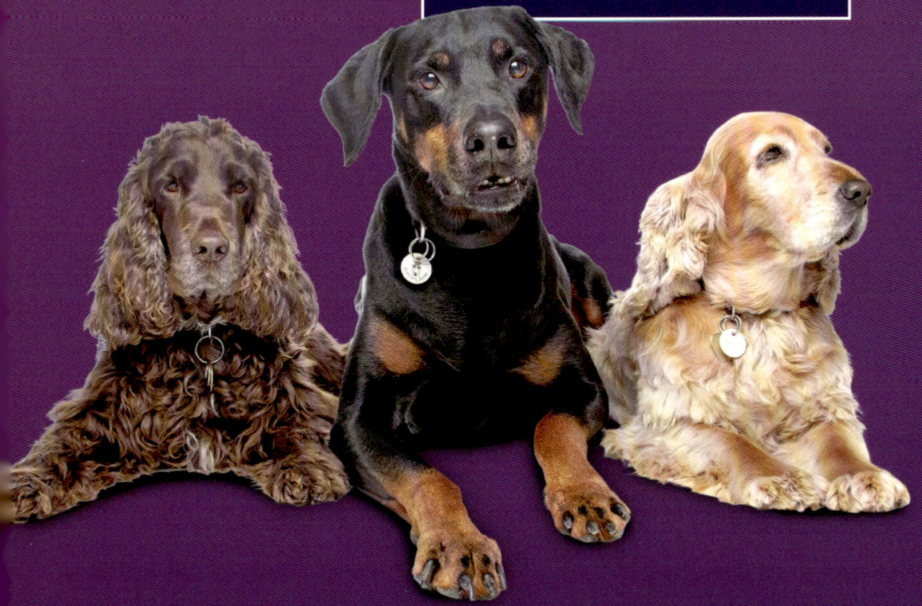

12 Autoimmune diseases tend to be persistent and long-lasting. Most are local or "organ-specific" and very few are systemic. The diagnosis is based on clinical data and the testing for autoantibodies and autoreactive lymphocytes by different immunological techniques.

ORGAN-SPECIFIC AUTOIMMUNE DISEASES (hypersensitivity mechanism associated with tissue damage)	
Hypothyroidism	Destruction of glandular cells of the thyroid mediated by autoreactive Tc cells (IV).
Diabetes mellitus type 1 (insulin-dependent)	Destruction of β cells of the pancreatic islets mediated by autoreactive Tc cells and auto-Ab (IV and II).
Canine polyneuritis	Destruction of the myelin sheath of the peripheral nerves mediated by autoreactive Tc cells (IV).
Autoimmune hemolytic anemia	Lysis of erythrocytes mediated by auto-Ab (II).
Autoimmune thrombocytopenia	Lysis of thrombocytes mediated by auto-Ab (II).
Pemphigus	Destruction of desmosomes (structures which bind cells of the epidermis with the epithelial basal layer) by auto-Ab (II).
SYSTEMIC AUTOIMMUNE DISEASES (hypersensitivity mechanism associated with tissue damage)	
Systemic lupus erithematosus	Damage in different body systems and tissues, produced by a large variety of auto-Ab: anti-nuclear (ANA), anti-erythrocytes and anti-thrombocytes (II and III).
Rheumatoid arthritis	Polyarthritis produced by auto-Ab against IgG ("rheumatoid factor") (III and IV).

IMMUNODEFICIENCIES AND IMMUNOSUPPRESSION

Immunodeficiency is the extended impairment in the response of the immune system, which leads to increased susceptibility to infections. It can be primary (congenital) or secondary (acquired).

Immunosuppression is the transient inhibition of the immune system, secondary to another disorder, and that disappears when the cause is removed.

PRIMARY IMMUNODEFICIENCIES

1 **Primary immunodeficiencies** are very rare and are a result of genetic mutation in different stages of the development of either innate or acquired immune systems. They are often detected in very young puppies once maternal immunity wanes, and do not have treatment. They are inherited and associated with certain breeds or pedigrees, especially in dogs.

2 More than 30 types of canine immunodeficiencies have been described, but the genetic basis of them is only known in few cases. The best known are shown in the figure on the next page.

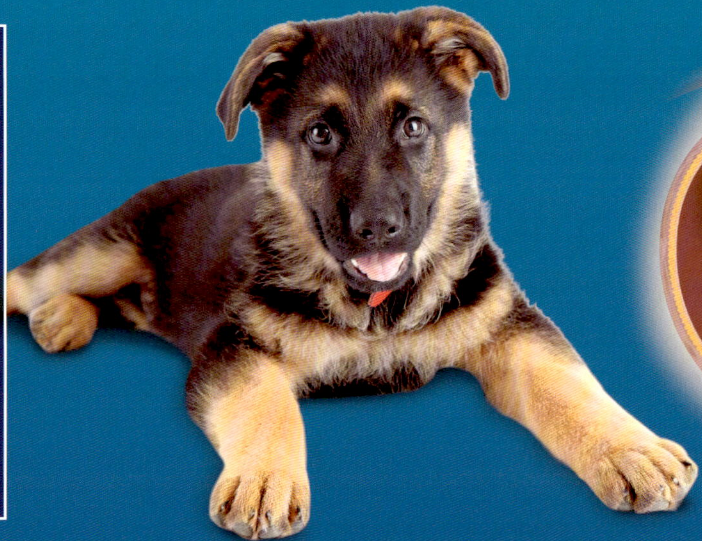

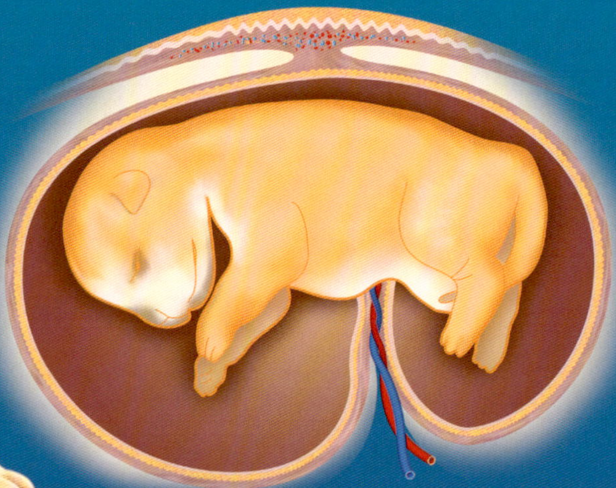

SECONDARY IMMUNODEFICIENCIES AND IMMUNOSUPPRESSION

3 **Secondary or acquired immunodeficiencies** are much more frequent. They appear in animals of any age, but especially in adults. Usually they are caused by certain infections, mainly of viral etiology (*e.g.*, feline immunodeficiency virus or FIV, see Chart 37). They are also associated with malnutrition, endocrine disorders, chronic stress, chronic inflammatory and neoplastic diseases, and the use of certain drugs such as glucocorticoids (see Chart 25).

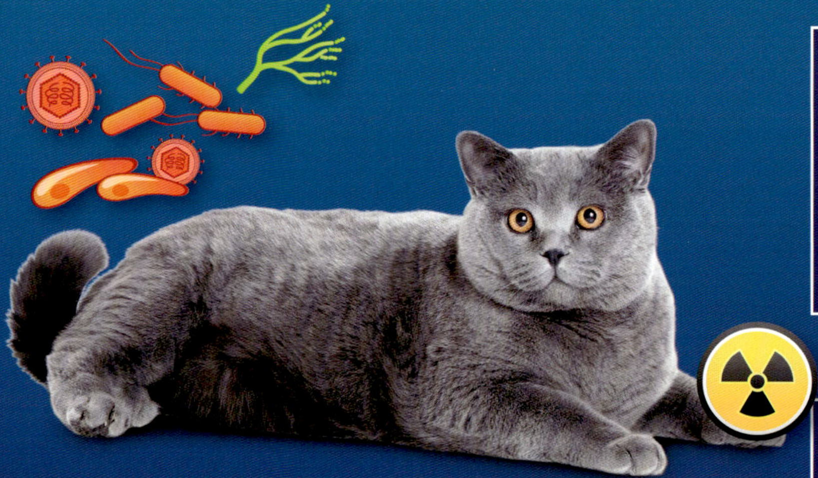

4 **Immunosenescence** is a physiological aged-related immunodeficiency. Senior cats and dogs have a decline in immune response, decreased CD4+ T cell counts, a reduction in CD4/CD8 ratio, predominance of memory T cells and a reduced primary response, but elevated serum levels of Ab.

5 **Immunosuppression** can be induced by "natural" causes (*e.g.*, canine distemper virus infection) or medically (*e.g.*, X-ray treatment for tumors, or administration of immunosuppressive drugs (see Chart 25).

Immunodeficiency should be suspected when animals have chronic, recurrent, or systemic infections that do not respond to treatment, caused by opportunistic microorganisms.

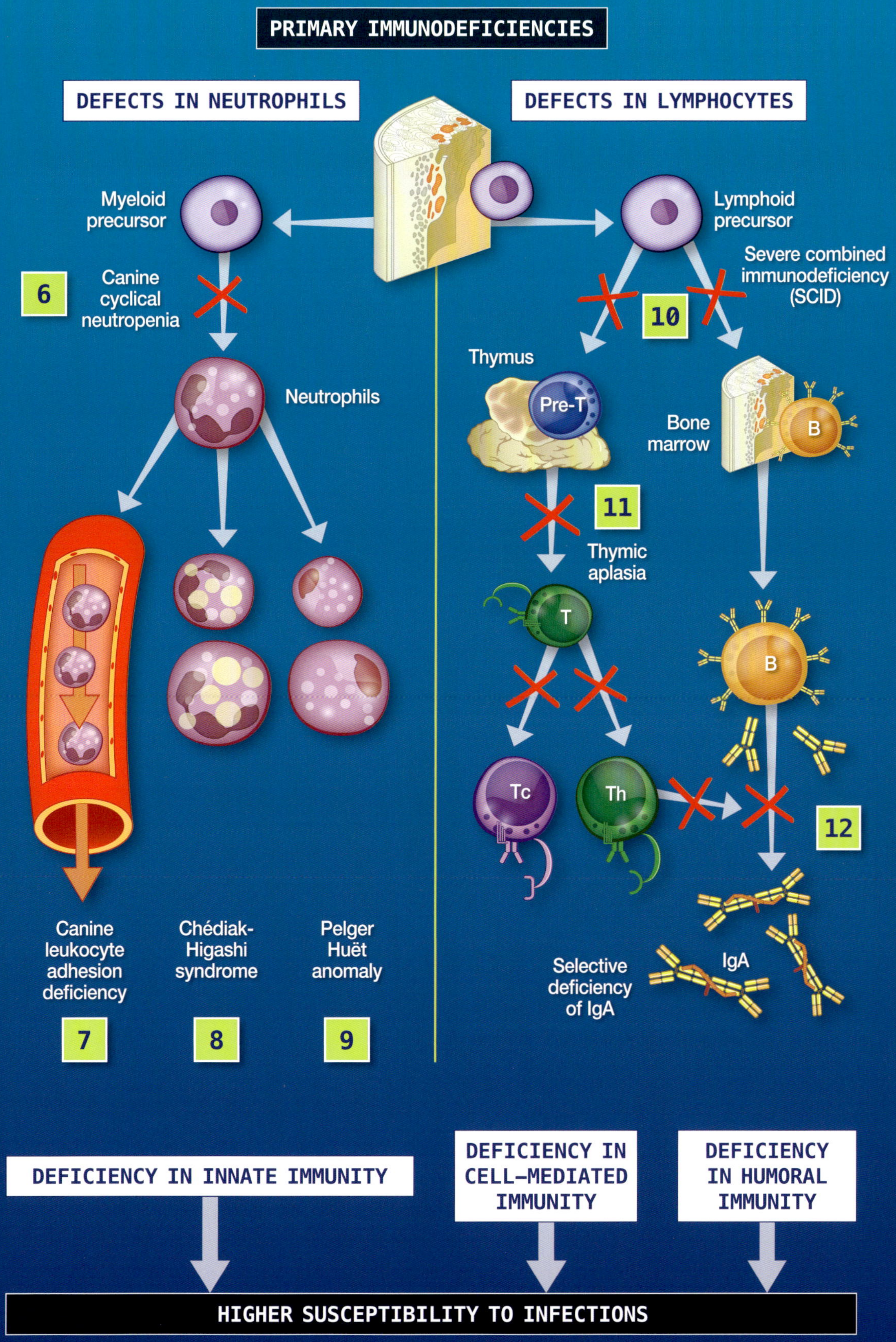

The best known primary immunodeficiencies are:

6 **Canine cyclical neutropenia.** It occurs approximately every 14 days, coinciding with episodes of infection. It has been described in grey Collies.

7 **Canine leukocyte adhesion deficiency.** Neutrophils do not express integrins CD18 and CD11b. This prevents their adherence to endothelial cells, their diapedesis, and migration to the focus of infection (see Chart 7). It has been described in Irish Setters.

8 **Chédiak-Higashi syndrome.** The granules of neutrophils are abnormally large and do not form the phagolysosomes (see Chart 8), so there is a reduced intracellular killing. It has been described in Persian cats.

9 **Pelger Huët anomaly.** It is characterized by a reduced segmentation of neutrophil nuclei, even though animals are clinically normal. It has been described in shorthair cats and dogs.

10 **Canine severe combined immunodeficiency (SCID).** It is the most severe alteration, since it affects both T and B cells, causing absence of cell-mediated immune response and of Ab production. A characteristic finding is lymphopenia. The SCID has been associated with a non-functional IL-2 receptor on T cells which prevents the activation of these cells (described in Basset Hounds and Welsh Corgis); or to a failure in the development of TCR and BCR in T and B cells, respectively (described in Jack Russell Terriers).

11 **Thymic aplasia.** It is characterized by a lack of mature T cells and is associated with the absence of body hair on the animals. It has been described in some breeds of hairless dogs and cats.

12 **Deficiency in one or more immunoglobulin classes.** It is the most common primary immunodeficiency in dogs and cats. It may be due to defects in either the B or the Th cells, which induce the Ig class switch. The most frequent is the **IgA deficiency**, described in German Shepherds, Shar-Peis, Beagles and Cocker Spaniels.

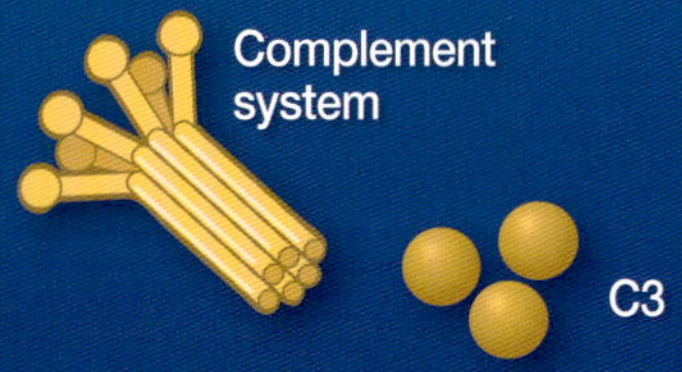

13 The deficiencies in some components of the **complement system** cause increased susceptibility to infections (*e.g.*, C3 deficiency in Britanny Spaniels, see Chart 4).

IMMUNODIAGNOSIS

Immunological techniques are used primarily for the diagnosis of infectious diseases, although they are also used to diagnose allergies, hypersensitivity reactions, autoimmune diseases and immunodeficiency, neoplastic diseases, etc. Diagnosis can be either direct or etiological (Ag detection), or indirect (detection of specific Ab against an Ag). Most of the techniques are based on *in vitro* Ag–Ab reactions. There are currently numerous commercial in-office kits easy and fast to use.

1

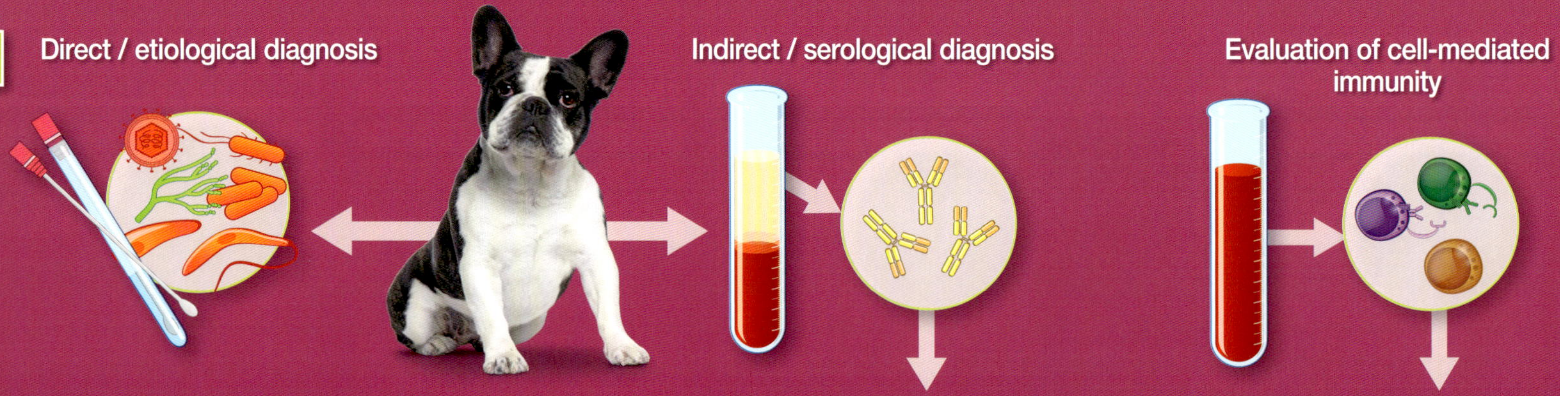

2 Ab TITER OF A SERUM

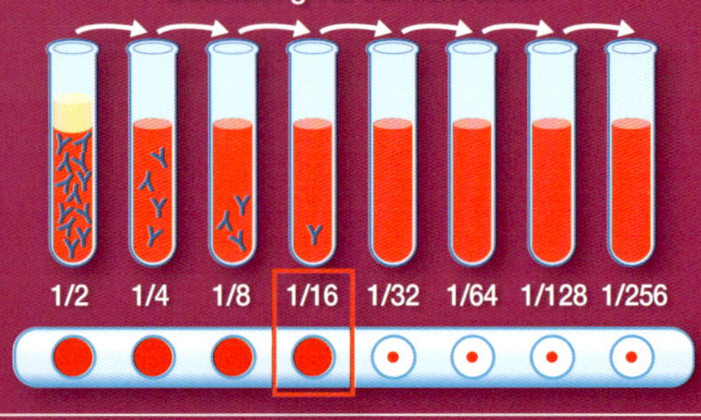

3

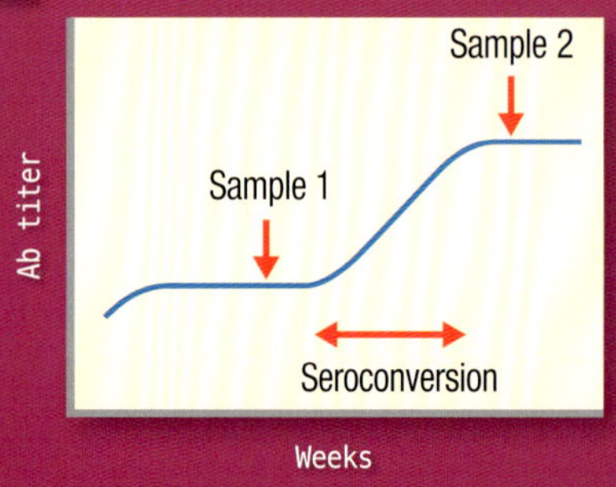

4 FLOW CYTOMETRY

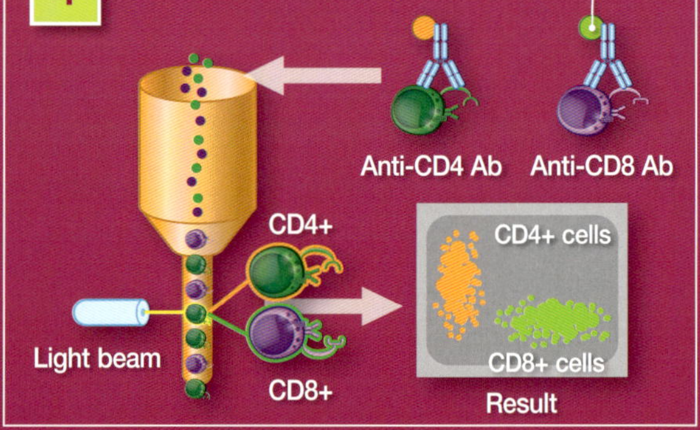

1 Direct immune diagnosis can be performed on any sample of the animal where the Ag may be present (blood, feces, secretions, biopsy of organs, etc.). Serum is often used for indirect immune diagnosis; for this reason, indirect diagnosis is called **serologic diagnosis or serology**. Ab may also be detected in whole blood and in other fluids such as saliva, vaginal exudate or milk.

2 The **titer of a serum** or of Ab is the concentration of specific Ab against an Ag. It is defined as the reciprocal of the highest dilution of a serum giving a positive reaction in an immunological test. The higher the titer, the higher the concentration of Ab in the sample.

3 **Seroconversion** is the 2 to 4-fold increase of the Ab titer between two serum samples taken 2-3 weeks apart. It implies an active infection. If the antibody titer is maintained or decreases it usually means that the animal is recovering from the infection.

4 **Flow cytometry** is used with whole blood or bone marrow aspirates, in order to evaluate the immune cell populations. It involves the use of monoclonal Ab labeled with fluorochromes for detecting cell surface Ag. One of its applications is the diagnosis of immunodeficiency (*e.g.*, CD4/CD8 ratio < 1.0 in cats).

5 Immunological techniques must have a high **sensitivity and specificity**. In general, highly sensitive tests tend to have low specificity and **vice versa**. In practice, the technique that offers the greatest sensitivity and specificity is the ELISA.

5 **SENSITIVITY AND SPECIFICITY OF A DIAGNOSTIC TEST**

Sensitivity: ability to detect very small concentration of Ag or Ab, and, thus, to detect most of the positive or infected animals.

Specificity: ability to detect only specific Ag or Ab.

False positive results	False negative results
• Ab that cross-react with other Ag. • Colostral Ab. • Vaccine-derived Ab.	• Very low Ab titer. • Absence of Ab (immunodeficient or immunosuppressed animal or immunotolerant animal). • Very early stages of the infection. • Disease which progresses very fast.

• Incorrect use of the test.
• Inappropiate sample or test.

6 TECHNIQUES THAT USE LABELED Ab

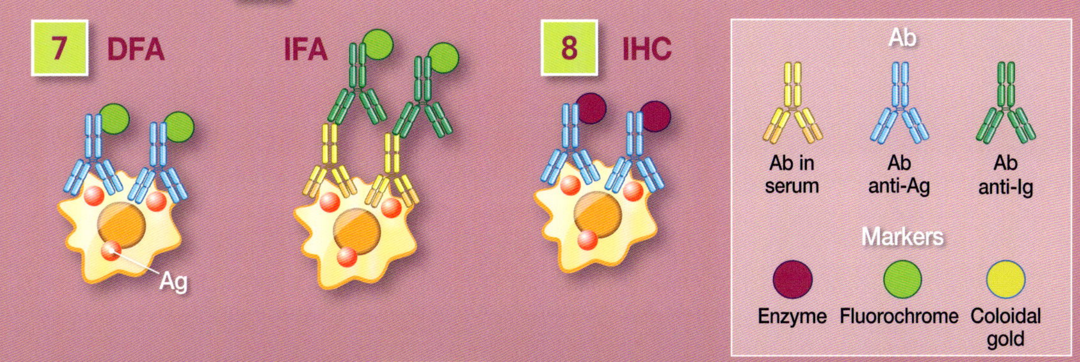

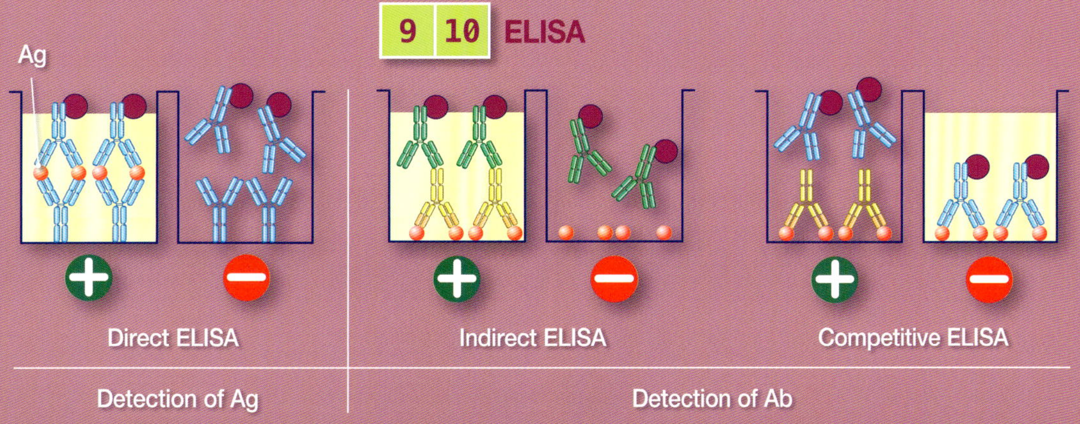

11 IMMUNOCHROMATOGRAPHY

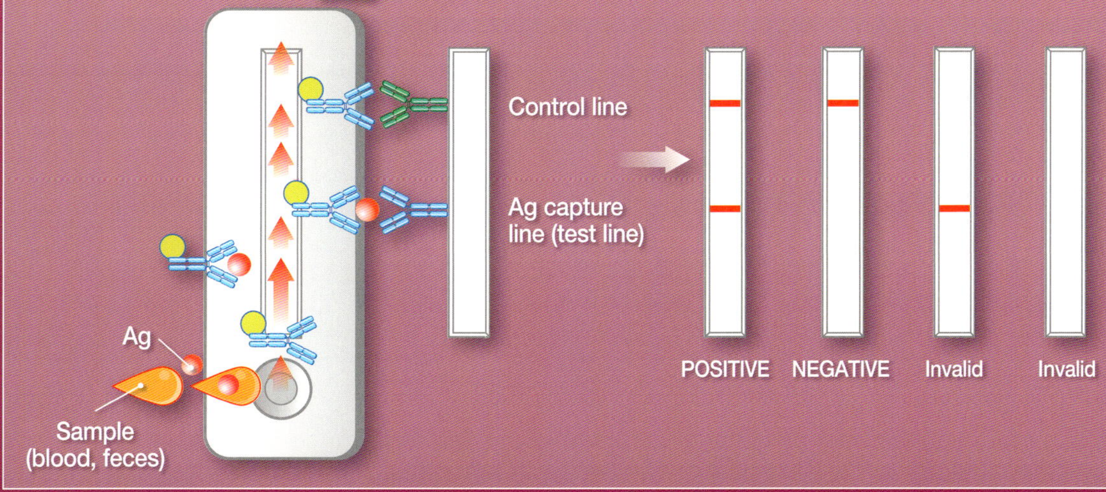

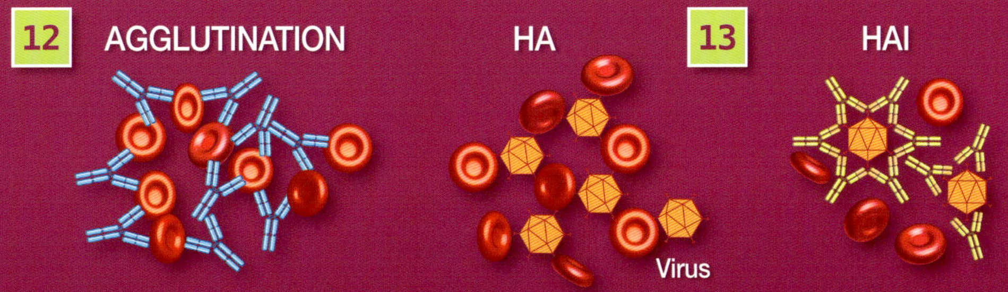

6 Most of the techniques use **Ab conjugates**, labeled with fluorochromes (immunofluorescence), enzymes (ELISA), or colloidal gold (immunochromatography).

7 **Direct immunofluorescence assays** (DFA) are used to detect Ag in infected or altered cells (*e.g.*, canine distemper virus). **Indirect immunofluorescence assays** (IFA) are used to detect and titer Ab when incubating increasing dilutions of sera on Ag positive cells (*e.g.*, canine leishmaniosis).

8 **Immunohistochemistry** (IHC) and **immunoperoxidase assays** (IP) are designed to detect Ag in histological sections of tissues (*e.g.*, infectious canine hepatitis, and feline infectious peritonitis). They are usually performed **post-mortem**.

9 **ELISA** is used to detect and quantify Ag (capture or sandwich ELISA) or Ab (indirect and competitive ELISA). It is a quantitative and automatable microplate technique (the optical density of the color, O.D., is determined by an ELISA reader). Commercial ELISA kits allow analyzing individual samples. It is the most widely used diagnostic test.

10 Currently there are many **kits or rapid immunoassay devices** based on the ELISA technique. A positive reaction is seen as a color circle or line ("dot-ELISA"). Either Ag or Ab or both may be detected (*e.g.*, Ag of feline leukemia virus and Ab against feline immunodeficiency virus, see Chart 36).

11 **Immunochromatography** (IC) is used in commercial in-office simple and fast devices, in which the sample flows quickly along a nitrocellulose strip. The positive reaction is seen as a colored line (*e.g.*, detection of coronaviruses and canine parvoviruses).

12 **Agglutination** is used for the detection of specific Ab, for determining the blood group, and for the diagnosis of autoimmune hemolytic anemia (Coombs test).

13 **Hemagglutination** (HA) and **hemagglutination inhibition** (HAI) assays are used to detect haemagglutinating viruses in samples (HA) (*e.g.*, canine parvovirus), and to titer Ab in sera (HAI), which specifically inhibit the reaction.

14 **Seroneutralization** (SN) is a technique for the titration of neutralizing Ab: viruses are incubated with increasing dilutions of serum on cell cultures, and if there are neutralizing Ab, the cytopathic effect of the virus is inhibited (*e.g.*, canine herpesvirus).

IMMUNOTHERAPY

The term immunotherapy includes all those treatments aimed at modulating the immune response in the animal. Some treatments are intended to decrease the immune response (immunosuppressants) in cases of excessive or inappropriate responses, such as autoimmunity and hypersensitivity. In other occasions it is necessary to administer immunostimulants to stimulate the immune system. This would be the case in immunodeficiency, and to improve the response to infectious agents.

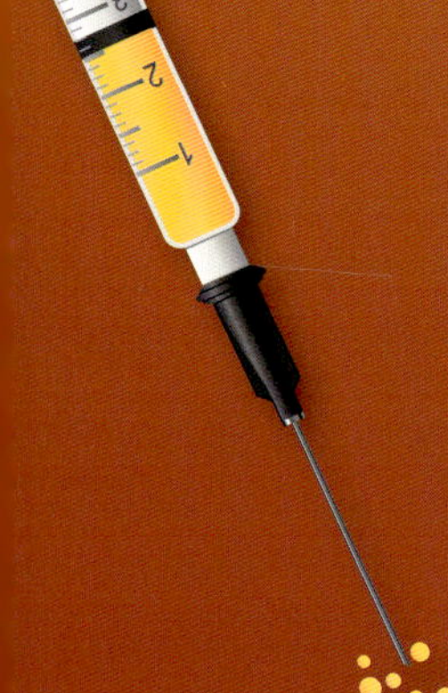

IMMUNOSUPPRESSIVE THERAPY

1 **Immunosuppressive therapy** is indicated when the immune response is excessive or inappropriate (see Charts 20 to 22), modifying, reducing or even abolishing the mechanisms that produce the disorder. The immunosuppressive drugs may affect different components of the immune system, so it is necessary to find a balance between the remission of the clinical signs and the risk of infections.

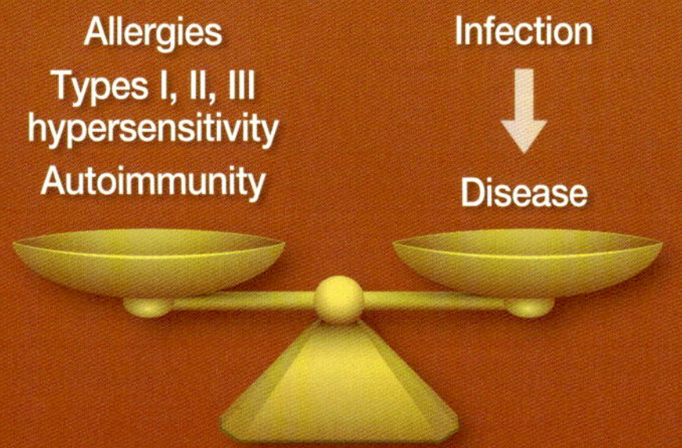

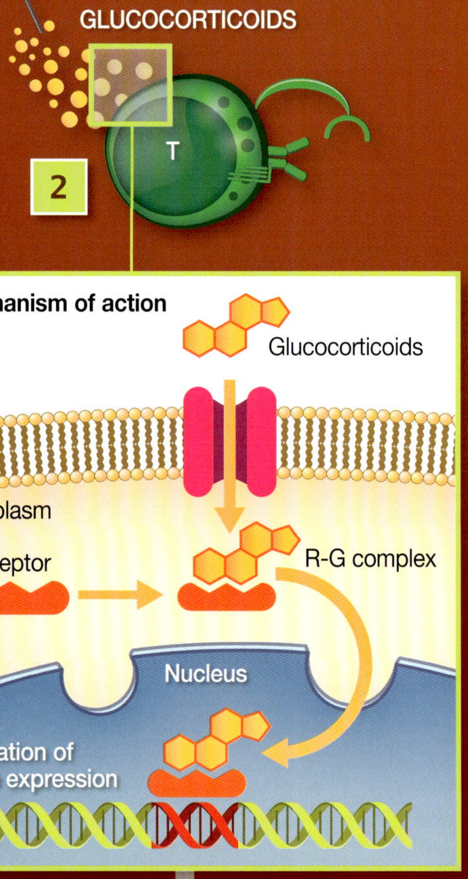

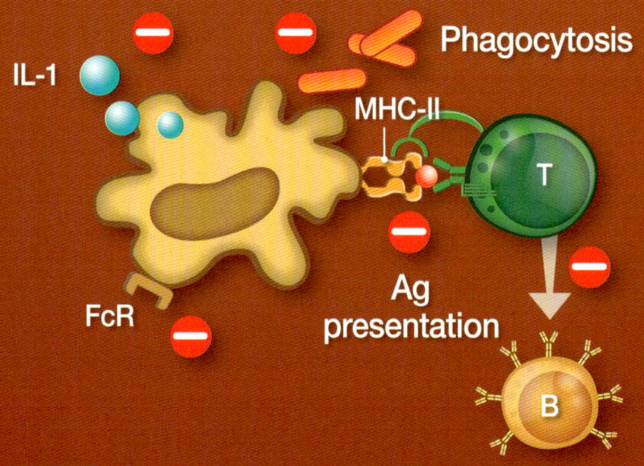

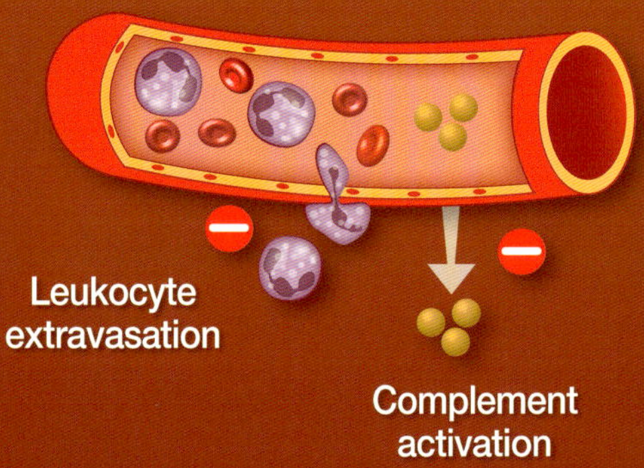

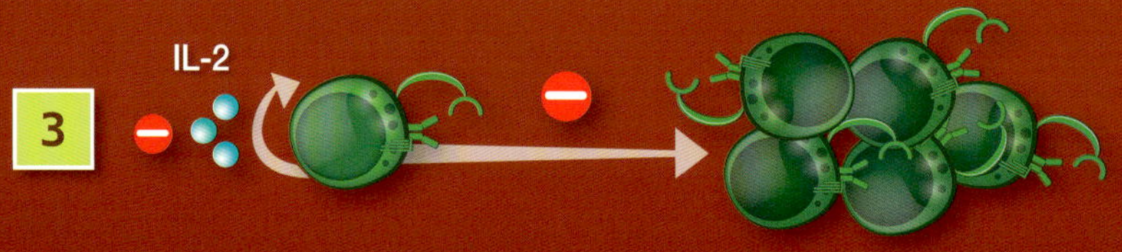

ANTI-INFLAMATORY AND IMMUNOSUPPRESSIVE EFFECTS

2 **Glucocorticoids** bind to cytoplasmic receptors, and this alters the gene expression. Their main role is the inhibition of the T cell function, but they also act on different cells and molecules of the immune system. **Prednisone** and **dexamethasone** are among the most commonly used glucocorticoids in dogs and cats. Cats are more resistant to the action of the steroids because of a lower expression of receptors, and a higher dose of the drug is required to achieve the desired effect.

3 Other immunosuppressant drugs used in dogs are **azathioprine** and **cyclophosphamide**; **chlorambucil** is used in cats. They have cytotoxic activity, which interferes with the multiplication of cells. **Cyclosporine** and **tacrolimus**, which block the synthesis of IL-2 by T cells (see Chart 9), may also be used.

4 Allergies (see Chart 20) can be prevented by **"allergy vaccines"**, a **desensitization** treatment specific for the allergen. This treatment consists in the administration of the allergen in very low, repeated and increasing doses. The mechanism of action is unclear, but it may be due to the production of IgG, that block the IgE binding sites (see Chart 20), or to the induction of tolerance to the Ag (see Chart 10).

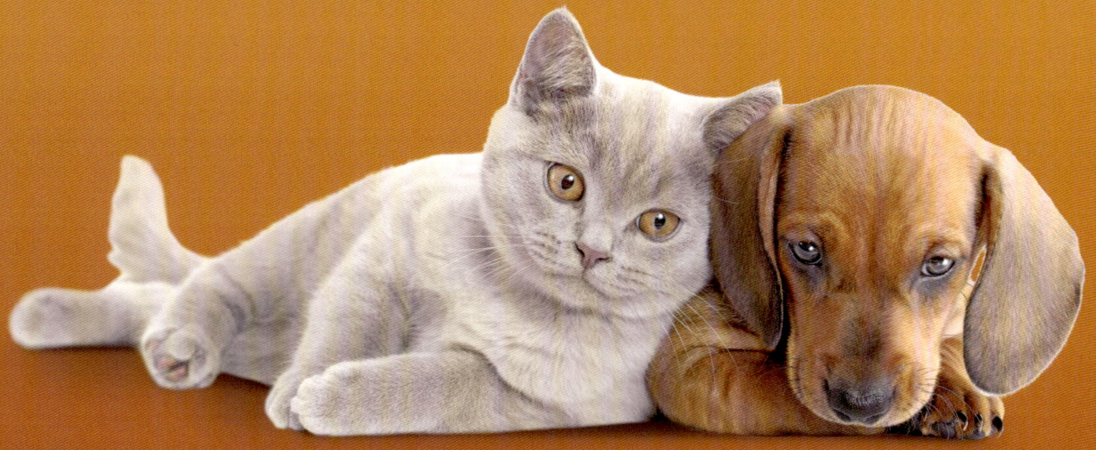

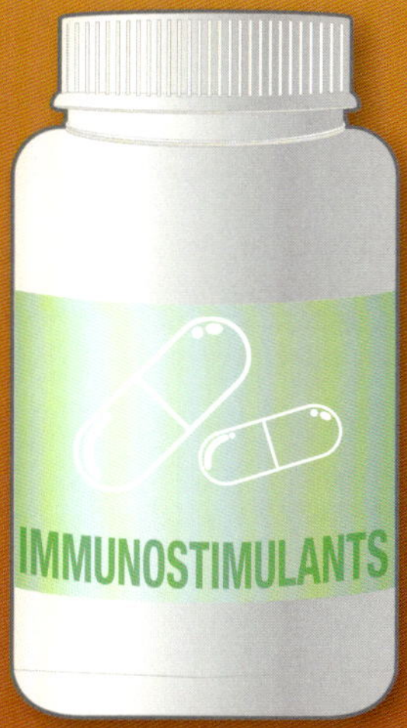

IMMUNOSTIMULANT THERAPY

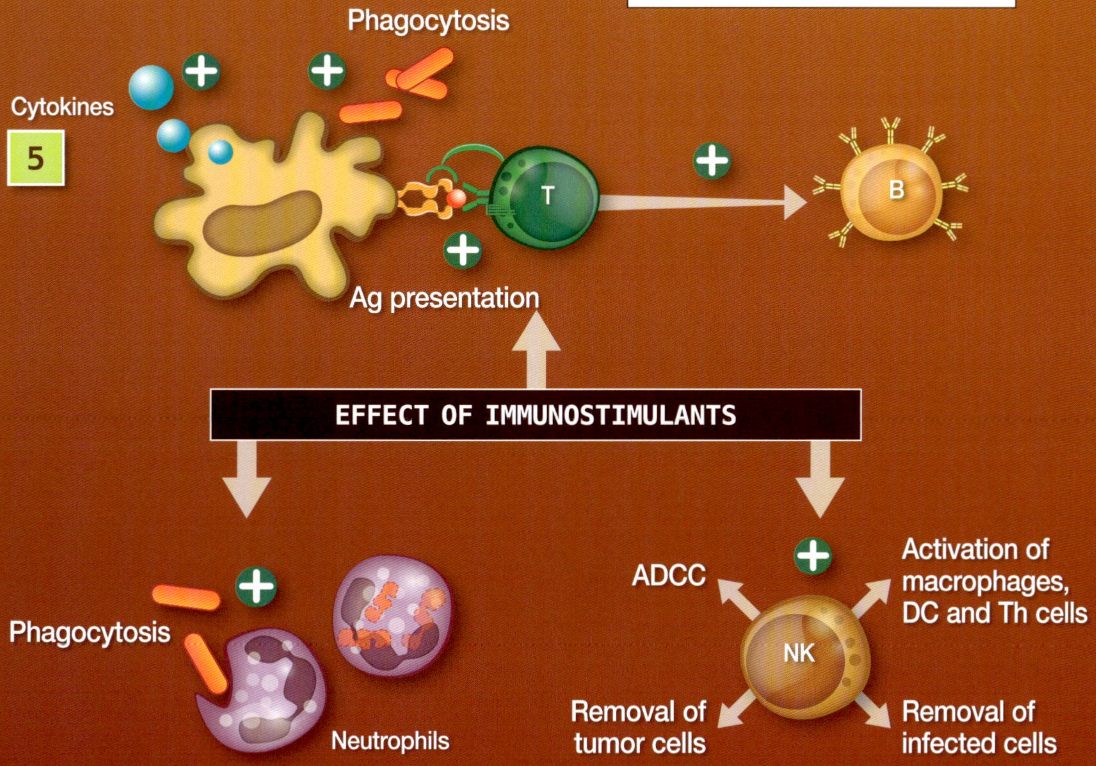

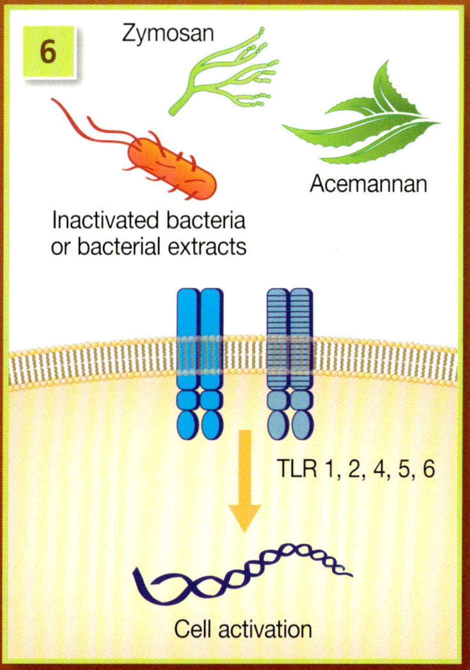

5 Stress and some infections cause **immunodeficiency** in the animal (see Chart 23), which increases its susceptibility to infections. In these cases, the administration of **immunostimulants**, which enhance the innate immune responses, is indicated (see Chart 4).

6 Some immunostimulant compounds are **plant extracts**, such as the acemannan (*Aloe vera*). Several **fungal products**, such as the β-glucans (*e.g.*, zymosan), and **bacterial products** (inactivated *Propionibacterium acnes*, extracts of *Mycobacterium* or *Staphylococcus aureus*) may also stimulate the immune system; in these cases, PAMP molecules may activate the complement and would also be recognized by the TLR of the cells of the innate immune system (see Charts 3 and 4).

7 Some **cytokines** are used in patients with immunodeficiency, and also as adjuvant therapy against infectious or neoplastic diseases. For example, feline **interferon-ω** may be administered to cats with retroviral (FIV, FeLV) or parvoviral infections, or feline **IL-2** may be applied locally after resection of sarcomas in cats.

Passive immunization

Passive immunization is the process by which immunoglobulins are transferred from one animal to another, usually of the same species, providing immediate humoral immunity. Passive immunity can be acquired **naturally**, as in the case of transfer of maternal Ab to the newborn through colostrum (see Chart 12); or **artificially**, as when a hyperimmune serum is administered to dogs with parvoviral infection or to prevent the effects of tetanus toxin.

GENERAL CHARACTERISTICS OF VIRUSES

Viruses are extremely small infectious agents, composed of a single type of nucleic acid, RNA or DNA, protected by a protein coat called capsid. Some viruses also have an envelope (a lipid bilayer, so they also have lipids) and, sometimes, the surface-most proteins possess carbohydrates (glycoproteins) (fig. 1).

1

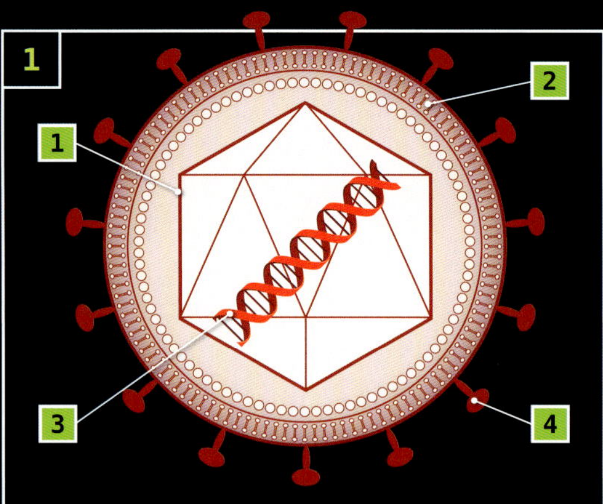

1 Protein capsid
2 Lipid envelope
3 DNA/RNA ss/ds single/fragmented linear/circular
4 Surface proteins (with carbohydrates)

While some viruses can circumvent the extracellular phase, none can avoid the intracellular phase. Therefore, the study of viruses always requires living cells.

Given their extreme simplicity and structural composition, viruses are unable to lead an independent life and absolutely require parasitizing cells, which are going to provide them with the molecules they lack, and allow their replication. Therefore, two phases are recognized in the life cycle of viruses (fig. 2):

1 **extracellular phase**, in which they act as inert particles without any metabolic activity; they only pass from cell to cell;

2 **intracellular phase**, in which they complete their replication cycle, and from which their pathogenic effect derives.

DNA AND RNA VIRUSES

Viruses may contain DNA or RNA. In the majority of families with DNA, the genome is double-stranded (ds; poxviruses, herpesviruses, adenoviruses, etc.). However, parvoviruses, which cause important diseases in dogs and cats, have single-stranded (ss) DNA. In the vast majority of RNA viruses, this is single-stranded.

Single-stranded RNA can be of positive sense (RNA+), when it is equivalent to messenger RNA and can be immediately translated by ribosomes; or of negative sense (RNA–), which needs to be converted into RNA by an RNA polymerase prior to translation (fig. 3).

GENETIC STABILITY

Viruses containing **DNA** as genetic material present **much less variability** than those which possess RNA, not only due to the greater stability of DNA *versus* RNA, but also because most of them use the cellular DNA polymerases to duplicate their genetic material (fig. 4). This enzyme has an editing function. Precisely due to this fidelity of DNA polymerase, the genomes of DNA viruses tend to be longer than those of RNA viruses.

2

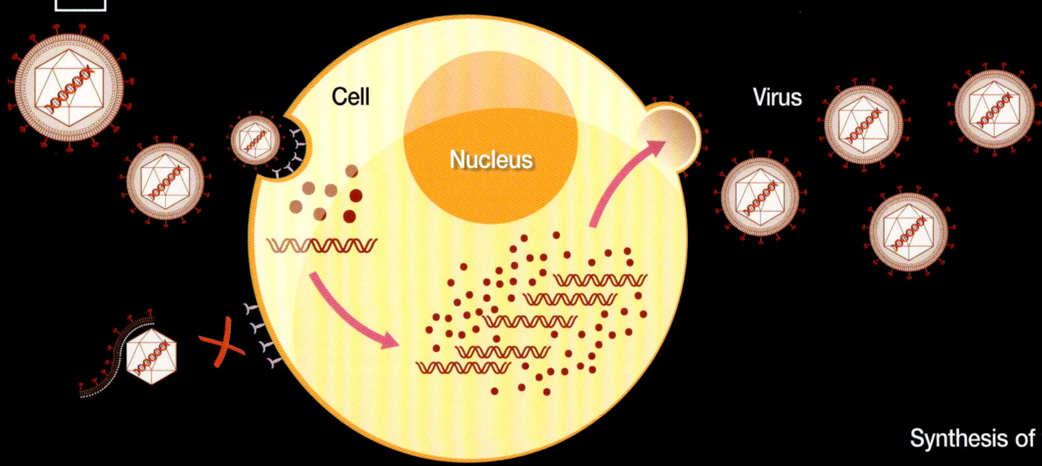

3

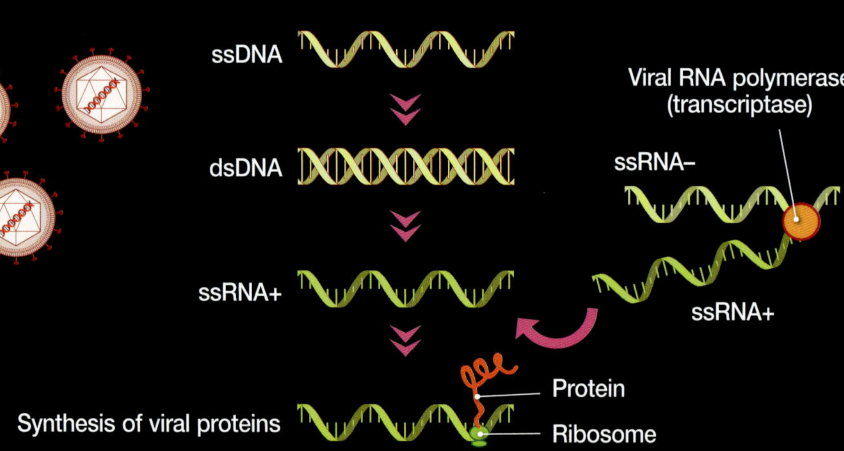

However, **RNA** viruses need to transcribe RNA into RNA, a process that is not done by the eukaryotic cell. The enzyme that carries out this transcription is called **RNA polymerase or transcriptase**, and is always viral (fig. 4). Transcriptases have no editing function, so they **introduce many mistakes** when transcribing RNA into RNA. In practice, it is observed that many mutations are not tolerated, because they annul the function of some protein essential for viral replication. The best tolerated mutations are those which affect structural proteins, and in particular, mutations in the outer proteins are favored, provided that they do not affect the recognition by the cell receptor. This means that it is harder for the immune system to react effectively against RNA viruses, and that vaccines against these viruses are more difficult to develop.

In RNA viruses, mutations affecting structural proteins are more common. For this reason, the effectiveness of the immune response is reduced, and it is difficult to develop vaccines.

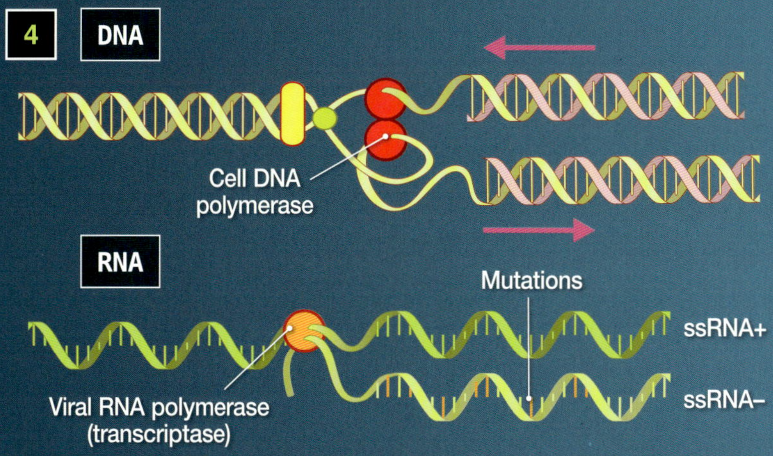

CONTROL

Since viruses are obligate intracellular parasites, they are difficult to fight inside the animal. **Antiviral drugs** have been designed mainly against the herpes viruses, orthomyxoviruses, and retroviruses. The first two groups of viruses can affect cats and dogs and the retroviruses produce the feline immunodeficiency and feline leukemia. In practice, the most commonly used antiviral drugs are precisely against the latter infections, due to their chronic and long-lasting nature. The most used anti-retroviral drug is zidovudine (ZDV), combined with lamivudine (3TC) and nevirapine (Nevi).

It is easier to destroy viruses when they are outside the animal. In this sense, **viruses that possess an envelope are more fragile** than those which do not, because the envelope is labile and easily lost, and with it, proteins that are recognized by the receptors (fig. 2). For this reason, the majority of diseases by enveloped viruses (orthomyxoviruses, retroviruses, herpes viruses) occur in winter, in high moisture conditions, or are transmitted over short distances (many of them through grooming, licking or bites). On the other hand, **non-enveloped or naked viruses are extremely resistant**, to the point of supporting the aggressive conditions of the gastrointestinal tract, and they can produce digestive diseases (parvoviruses, adenovirus which produces canine infectious hepatitis).

Antibiotics are totally ineffective against viruses, since they are designed to block specific phases of the biology of bacteria.

Main viral diseases in the dog and the cat, family to which the producing virus belongs and presence/absence of envelope and type of nucleic acid of the virus.

Main diseases	Family	Envelope	Type of virus	ss/ds	Type
Feline poxvirus infection	Poxvirus	With	DNA	ds	Single
Feline viral rhinotracheitis Hemorrhagic disease in dog puppies[2]	Herpesvirus				
Canine infectious hepatitis Canine infectious tracheobronchitis[3]	Adenovirus	Naked			
Canine oral papilloma	Papillomavirus				
Canine parvovirosis Feline panleucopenia	Parvovirus			ss	Single
Canine distemper Canine infectious tracheobronchitis[3] Canine parainfluenza	Paramyxovirus	With	RNA	ss–	Single
Rabies	Rhabdovirus				
Dog and cat influenza	Orthomyxovirus				Fragmented
Feline infectious peritonitis Canine coronavirosis	Coronavirus			ss+	Single
Rhinitis in dogs and cats[2]	Picornavirus	Naked			
Feline calicivirosis	Calicivirus				
Feline immunodeficiency Feline leukemia	Retrovirus	With	RNA→ADN		Diploid

[1] ss: single-stranded; ds: double-stranded; +: positive sense; –: negative sense;
Single: a single molecule of nucleic acid; Fragmented: nucleic acid distributed in fragments; Diploid: two identical molecules of RNA.

[2] The disease has a low incidence in Europe.

[3] In association with other pathogens to form an etiological complex.

CANINE DISTEMPER

ETIOLOGY

Canine distemper virus belongs to the family *Paramyxoviridae* (enveloped ARN virus), genus *Morbillivirus*.

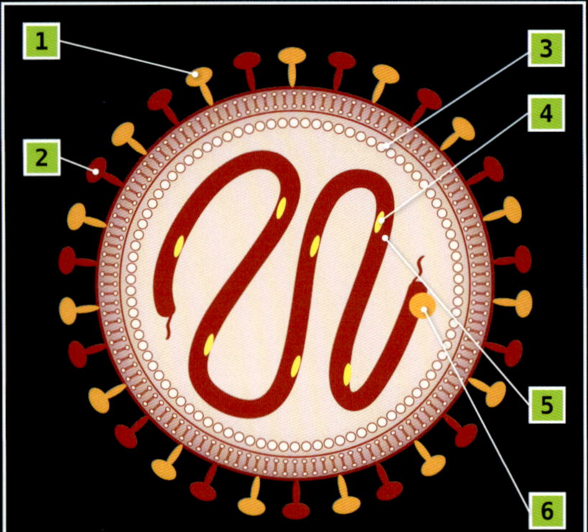

1 Fusion protein (F)
2 Hemagglutinin (H)
3 Matrix (M)
4 Transcriptase (P)
5 Nucleocapsid (N)
6 Polymerase (L)

STRUCTURE OF THE VIRUS

Two relevant proteins for the development of the protective immune response are located on the surface of the viral particle:

- **Hemagglutinin (H):** viral molecule recognized by the cellular receptors.
- **Fusion protein (F):** related to the penetration of the virus in the host cell.

The internal proteins are named:

- N (nucleocapsid).
- P (transcriptase).
- L (polymerase).
- M (matrix).

Canine distemper virus is very labile from a physico-chemical point of view.

DIFFERENCES BETWEEN THE CIRCULATING VIRAL STRAINS THROUGHOUT THE WORLD

- **Genetic and antigenic:** they affect viral neutralization and the antibody titer induced in the host during the infection.
- **In pathogenicity:** associated with different tissue tropisms and disease severity.

Canine distemper virus infects diverse cell types in different tissues, organs and systems: epithelial, mesenchymal, neuroendocrine and hematopoietic.

MECHANISMS OF INFECTION

- The virus can codify proteins which may integrate in the infected cellular membrane, rendering it susceptible to cytolysis.
- The virus is able to induce cellular fusion in order to spread to other cells, thus evading the extracellular environment.

EPIDEMIOLOGY

SPECIES SUSCEPTIBLE TO THE INFECTION

- **Carnivorous:** *Canidae* (dog, wolf, fox), *Felidae* (lion, ocelot, jaguar), *Aleiuridae* (panda bear), *Ursidae* (bear), *Mustelidae* (ferret, mink), *Procyonidae* (raccoon, coatimundi) and *Viverridae* (mongoose, genet).
- **Marine mammals:** seal, porpoise, dolphin, etc.

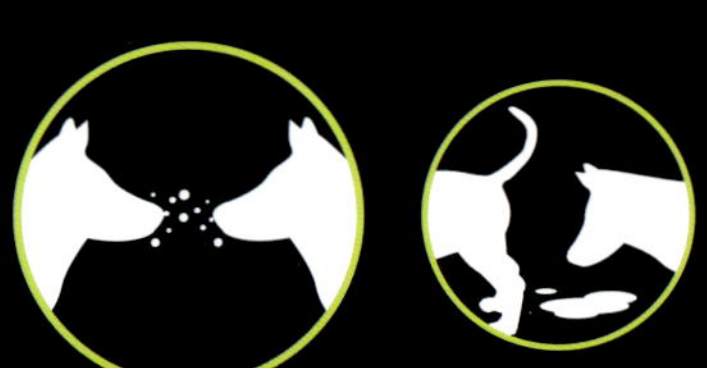

CLINICAL OUTCOME

The clinical outcome depends to a great extent on:

- Age: greater incidence in young animals although it can affect dogs of all ages.
- Virulence, tropism and viral load of the infective viral strain.

Infected animals can shed viruses through all body secretions and fluids (up to 90 days post-infection in persistent infections).

Due to the extended shedding periods, the virus is very ubiquitous and circulates persistently in the canine population, where more than 50 % of the infections may go undetected.

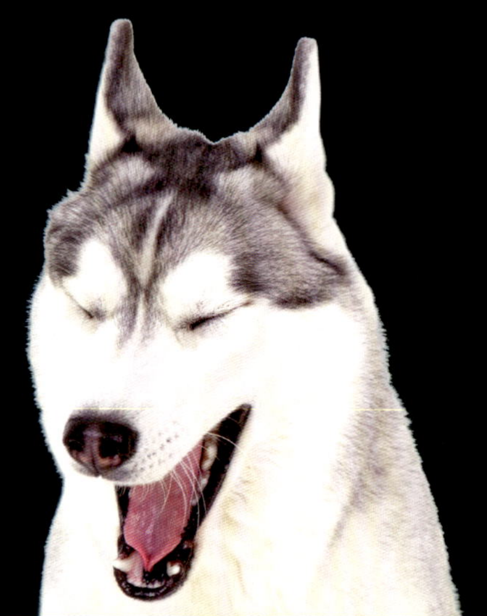

The infection is transmitted mostly through aerosol droplets.

PATHOGENESIS

1 Viruses enter via aerosol droplets and they initially replicate in tonsils and bronchial lymph nodes.

2 Later they migrate, associated with macrophages and monocytes, to lymphoid tissues in other locations such as the intestine and liver (viremia: 2nd-4th day post-infection).

3 Beginning of the humoral immune response (1st week post-infection). Three situations:

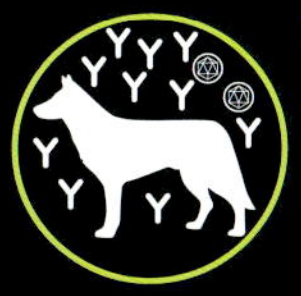

3a **Animals with high antibody titers** (50 % of cases): elimination of the infection without development of clinical manifestations.

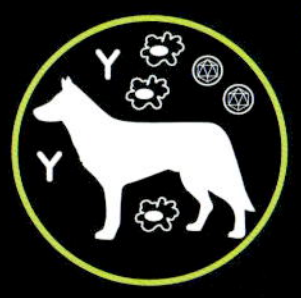

3b **Animals with low antibody titers but with suitable cell-mediated immune response:** gradual removal of the virus from most tissues (possibility of persistence in skin and CNS). Development of mild manifestations of the disease.

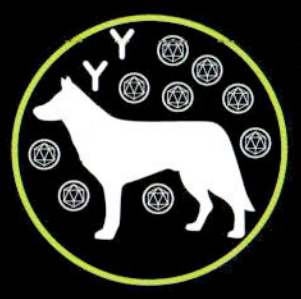

3c **Failure of the immune response:** the virus persists in various tissues and a severe disease develops with multisystemic manifestations. Only a scarce number of animals are affected.

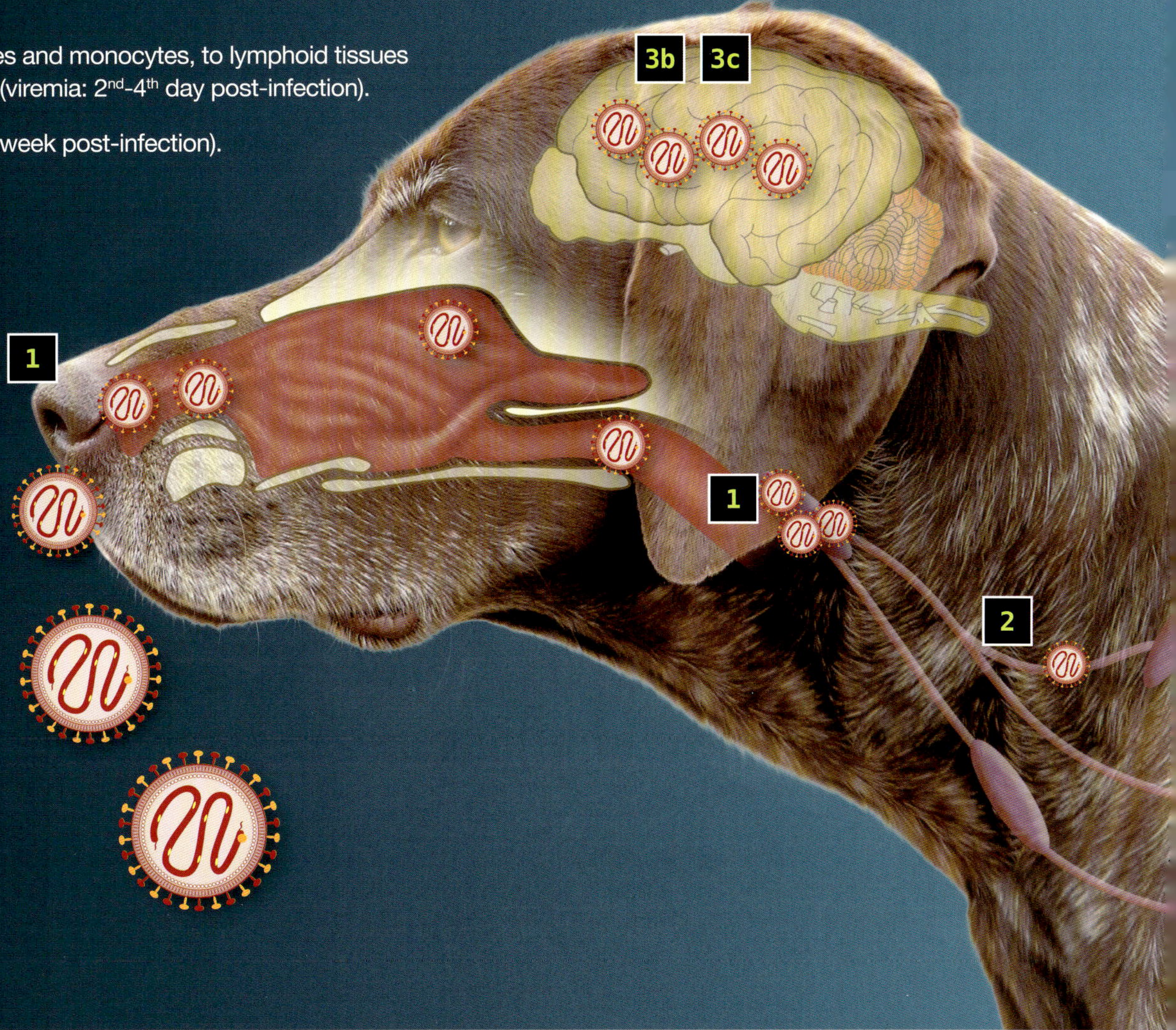

PATHOGENIC MECHANISMS AND CONSEQUENCES OF THE INFECTION

- Viral replication **in lymphoid tissues** during the early phase of the infection produces cellular depletion in lymphoid organs with decreased T cell (CD4+ and CD8+) counts, apoptosis of lymphoid cells and immune depression.
- The **invasion of the CNS by the virus** (by the hematogenous or neural routes) occurs when viremia is elevated and depends on the immune response. In the early phase it causes multifocal necrosis, demyelination and infiltration of T CD8+ cells, with upregulation of the synthesis of proinflammatory cytokines. **In young and immunodepressed** dogs these alterations cause **acute encephalitis.**
- In some animals a **chronic infection** can develop, with myelin loss due to Type IV hypersensitivity (delayed hypersensitivity, see Chart 21) and to the cytotoxic action of T CD8+ cells, which originate **subacute or chronic encephalitis**.
- In rare occasions **old dog encephalitis** (ODE) may be observed in dogs with **chronic progressive inflammatory distemper**.

Canine distemper virus can produce demyelination, gliosis and astrocytosis in the CNS.

DIAGNOSIS

Differential diagnosis: canine distemper needs to be distinguished from canine infectious respiratory disease and infectious canine hepatitis.

Technique	Samples	Observations
Viral detection (DFA, IC y RT-PCR)	• *In vivo:* respiratory discharges or tracheal washes, conjunctiva, urine, cerebrospinal fluid (CSF) and biopsy of the footpads. • *Post-mortem:* lung, urine bladder, CNS, and lymphoid tissue.	• The most used. • Commercial IC available.
Serology (IFA and ELISA)	Serum and CSF.	• It is necessary to assess seroconversion. • Commercial IFA and ELISA available.

It is not possible to diagnose whether an animal is infected solely through serology or through viral detection: it is necessary to value the patient.

In order to establish a presumptive clinical diagnosis it is necessary to consider the anamnesis, age, clinical signs and vaccine status of the animal.

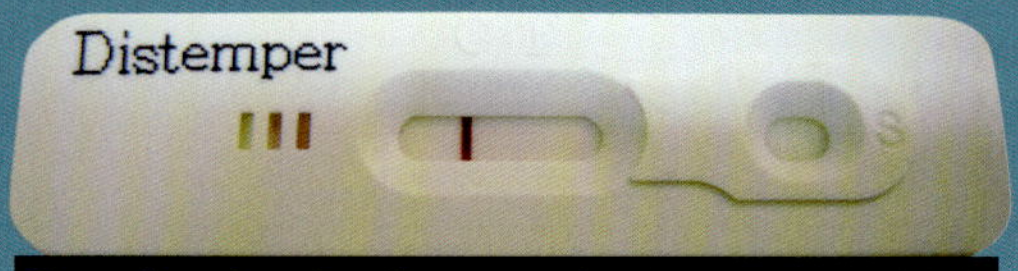

Detection of canine distemper virus by a commercial IC

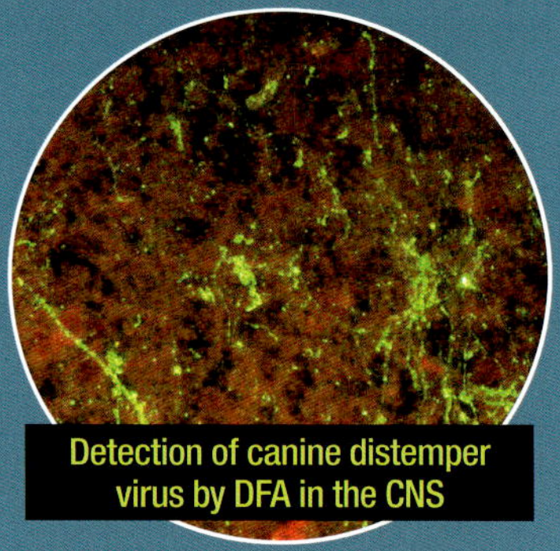
Detection of canine distemper virus by DFA in the CNS

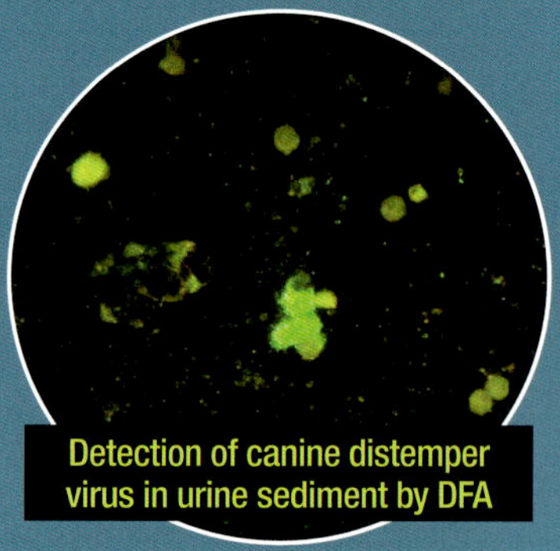
Detection of canine distemper virus in urine sediment by DFA

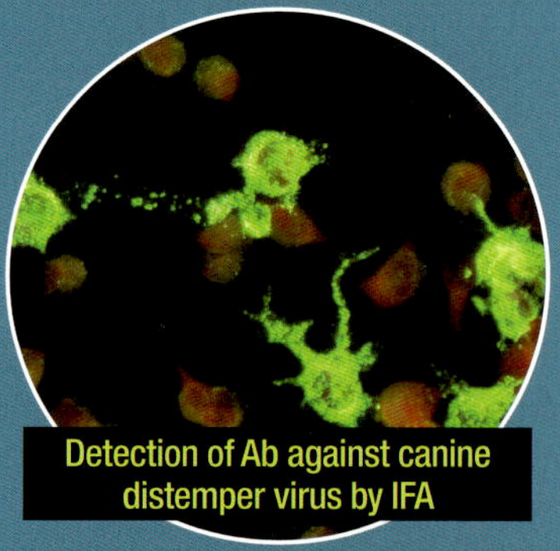
Detection of Ab against canine distemper virus by IFA

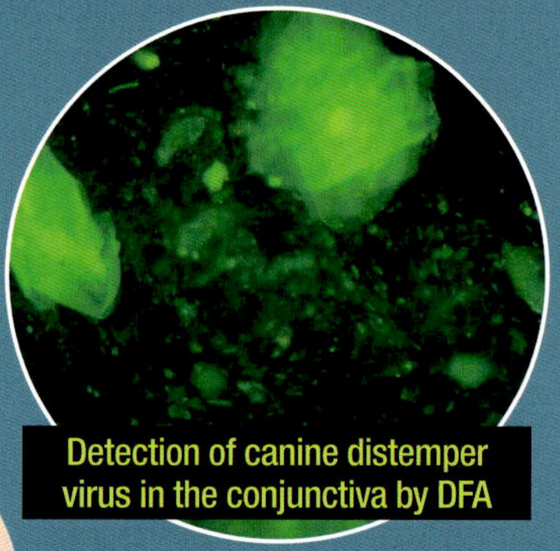
Detection of canine distemper virus in the conjunctiva by DFA

TREATMENT

Treatment is symptomatic and supportive and can include:

- **Antibiotics** to treat the respiratory secondary bacterial infections.
- **Fluid therapy** to combat dehydration.
- **Vitamin B complex** to obtain a suitable regulation and metabolism of neurotransmitters.
- **Anti-inflammatory drugs and anticonvulsants** to palliate the inflammation and the neurological signs.

In spite of the treatment, some animals with severe neurological syndrome do not recover or display long-lasting sequels.

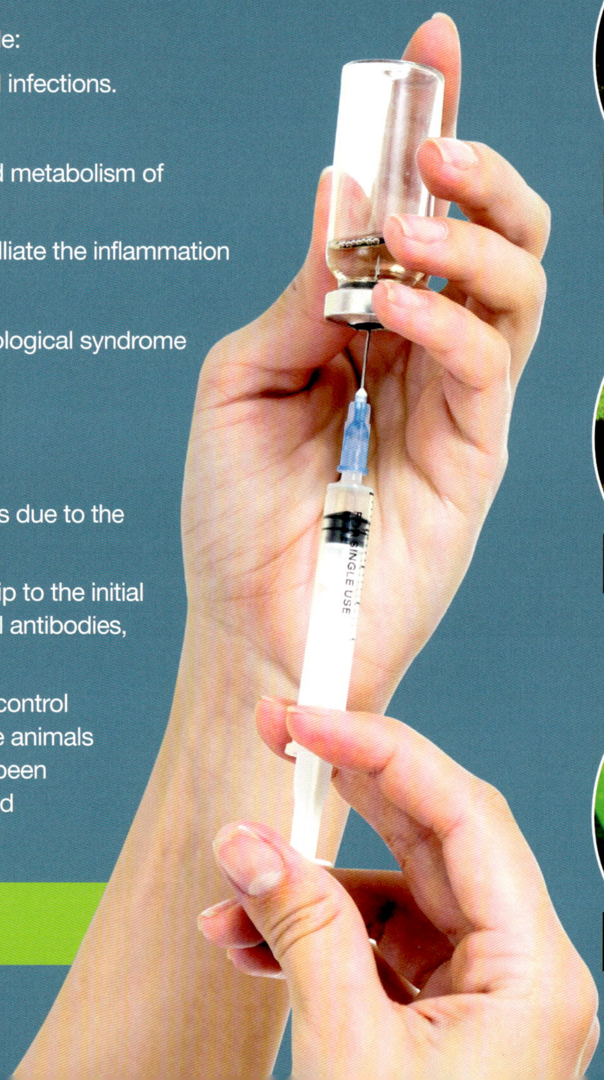

PREVENTION AND CONTROL

Canine distemper has been described in vaccinated dogs due to the development of nonprotective partial immunity.

If there is vaccine failure it must be analyzed in relationship to the initial immunological status of the animal (presence of maternal antibodies, see Chart 12) and to the vaccine schedule followed.

When the disease appears in populations it is difficult to control and in many cases it is possible to consider removing the animals and gradually reintroducing them after the kennels have been disinfected, as well as modifying the sanitary program and the management of the population.

The vaccines against canine distemper are attenuated and polyvalent.

CLINICAL SIGNS AND LESIONS

INITIAL SIGNS

- Fever.
- Anorexia.
- Depression.
- Leukopenia.
- Mild respiratory distress that often complicates quickly (the nasal discharge changes from clear to mucopurulent due to secondary bacterial complications).

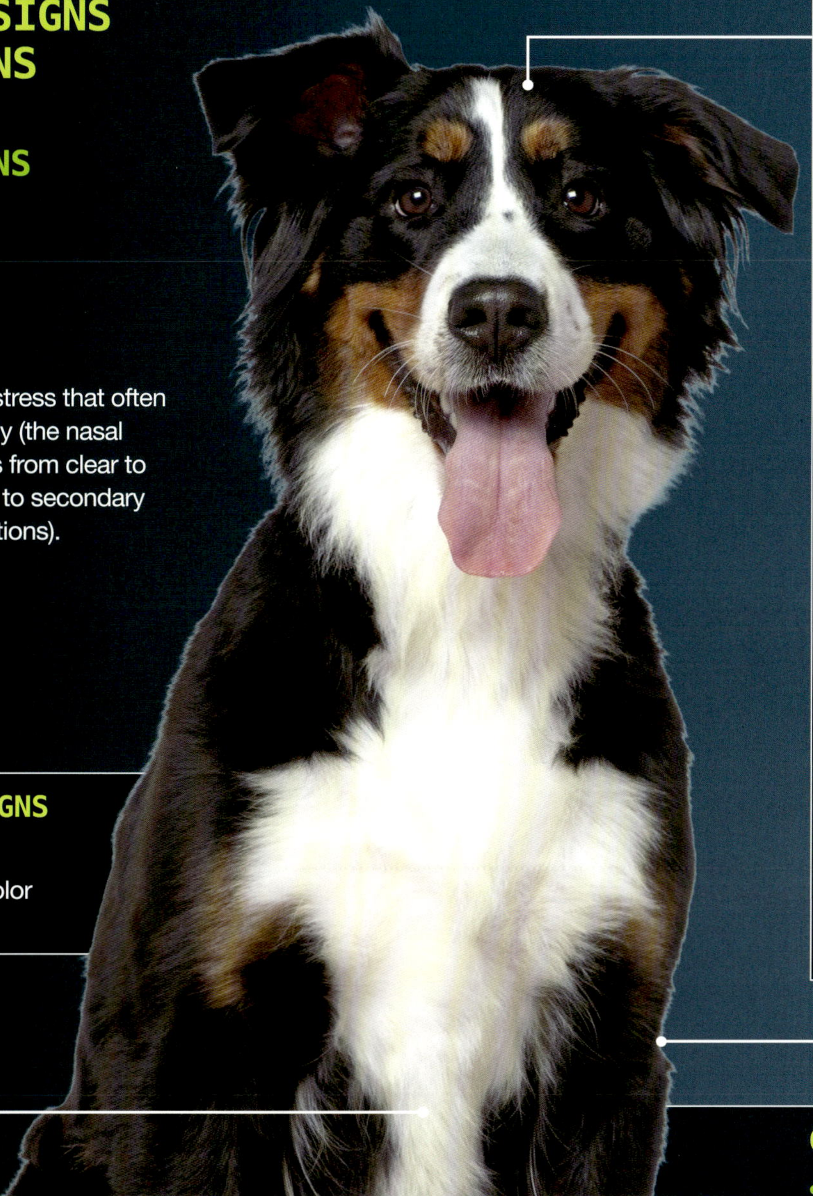

DIGESTIVE SIGNS

Decrease in the consistency and color of stools.

NEUROLOGICAL SIGNS

The neurological manifestations vary based on the area of the CNS affected by the replication of the virus:

- **Associated to the meninges:** cervical stiffness and hiperestesia.
- **Associated to the cerebellum and temporary lobe:** ataxia, sensorial diminution, myoclonus and seizures.
- **Associated to the spinal cord:** paresis to paralysis, myoclonus and abnormal proprioception.

In very young animals without immunity or with partial immunity, cranial or peripheral neuropathies may be observed, especially optic neuritis.

The nervous signs observed vary from a simple tremor to a severe syndrome with convulsions.

The nervous signs can appear delayed with respect to the rest of the signs.

Deaths associated with canine distemper are usually a result of neurological alterations.

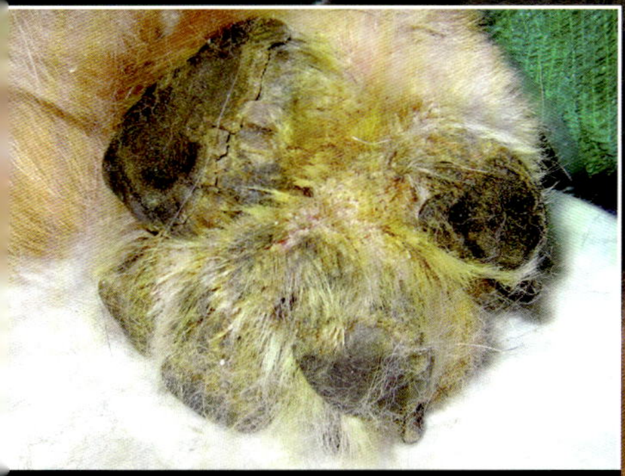

Hyperkeratosis of footpad

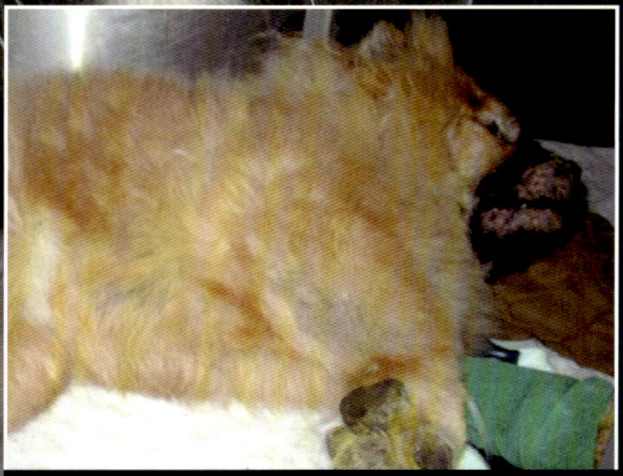

Systemic distemper

CUTANEOUS SIGNS

- **Impetigo:** usually, an indicator of a more benign prognosis of the infection.
- **Hyperkeratosis of the nose and footpads (hardpad disease):** frequently associated with neurotropic viral strains.
- **Neonatal infections:** they can be unapparent or produce various alterations. The most characteristic manifestation of these infections is the loss of dental enamel.

The most important lesions are located in the respiratory system, where secondary pneumonia develops.

INFECTIOUS CANINE HEPATITIS

ETIOLOGY

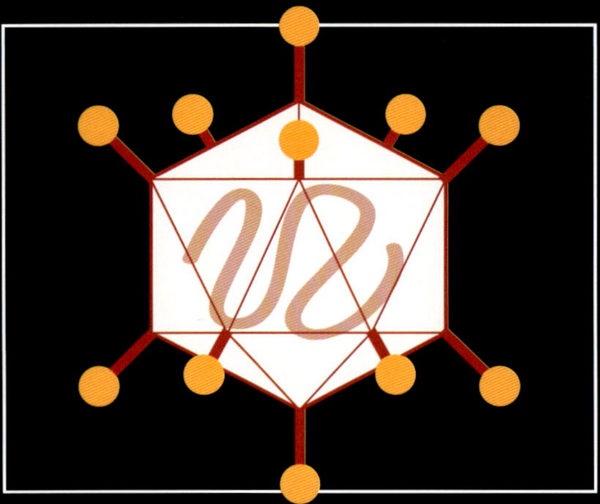

Infectious canine hepatitis is caused by a virus of the family *Adenoviridae* (non-enveloped DNA viruses), genus *Mastadenovirus*, called canine adenovirus type-1 (CAV-1).

This virus is resistant to environmental conditions and to various disinfectants.

There is antigenic homology between canine adenoviruses type-1 and type-2 (canine respiratory disease), resulting in a partial cross-protective immunity.

PATHOGENESIS

1 After oronasal contact, the virus multiplies in the tonsils and the cervical lymph nodes.

2 Viremia develops from the third day post-infection. It spreads the virus to the endothelium, liver and kidney (major target tissues and organs).

3 Approaching the 5th day post-infection, the virus may reach the lung, lymphoid tissue and CNS.

4 The replication of the virus induces cell necrosis and stimulates a rapid immune response (around the 7th day post-infection it is already possible to detect antibodies).

5 The formation of immune complexes can amplify the tissue damage and prolong some lesions and even make them chronic (interstitial nephritis and uveitis) (see Chart 21).

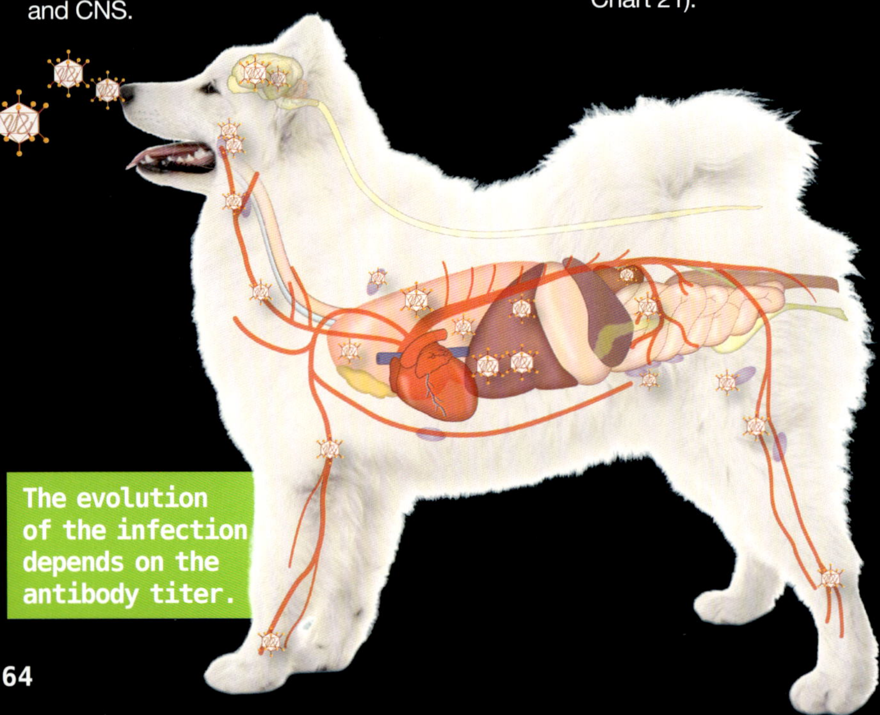

The evolution of the infection depends on the antibody titer.

The presence of high antibody titers promotes the removal of viruses from tissues and the general recovery which includes the fibrosis of the liver lesions.

Animals with low antibody titers develop acute hepatitis and in some cases the viral infection continues expanding causing general organ failure, hepatic encephalopathy, disseminated intravascular coagulation and death.

EPIDEMIOLOGY

SUSCEPTIBLE SPECIES

The disease occurs mostly in carnivores of the families *Canidae* (dog, wolf, fox, coyote) and *Mephitidae* (skunk). Other susceptible species when infected develop mild clinical signs. Thus, in cat and raccoon it produces only corneal edema.

SHEDDING

The virus is shed intermittently through all the secretions and body excretions.

The shedding through urine can be extended for several months.

Today the presentation of the disease is sporadic and mainly affects puppies.

TRANSMISSION

Mainly by oronasal direct contact.

Indirect transmission through contaminated objects and iatrogenic route are also significant.

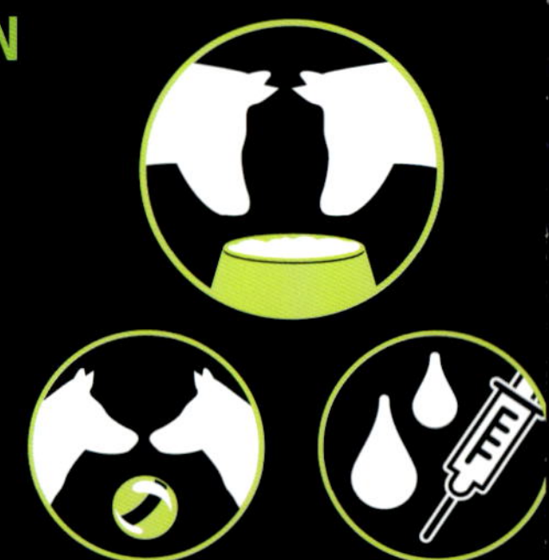

CLINICAL SIGNS AND LESIONS

PERACUTE FORM

It is rare and occurs in young animals lacking sufficient immunity. Short course (1 to 3 days).

Development of **hemorrhagic alterations** evident in conjunctiva and mucous membranes, accompanied by vomiting, diarrhea, abdominal pain, stupor and death.

LESIONS OBSERVED

Systemic hemorrhages.

ACUTE FORM

- **Initially:** hyperthermia, hypertrophy of superficial lymph nodes, inflammation of the larynx and pharynx and respiratory non-productive cough, mild diarrhea, listlessness and reluctance to move.
- **As the course of the disease progresses:** weight loss and deterioration of body condition, abdominal distension with hepatomegaly, hemorrhagic diathesis, and edema (most evident in subcutaneous tissue).
- **Neurological manifestations**, like disorientation, stupor and coma due to the development of a hepatic encephalopathy, may occur.

LESIONS OBSERVED

Mild jaundice, congestion and hepatic necrosis and edema, hemorrhage and inflammation in renal epithelia and glomeruli and in other endothelia.

The characteristic uveitis **("blue eye disease")** usually appears around two weeks after the onset of the subclinical infections without causing sequels.

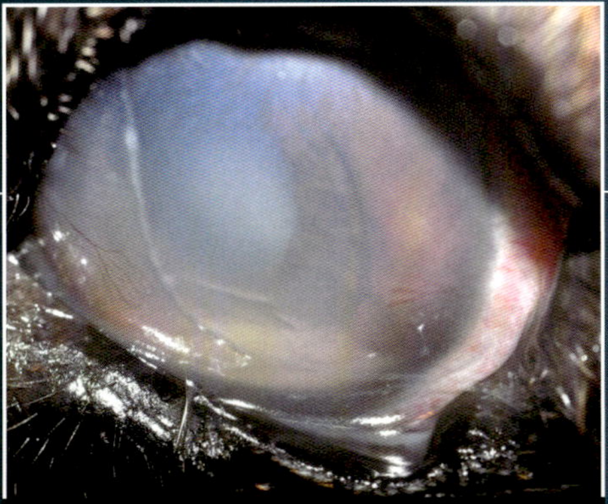

Uveitis

DIAGNOSIS

DIFFERENTIAL DIAGNOSIS

Age, prior clinical history and vaccination status have to be taken into account.

In the peracute form canine infectious hepatitis must be distinguished from poisoning causing hemorrhages.

LABORATORY DIAGNOSIS

Techniques	Samples	Observaciones
Viral detection (PCR, DFA, IHC)	• *In vivo:* blood, urine and ocular, nasal and genital discharges. • *Post-mortem:* liver, kidney, lung, lymphoid tissue, etc.	
Serology	Serum.	It is necessary to assess seroconversion.

TREATMENT

The treatment is symptomatic and consists of:

1. **Fluid therapy** (with glucose and vitamin B complex) to prevent shock, hypoglycaemia, and encephalopathy.
2. **Blood or plasma transfusion** to replace clotting factors and platelets.
3. **Vitamin K** to treat hemorrhages.
4. **Antibiotics** to prevent secondary bacterial infections.

Convalescent animals should be fed with low-protein diets.

PREVENTION AND CONTROL

Vaccines are attenuated, contain canine adenovirus type-2 and protect partially against infectious canine hepatitis and canine infectious respiratory disease.

Only healthy and properly dewormed dogs should be vaccinated.

In case of sporadic disease it is necessary to:

1. Intensify the hygiene measures.
2. Prevent the iatrogenic and indirect infections.

CANINE LEPTOSPIROSIS

ETIOLOGY

Leptospira are spirochetes (thin, helical bacteria with axial filaments or endoflagella which allow them to be mobile) included in the family *Leptospiraceae*, genus *Leptospira*, which multiply by binary fission.

They are zoonotic agents.

Eight pathogenic species, which are classified into serogroups and serovars on the basis of their antigenic differences, have been described.

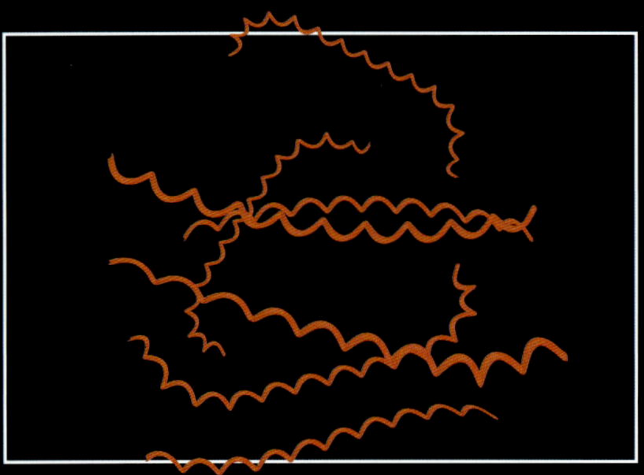

MOST IMPORTANT PATHOGENIC SPECIES AND SEROVARS FOR DOGS

1. *L. interrogans* serovars Canicola, Australis, Autumnalis, Bratislava, Hardjo, Icterohaemorrhagiae, Pomona and Grippothyphosa.
2. *L. kirschneri* serovars Pomona and Grippothyphosa.

Leptospira can survive in damp soils, stagnant water and effluents (non-acidic pH) for weeks.

FACTORS THAT CONTRIBUTE TO THE SURVIVAL OF LEPTOSPIRA OUTSIDE THE HOST

- Cell aggregation.
- Biofilm formation.

EPIDEMIOLOGY

Animal reservoirs are usually wildlife mammals, especially rodents.

SHEDDING

Leptospires colonize the body and are shed from the nephritic tubules in a large number of species of mammals.

Leptospira may be shed intermittently for several months.

TRANSMISSION

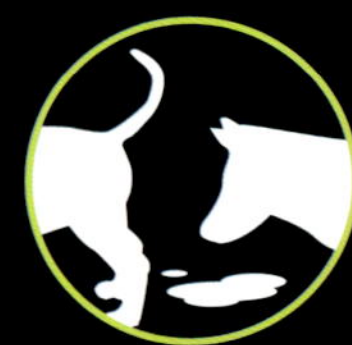

The main source of infection is the urine of infected animals.

The active entry in the new host is through mucous membranes or skin abrasions.

HIGHER PREVALENCE IN:

- Summer and fall months.
- Hunting dogs.
- Dogs living in rural areas or in kennels or shelters.

PATHOGENESIS

- Leptospira penetrate by contact through the skin and mucous membranes through active movements of rotation and gliding. They cross tissues and invade the bloodstream (leptospiremia) in a few hours, establishing a rapid systemic infection. Around three days post-infection they infect multiple organs, mainly liver and kidney.
- During the early phase of infection, they multiply efficiently and are able to evade the innate response of the host (resistent to the activation of the complement through the alternative pathway, see Chart 4).
- The immune response and lysis of the leptospira induce an intense stimulation of pro-inflammatory cytokines that mediate and amplify tissular and vascular damage, causing bleeding, thrombocytopenia and coagulopathy.
- If the immune response is not effective, leptospira can persist in the nephritic tubules from the 1st - 2nd week post-infection.

There are serovars, such as Grippothyphosa, capable of inducing chronic hepatic alterations.

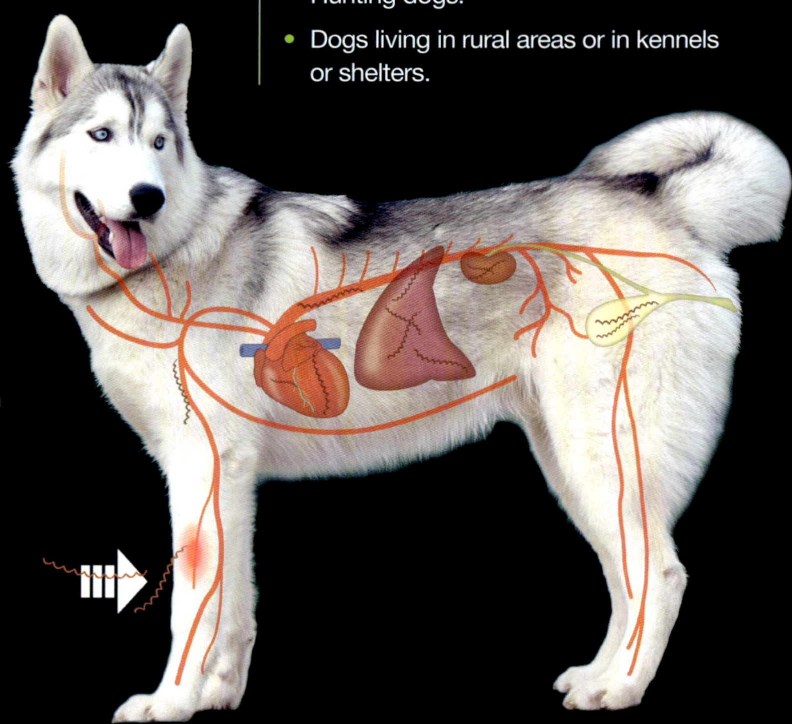

CLINICAL SIGNS AND LESIONS

ACUTE FORM

It occurs especially in puppies without immunity.

Signs may include:

- Fever.
- Muscle weakness and pain.
- Adynamia.
- Jaundice.
- Vomiting.
- Epistaxis.
- Petechiae.
- Oliguria.

SUBACUTE OR CHRONIC FORM

It is the most frequent form.

- It can occur with fever, anorexia, vomiting, abdominal and muscle pain, polyuria, polydipsia, liver failure, jaundice, ascites, renal insufficiency, interstitial nephritis, uremia and internal bleeding.
- Other alterations, which may include ocular, mostly uveitis, and respiratory alterations, occur occasionally.

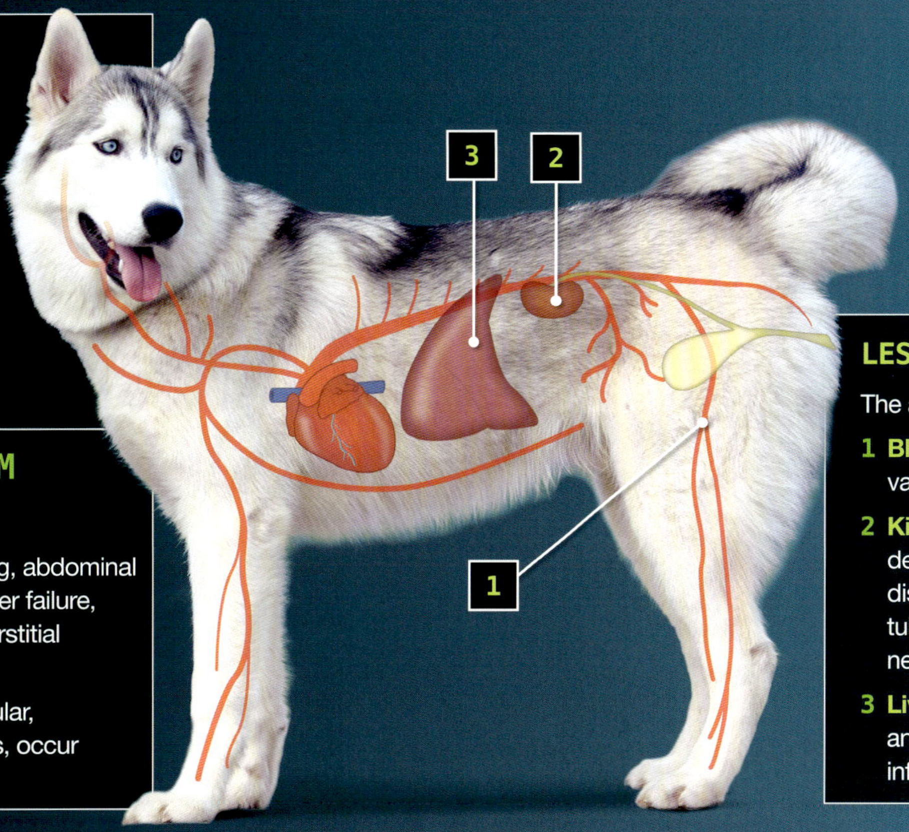

LESIONS

The are located in:

1. **Blood vessels:** vasculitis.
2. **Kidney:** inflammation-degeneration, discoloration and tubulointerstitial nephritis.
3. **Liver:** focal necrosis and chronic inflammation.

DIAGNOSIS

CLINICAL DIAGNOSIS

The presence of acute fever, hepatic or renal dysfunction of unknown etiology, uveitis and pulmonary hemorrhage can orientate the diagnosis.

LABORATORY DIAGNOSIS

Techniques	Samples	Observations
Bacterial isolation	Blood and urine (sterile collection).	• Samples must be collected during the febrile period. • Slow and difficult technique, it requires especial media and must be done in an approved laboratory with biosafety measures.
Bacterial detection (PCR and IHC)	Blood, urine and tissues (kidney and liver).	There may be false negative results and it is unable to differentiate pathogenic from non-pathogenic serovars.
Serology (microagglutination - MAT)	Serum.	• The most widely used. • It is necessary to assess seroconversion.

TREATMENT

Antibiotics to treat leptospirosis.

Various antibiotics, especially doxycycline, may be used provided they are administered at the onset of the disease and for an extended period (at least two weeks) to completely eliminate leptospira from the kidney.

PREVENTION AND CONTROL

There are inactivated and subunit vaccines of the serovars Icterohaemorrhagiae and Canicola, both in a monovalent and multivalent presentation. An additional vaccine contains also serovar Grippothyphosa.

Vaccines only protect against the homologous serovars.

Vaccination prevents or attenuates the clinical manifestations, but does not prevent infection and excretion of leptospira through the urine.

Other preventive measures include avoiding contact with farm effluents and with animal reservoirs.

The dog, because of its coexistence with man, should be considered a potential source of leptospira.

INFECTIONS CAUSED BY CANINE PARVOVIRUSES

ETIOLOGY

Canine parvoviruses belong to the family *Parvoviridae* (non-enveloped small size DNA viruses).

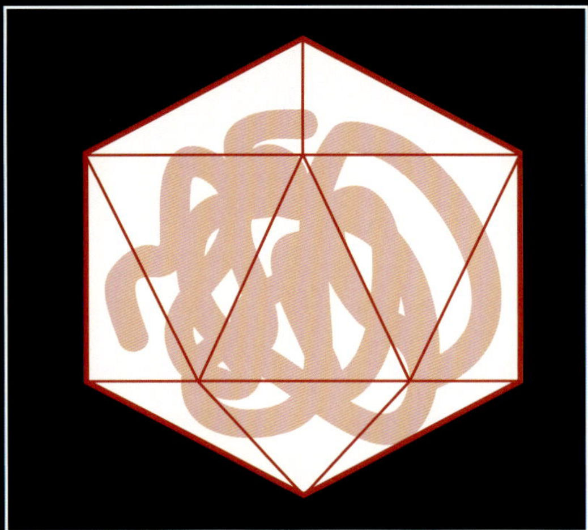

Canine parvovirus type-2 has undergone a rapid development over the past 35 years.

Parvoviruses are haemagglutinating particles which are highly resistant, both to physico-chemical agents and to environmental factors.

Parvoviruses need cellular factors expressed during the S phase of the cell cycle to complete their replication cycle. This determines the type of target cells, which are preferably located in tissues with high mitotic index (rapidly dividing), such as the intestine and the lymphoid tissue.

Canine parvoviruses (E.M.)

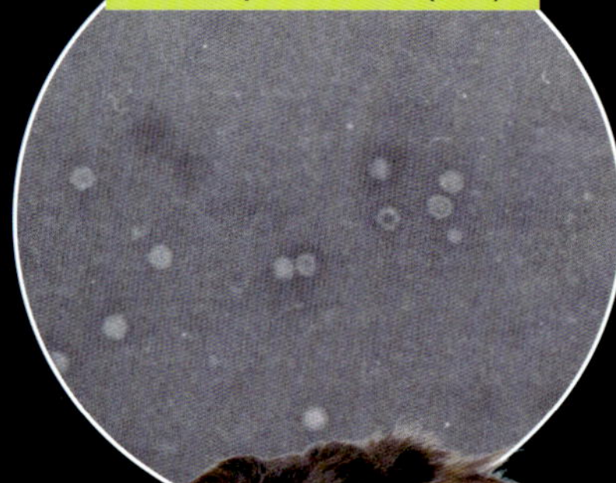

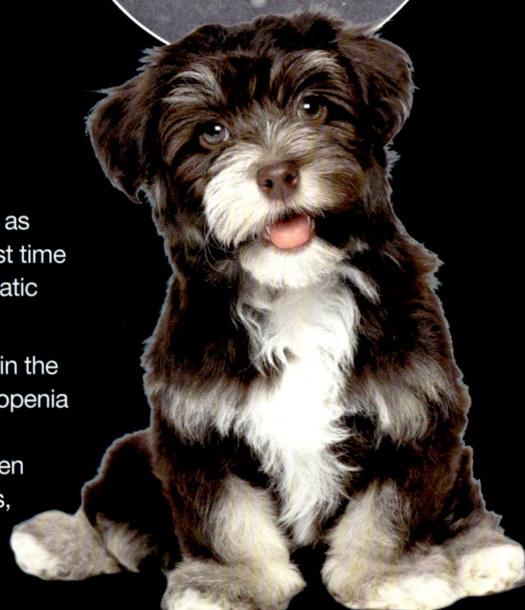

TYPES OF CANINE PARVOVIRUSES (CPV)

1. **Canine parvovirus type-1 (CPV-1):** considered as a non-pathogenic virus, was detected for the first time in 1967 while studying samples from asymptomatic animals.
2. **Canine parvovirus type-2 (CPV-2):** it emerged in the 1970s derived, possibly, from the feline panleukopenia virus, and initially circulated quietly in the canine population. In 1978 it was associated with sudden deaths due to myocarditis in very young animals, and bloody diarrhea. Subsequently, several antigenic variants emerged from this virus.

70's	1978	1980	1984	2000
CPV-2 emerges	CPV-2 is associated with sudden deaths	CPV-2a substitutes CPV-2 globally	CPV-2b is first described	CPV-2c is first described

EPIDEMIOLOGY

The infection is transmitted by the fecal-oral route.

CPV can cause disease in domestic and wild canines, and some of its variants also affect domestic cats.

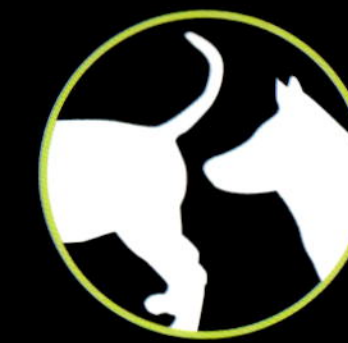

Infected dogs shed canine parvoviruses exclusively during the first week post-infection.

The disease usually affects puppies between 6 and 16 weeks of age. However, since 2006 mortality has also been seen in adults.

Infected dogs shed canine parvoviruses exclusively during the first week post-infection.

CLINICAL FORMS

- **Myocardial:** associated with sudden deaths due to myocarditis in very young puppies born from mothers who have no immunity.
- **Enteric:** characterized by hemorrhagic diarrhea.

THE CLINICAL OUTCOME DEPENDS ON:

- Age, immune status and breed of the dog.
- Viral load, variant and strain of canine parvovirus.

The disease may be more prevalent in dog populations.

PATHOGENESIS

Parvoviruses first replicate in the lymphoid tissue associated with the oropharynx, and subsequently, in other lymphoid organs, such as the thymus, spleen, bone marrow and lymph nodes.

Viremia is early and of short duration (between the 2nd and 4th day post-infection).

The replication of canine parvoviruses in lymphoid tissues causes transient leukopenia and immunosuppression.

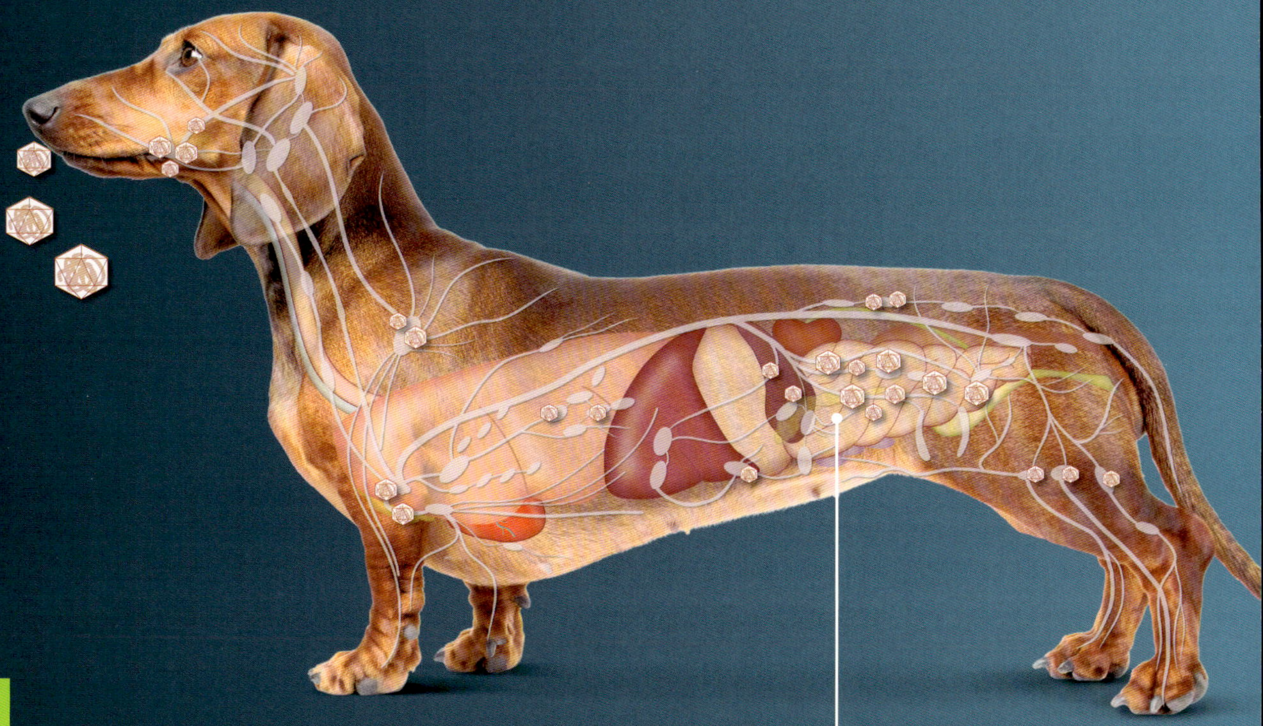

ENTERIC FORM

Canine parvoviruses quickly reach the small intestine, especially the jejunum and ileum.

Target cells are located in the intestinal crypts.

Viral replication in the crypts induces cell death and secretory deficit. Thus, replacement of the cells situated in the apex of the intestinal villi is arrested. These cells, which desquamate physiologically, are responsible for the absorption of nutrients and produce a secondary malabsorption syndrome. Intestinal overload and increased peristalsis elicit diarrhea which may be hemorrhagic since its inception.

The presence of concurrent infections, such as those caused by the canine coronaviruses, increases the severity of enteritis.

MYOCARDIAL FORM

It is caused by the necrosis of myocardial cells still in development (non-suppurative myocarditis) during the first 8 weeks of life.

Presently, the myocardial form is very rare due to vaccination.

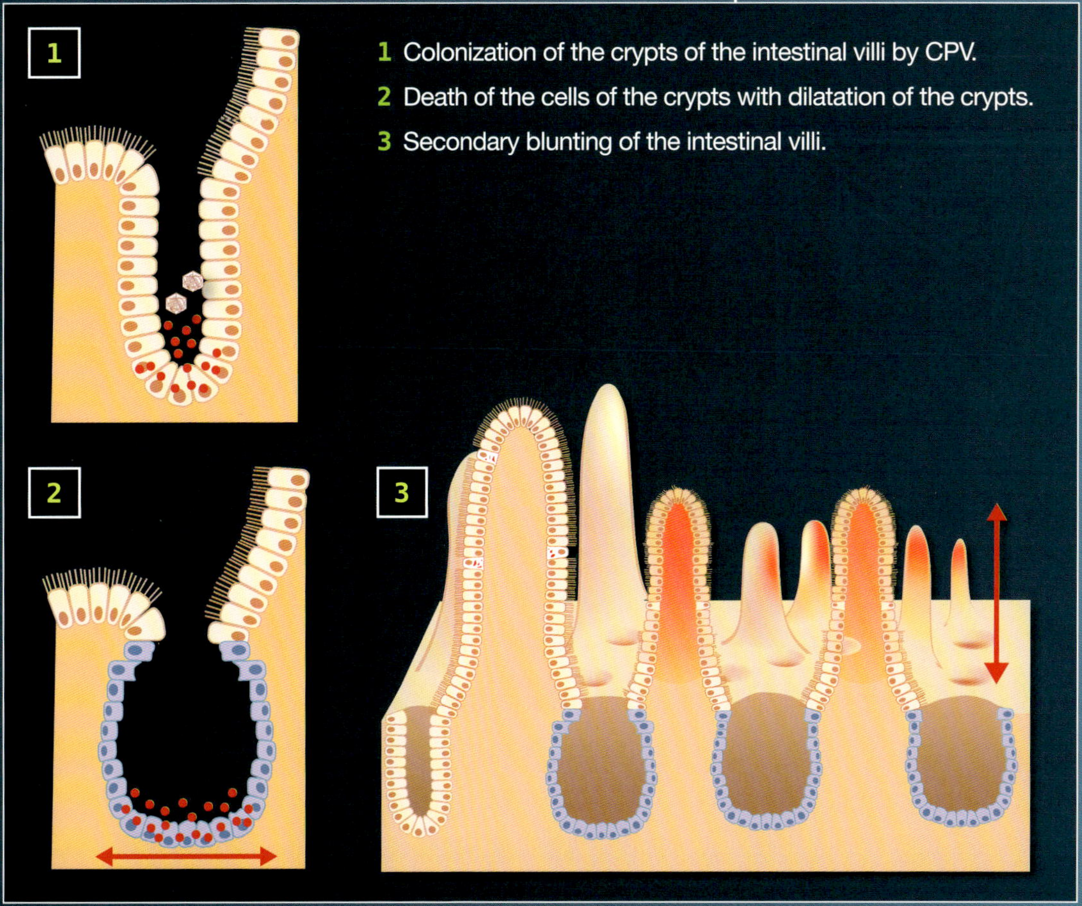

1 Colonization of the crypts of the intestinal villi by CPV.
2 Death of the cells of the crypts with dilatation of the crypts.
3 Secondary blunting of the intestinal villi.

DIAGNOSIS

- The epidemiological background, age and profile of the animal have to be taken into account in the differential clinical diagnosis.
- In some cases it is advisable to use diagnostic imaging to rule out the presence of foreign bodies or intussusception.
- The suspicion of parvovirosis is easy to confirm when acute bloody diarrhea is present. However, when the diarrhea is less specific, other enteric pathogens should be considered.
- For laboratory diagnosis it is essential that stools are shipped early after the onset of diarrhea (due to the short period of viral replication in the intestine).

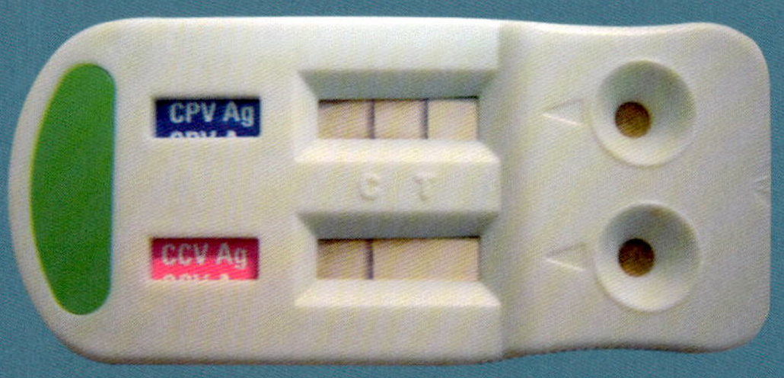

Commercial IC for the combined detection of parvovirus and canine coronavirus

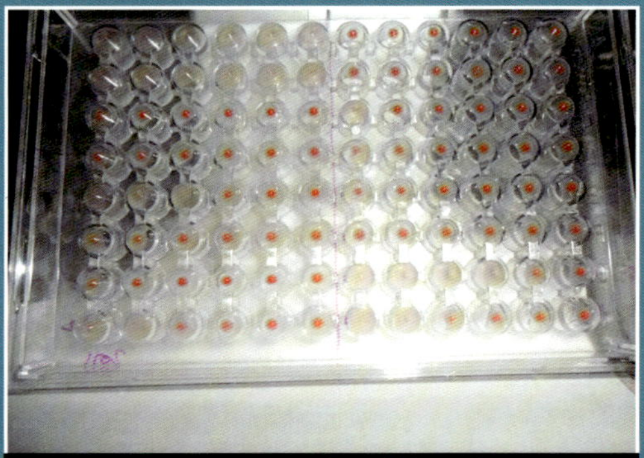
HAI for the detection of Ab against canine parvovirus

Techniques	Samples	Observations
Viral detection (IC, PCR and HA)	Stools.	IC commercially available (the most widely used technique for screening, especially in combination with canine coronaviruses).
Serology (ELISA and HAI)	Serum.	• It is necessary to assess seroconversion. • Commercial in-office ELISA available.

TREATMENT

The rapid establishment of intravenous therapy is crucial to correct dehydration and avoid the hypovolemic shock.

- **Fluid therapy** to correct dehydration and avoid shock. In a first phase crystalloid isotonics and colloids are used, which can be combined with the transfusion of plasma or whole blood, to continue with a supportive level of fluid therapy.
- **Antibiotics, antiemetics and antisecretory drugs** are recommended according to the profile of the patient and the presence or absence of fever.
- **Interferon-ω** to reduce mortality and severity of the enteric manifestations.

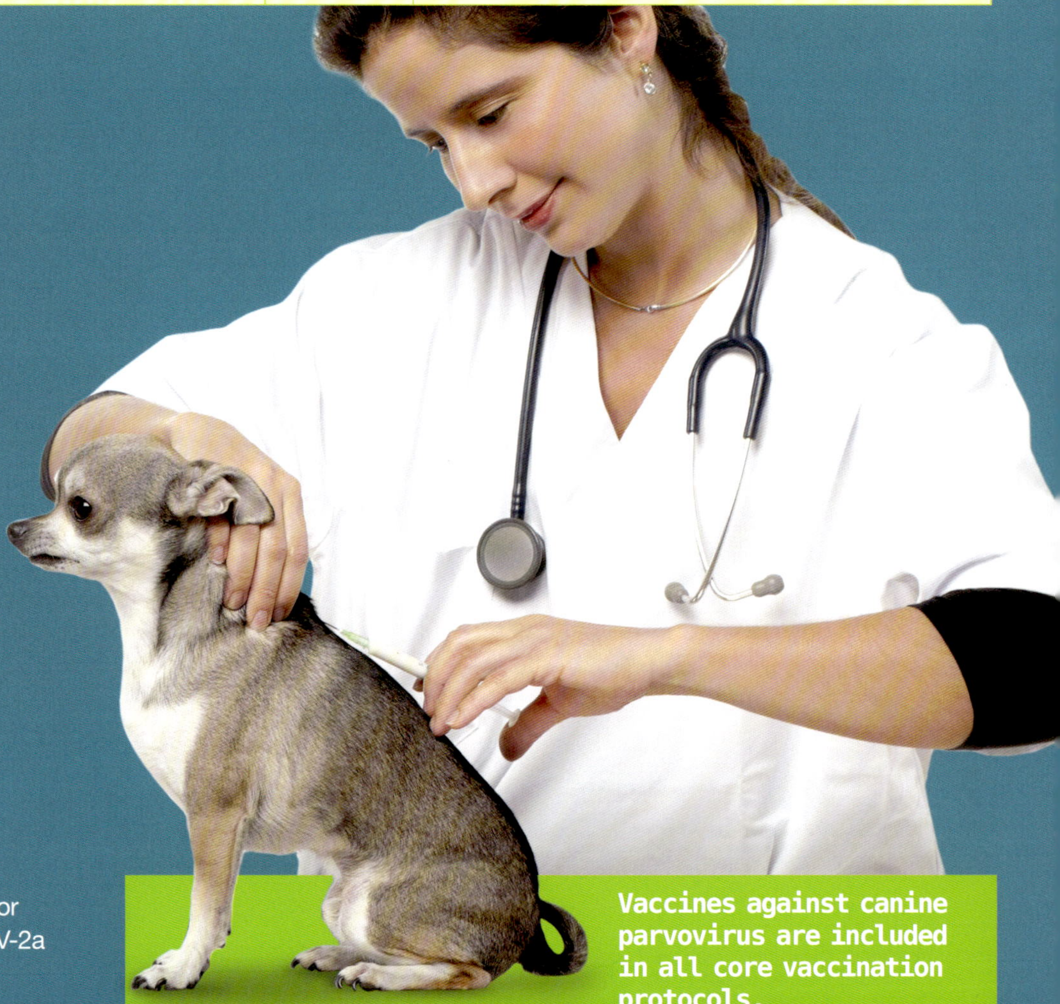

VACCINES

Vaccines against parvoviral diseases are attenuated, mono or multivalent, and include various doses, variants (CPV-2, CPV-2a or CPV-2b) and strains of canine parvovirus.

In general, vaccines induce a strong and lasting immunity.

Vaccines against canine parvovirus are included in all core vaccination protocols.

CLINICAL SIGNS AND LESIONS

ENTERIC (INTESTINAL) FORM

CLINICAL SIGNS

The enteric form is acute, and occurs in puppies and in a small number of adults.

Early clinical signs include very severe depression, prostration and, occasionally, vomiting.

These signs are quickly followed (within a few hours) by diarrhea which may be hemorrhagic from the beginning. Diarrhea is continuous and induces a rapid loss of body condition and severe dehydration.

The clinical evolution is short (between 3 and 5 days).

If the adequate intravenous treatment is not started promptly, the puppies become dehydrated rapidly and often die.

LESIONS

Lesions are initially located in the jejunum and ileum and progress to the first sections of the colon.

Common lesions seen:

- Very marked Peyer's patches.
- Congestive to hemorrhagic intestinal serosa and mucosa.
- Hemorrhagic content inside the intestine.

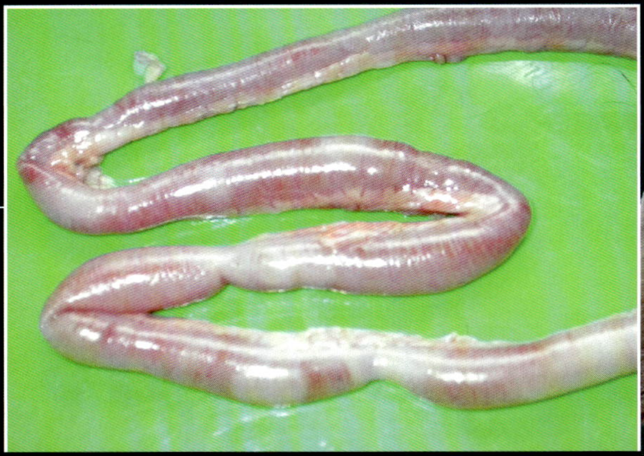

Small intestine: distinct Peyer's patches and congestive and hemorrhagic serosa

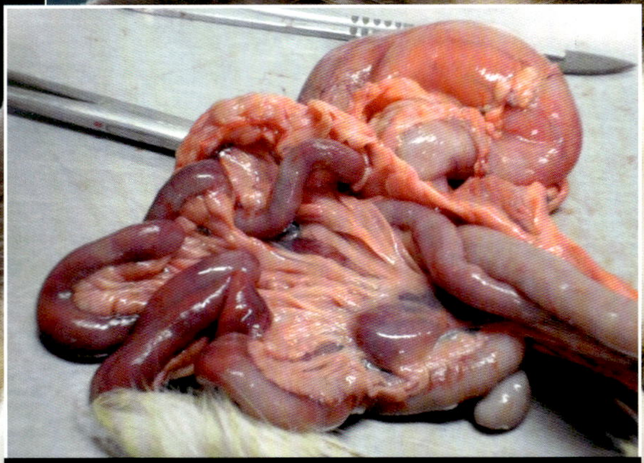

Small intestine: distinct Peyer's patches and congestive serosa

MYOCARDIAL FORM

It is rare and occurs in puppies a few weeks old born from mothers who provide no immunity.

In some puppies this form can cause sudden death, and in other puppies it occurs acutely with dyspnea, tachycardia, thready pulse, pale or cyanotic mucosa and, often, death.

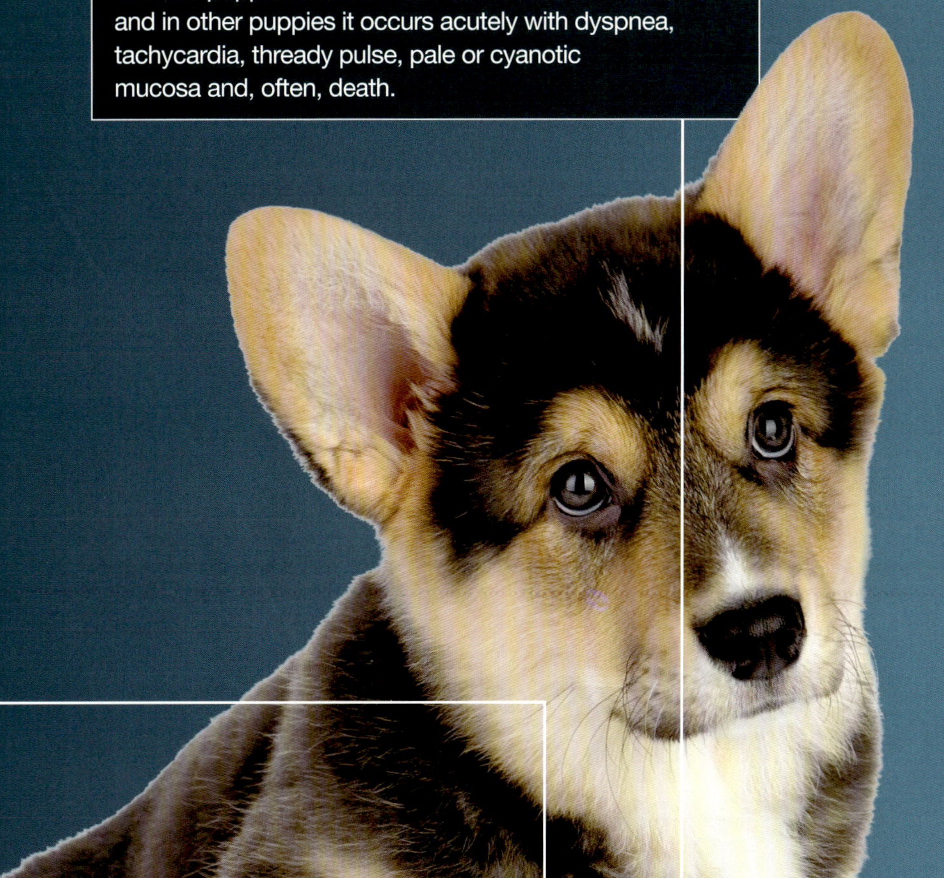

INFECTIONS CAUSED BY CANINE CORONAVIRUSES

ETIOLOGY

Coronaviruses belong to the family *Coronaviridae* (enveloped RNA viruses).

Coronaviruses are classified into groups and subgroups on the basis of their antigenic and genetic differences.

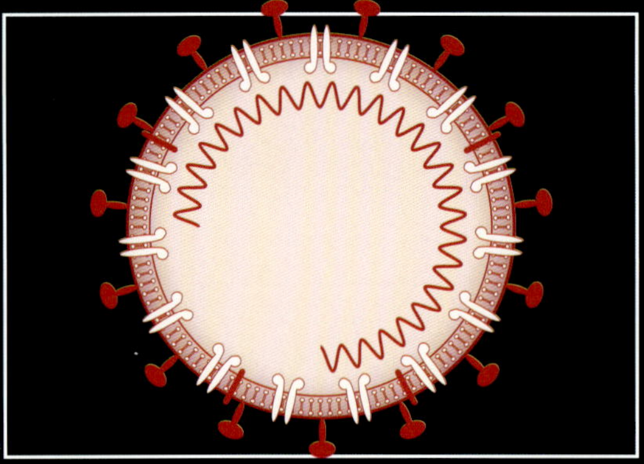

SUBGROUP 1A INCLUDES:

- Canine coronavirus.
- Feline coronavirus.
- Porcine transmissible gastroenteritis virus.
- Porcine respiratory coronavirus.

Currently, it is considered that these viruses are of the same species that has evolved in different hosts.

Canine coronaviruses are classified into two genotypes: I and II, both associated with digestive manifestations.

Recently, some strains of genotype II have been associated with a systemic disease **(pantropic canine coronavirus)**.

PATHOGENESIS

1 There is no viremia and the infection is only locally disseminated.

2 Target cells are the cells lining the apex of the intestinal villi. The multiplication of the virus in them produces cell death, desquamation and primary shortening (blunting) of the villi.

3 Canine coronaviruses replicate in the jejunum and ileum, triggering a syndrome of malabsorption. This is due to altered transport and exchange of ions and water, and to the accumulation and overload in the intestinal lumen, in addition to the loss of the apex cells responsible for the absorption of nutrients. These alterations lead to increased peristalsis, hypersecretion and diarrhea.

4 Pantropic strains are able to colonize other tissues, besides the intestine.

5 The development of the humoral immune response in primary infections is slow (around day 15 post-infection) and does not confer protection.

Recovery is related to the development of a local (in the tissue) specific immune response.

Canine enteric coronaviruses enter orally and directly colonize the small intestine.

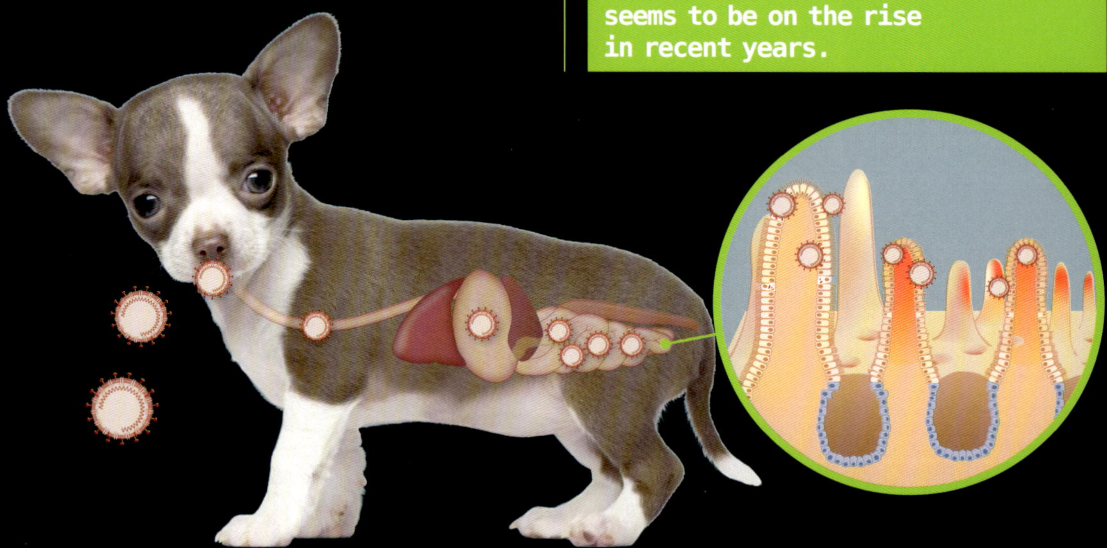

EPIDEMIOLOGY

SHEDDING

Viruses are shed through feces intermittently until two weeks post-infection.

TRANSMISSION

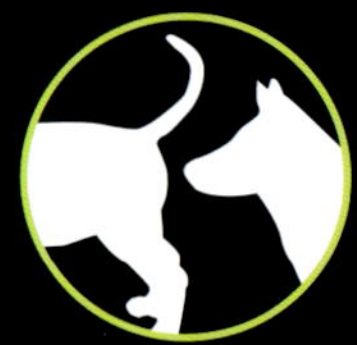

Fecal-oral.

THE CLINICAL OUTCOME DEPENDS UPON:

- **Age:** the disease occurs mostly in puppies between 6 and 16 weeks of age.
- **Exposure route, viral load and strain.**
- **Immune status of the animal.**

Gastrointestinal tract-associated coronaviruses induce less severe alterations and behave like ordinary enteric viruses.

Pantropic strains are associated with severe systemic outcomes in very young puppies.

It is relatively common to observe mixed infections by canine parvovirus and coronavirus.

The prevalence of the infection seems to be on the rise in recent years.

CLINICAL SIGNS AND LESIONS

DIGESTIVE FORM

The severity of digestive clinical signs is related to the presence of concurrent infections. In general, clinical signs include vomiting, loss of appetite, depression, decreased stool consistency and yellowish diarrhea, which can complicate and progress from mucous to bloody.

Animals recover towards day 7-10 post-infection if there are no concurrent infections.

Enteritis may recur if the animal remains in a contaminated environment and is re-exposed to the pathogen.

Mortality is very low when canine enteric coronavirus is the only pathogen.

LESIONS

- Sections of small intestine are enlarged and contain liquid.
- Congestive serosa and hemorrhagic mucosa.

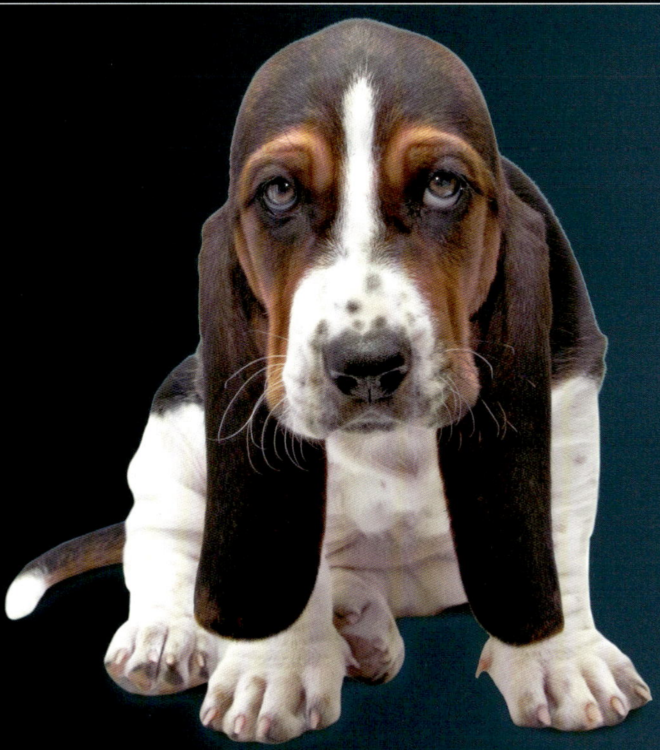

SYSTEMIC FORM

Clinical signs may include fever, lethargy, anorexia, vomiting, hemorrhagic diarrhea, nervous signs and high mortality in puppies.

DIAGNOSIS

CLINICAL DIAGNOSIS

It depends on the presentation, outcome and severity of the diarrhea.

DIFFERENTIAL DIAGNOSIS

The presence of other parasitic and viral agents has to be ruled out, especially canine parvovirus.

LABORATORY DIAGNOSIS

Techniques	Samples	Observations
Viral detection (IC and ELISA)	Stools (from the first days of diarrhea).	IC diagnostic kit is commercially available for coronavirus and parvovirus.
Serology (ELISA and seroneutralization)	Serum.	• Commercially available ELISA. • It is necessary to assess seroconversión.

TREATMENT

Fluid therapy by intravenous infusion to correct dehydration and avoid the hypovolemic shock.

The treatment of enteric illnesses caused by the canine coronavirus is **supportive** and **urgent**, similar to treatment for canine parvoviral infections.

PREVENTION AND CONTROL

VACCINATION

Vaccines against canine coronaviruses are inactivated and polyvalent.

Vaccines induce antibody production, but the antibody titer does not correlate directly with the level of protection.

PREVENTION IN DOG POPULATIONS

- Provide good hygiene conditions.
- Group animals by age range.
- In the presence of diarrhea outbreaks it is necessary to implement extreme disinfection measures.

CANINE INFECTIOUS RESPIRATORY DISEASE

Infections by canine parainfluenza virus, *Bordetella bronchiseptica* and canine adenoviruses.

ETIOLOGY

The main agents responsible for canine respiratory disease are:

1 **Canine parainfluenzavirus**: they belong to the family *Paramyxoviridae* (enveloped RNA viruses), genus *Paramyxovirus*.

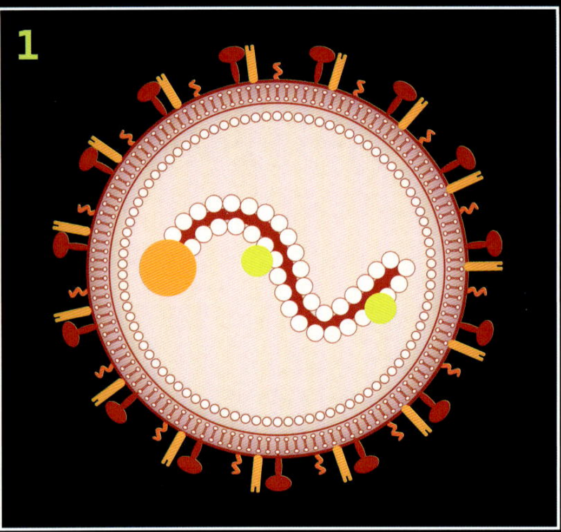

2 **Canine adenovirus type 2 (CAV-2)**: classified in the family *Adenoviridae* (non-enveloped DNA viruses), genus *Mastadenovirus*.

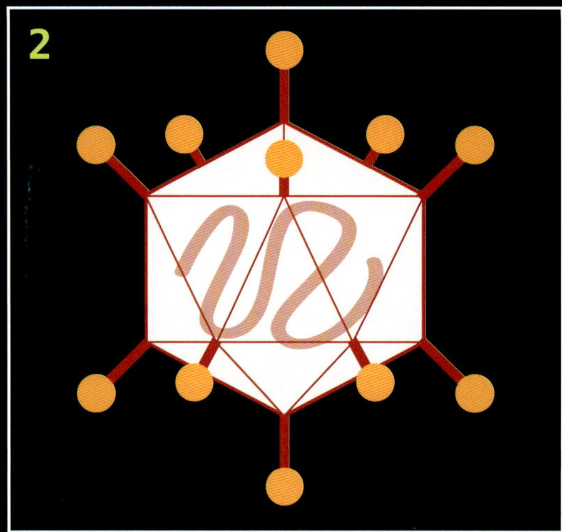

3 ***Bordetella bronchiseptica***: a gram-negative coccobacillus, mobile by flagella, it possesses fimbriae and produces toxins. It is an obligate parasite of the upper respiratory tract of dogs, cats, pigs, rabbits and rodents, and is capable of producing respiratory diseases in these species.

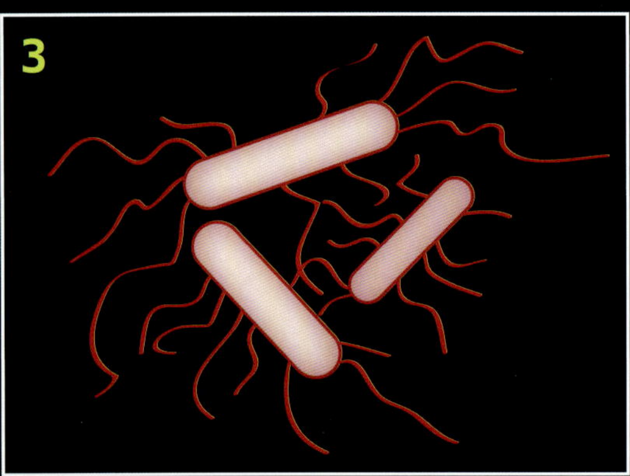

4 ***Mycoplasma***: are small bacteria that lack cell wall, belonging to the class *Mollicutes*.

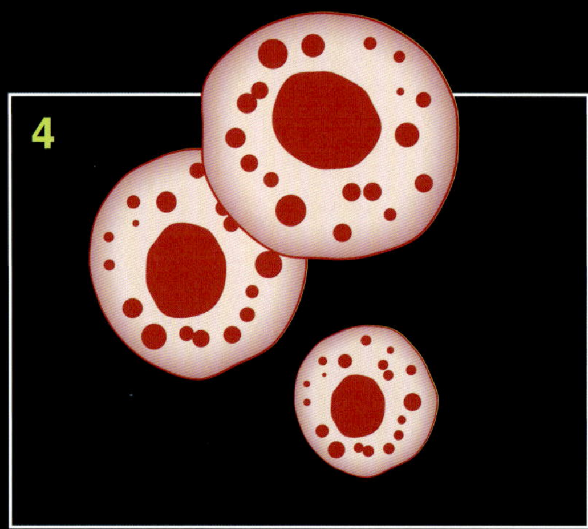

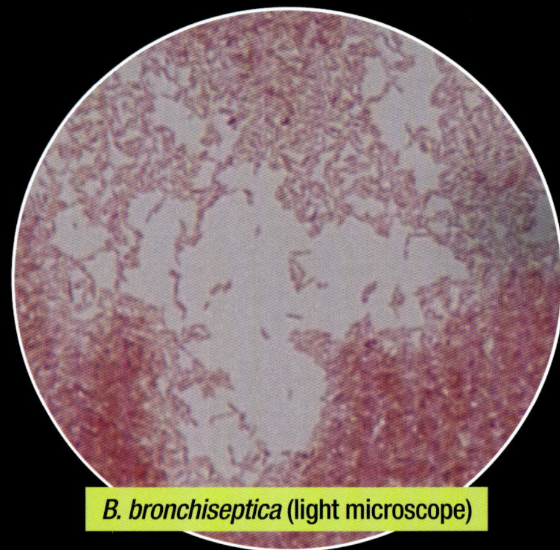

B. bronchiseptica (light microscope)

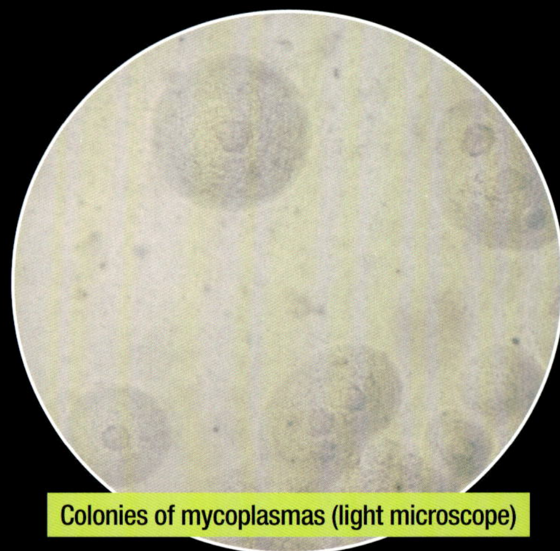

Colonies of mycoplasmas (light microscope)

Other pathogens can also participate in the canine respiratory disease, also known as canine infectious tracheobronchitis or "kennel cough". Some of these are canine distemper virus, canine herpesvirus type 1, influenzavirus and pantropic respiratory strains of canine coronavirus.

In addition, various bacteria can act as secondary invaders

EPIDEMIOLOGY

SHEDDING

The pathogens which produce this disease are present in the respiratory secretions of infected animals.

TRANSMISSION

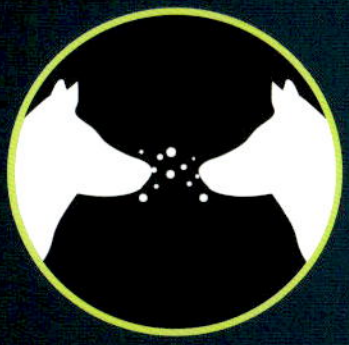

By airborne droplets.

PRESENTATION

Canine respiratory disease occurs suddenly and spreads rapidly among dogs housed in populations such as breeding kennels or shelters, and can affect all animals in the group.

The disease is more severe in young animals and when a greater number of agents are involved.

MAIN RISK FACTORS IN THE POPULATIONS

- Extreme temperature and poor ventilation.
- High animal density.
- High microbiological load in the environment.
- Poor hygiene and disinfection measures.

The emergence of the disease tends to be seasonal, coinciding with low temperatures and wide temperature variations. It may also coincide with a recent history of vaccination, especially in young animals.

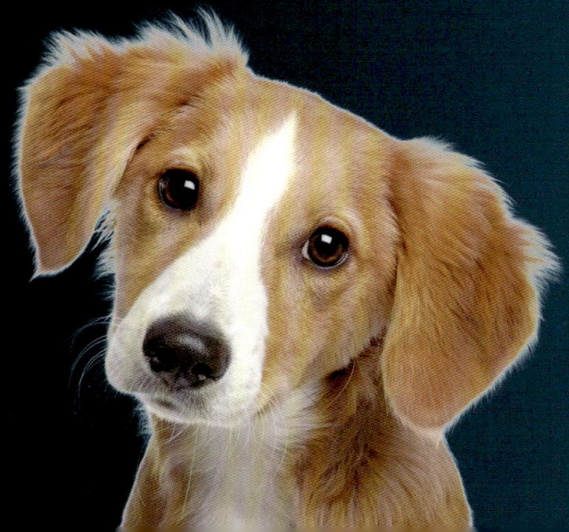

PATHOGENESIS

- **Canine parainfluenza viruses** usually colonize only the upper respiratory tract transiently and in a self-limiting way.
- **Canine adenovirus type 2** usually replicates between the upper respiratory tract and the bronchiolar epithelium, with a capability of causing pneumonia.
- ***B. bronchiseptica*** adhere to the cilia of the trachea and bronchi through their fimbriae and multiply quickly. They increase their numbers until the first two weeks post-infection and decrease thereafter.

  Mechanisms of pathogenicity:

  - Toxin production (dermonecrotic and tracheal).
  - Inhibition of phagocytosis.
  - Paralysis of the ciliary movement: this favors colonization by other bacteria that would not have the capacity to adhere to the cilia of the trachea and bronchi of dogs.
- ***Mycoplasma*** originate an inflammatory process of the respiratory tract and, occasionally, can cause pneumonia.

Viruses are only isolated the first days or weeks post-infection, while the excretion of *B. bronchiseptica* and *Mycoplasma* can last up to 3 months.

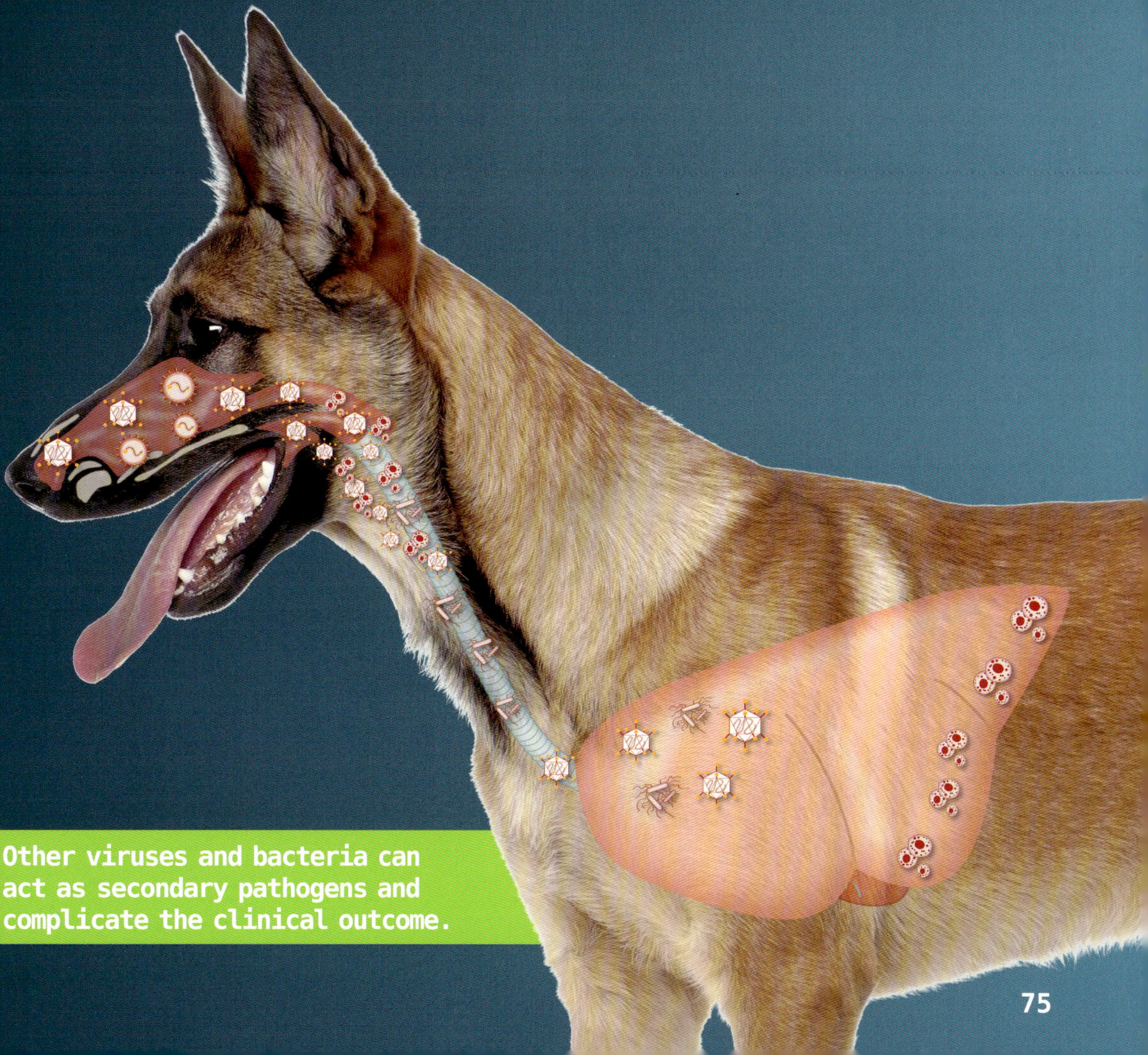

Other viruses and bacteria can act as secondary pathogens and complicate the clinical outcome.

CLINICAL SIGNS AND LESIONS

The disease starts with sudden onset of nasal catarrh, paroxysmal cough and fever, and the outcome can be either mild or severe.

CLINICAL FORMS

SEVERE FORM

- It occurs in very young animals or those with malnutrition.
- The clinical signs include increasingly dry, painful cough or with mucous, accompanied by nasal and ocular discharges and bronchopneumonia.
- The destruction of the ciliated respiratory epithelium promotes the emergence of secondary bacterial infections. If this is the case, it can produce mortality in a small percentage of dogs due to severe dehydration and multisystemic clinical signs.

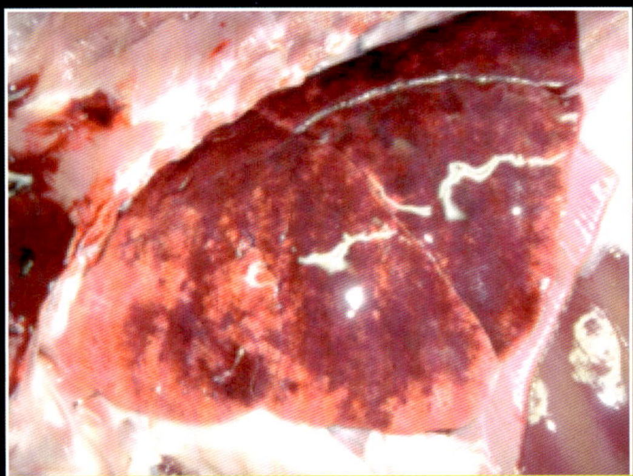

Pneumonia caused by *B. bronchiseptica*

MILD FORM

- Is characterized by harsh, dry cough and the production of characteristic laryngeal sounds, commonly known as "honking".
- Occasionally, the cough can induce retching.
- Clinical signs usually do not last more than two or three weeks.

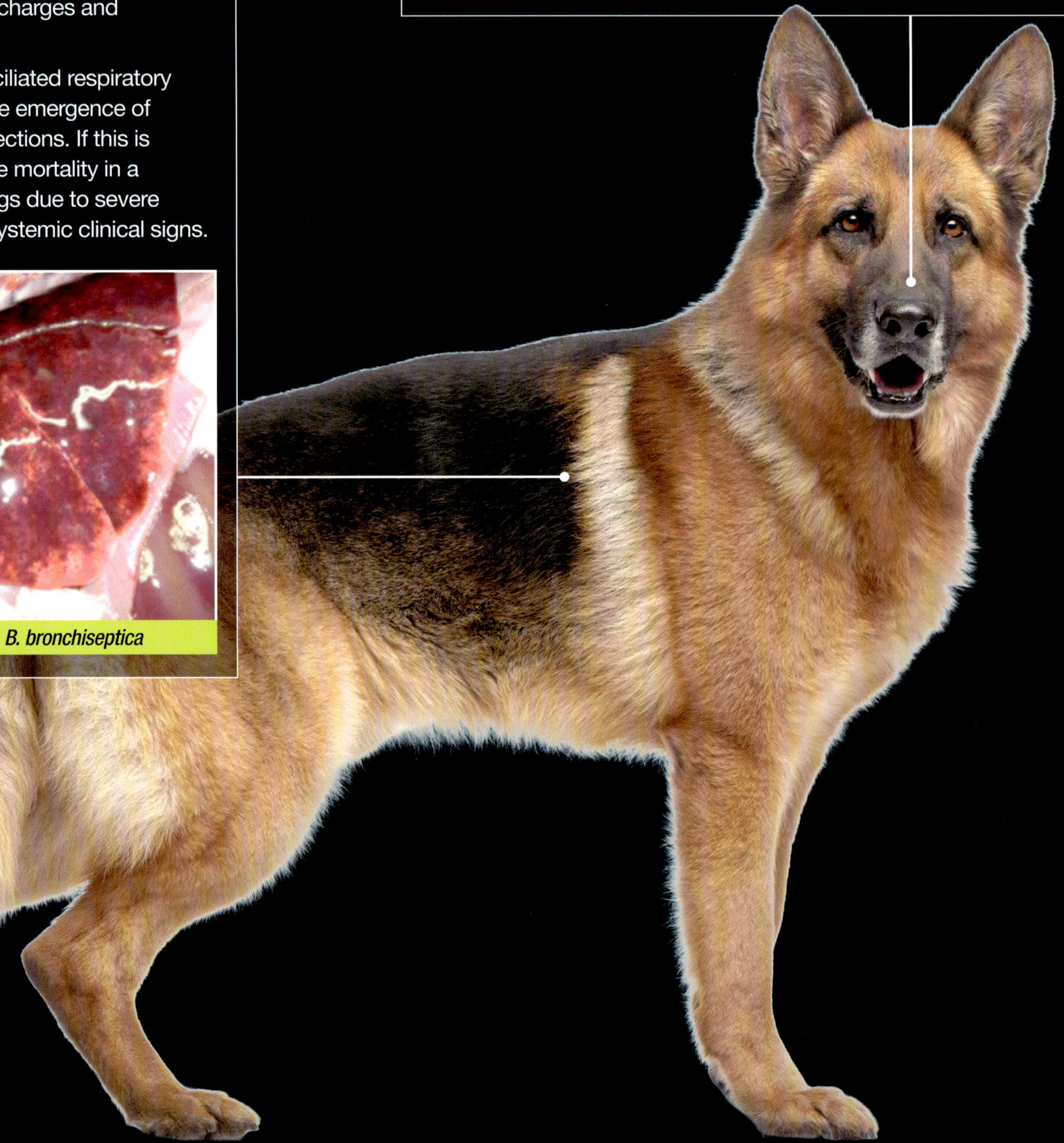

DIAGNOSIS

CLINICAL DIAGNOSIS

Though other illnesses of different etiology can produce respiratory clinical signs, the sudden onset, the rapid diffusion, high morbidity and the epidemiological context allow for a suspicion of canine respiratory disease.

The possible involvement of multiple agents hinders the etiologic diagnosis.

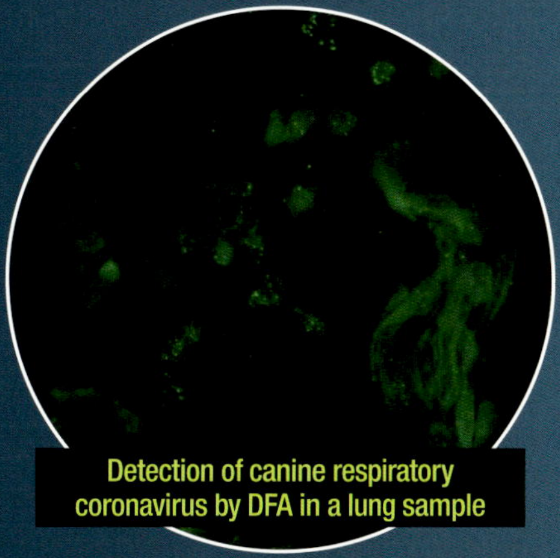

Detection of canine respiratory coronavirus by DFA in a lung sample

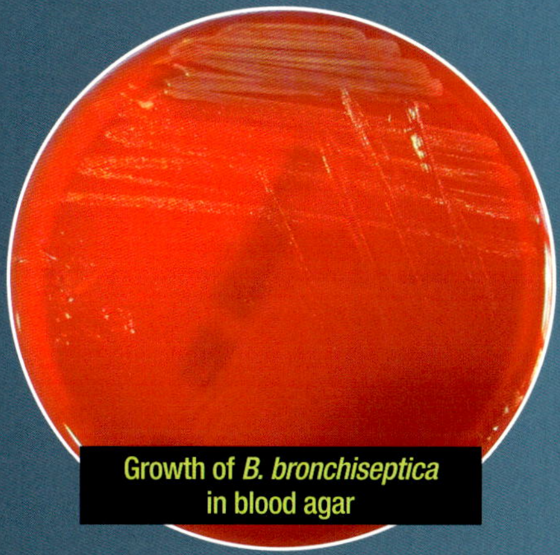

Growth of *B. bronchiseptica* in blood agar

LABORATORY DIAGNOSIS

Different techniques are available to identify the various viruses associated with this disease.

In many cases, and for practical reasons, only the bacteriological diagnosis to identify *B. bronchiseptica* and possible secondary bacteria and their corresponding antibiogram is ordered from the laboratory.

Samples	Multiplex PCR	Single PCR	Commercial IC for virus detection	DFA	Serology
Nasal discharge	+	+	+	+	−
Tissues	−	−	−	+	−
Serum	−	−	−	−	+
Observations	The most useful.		Adenoviruses and canine distemper virus.		

TREATMENT

- In mild cases: the disease remits spontaneously by **improving health, hygiene and environmental conditions** of the surroundings of the animals, and by providing a quiet, dry and clean environment.
- **Cough suppressants**, if coughing persists.
- **Mucolytics** and **expectorants** if coughing persists and is productive, to avoid the accumulation of exudates in the lower respiratory tract.
- **Bronchodilators** and **anti-inflammatory medications** to improve respiratory function.
- **Antibiotics** to treat infections by *B. bronchiseptica*.

The most commonly used antibiotics belong to the groups of tetracyclines and beta-lactam.

When treating individual animals, it is more efficient to administer antibiotics and drugs in the form of aerosols than parenterally.

Antibiotic therapy should only be applied to dogs with serious or persistent clinical signs.

VACCINES

Vaccines against *B. bronchiseptica*, canine parainfluenzavirus, and canine adenovirus type 2 are multivalent, attenuated (the majority) or inactivated. They can be injected (most often) or, in the case of *B. bronchiseptica* and canine parainfluenza virus, also administered intranasally.

They are useful mainly in young animals to reduce the clinical incidence of the disease.

They are mostly intended for canine populations (breeding kennels and shelters).

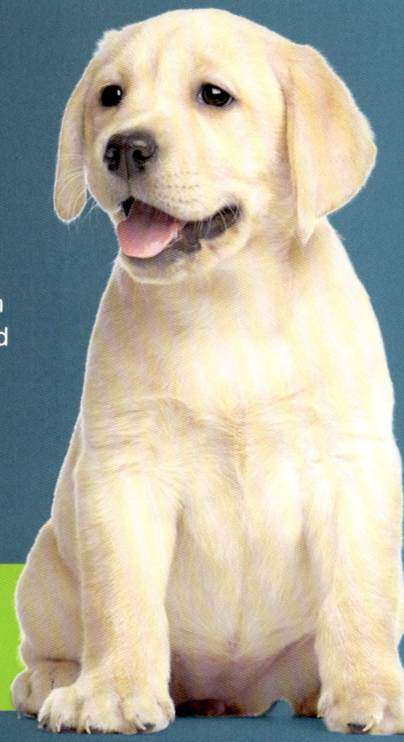

INFECTIONS CAUSED BY CANINE HERPESVIRUS

ETIOLOGY

Canine herpesvirus type 1 belongs to the family *Herpesviridae* (enveloped DNA virus), subfamily *Alphaherpesvirinae*, where most of the herpesviruses pathogenic for different species of domestic animals are classified.

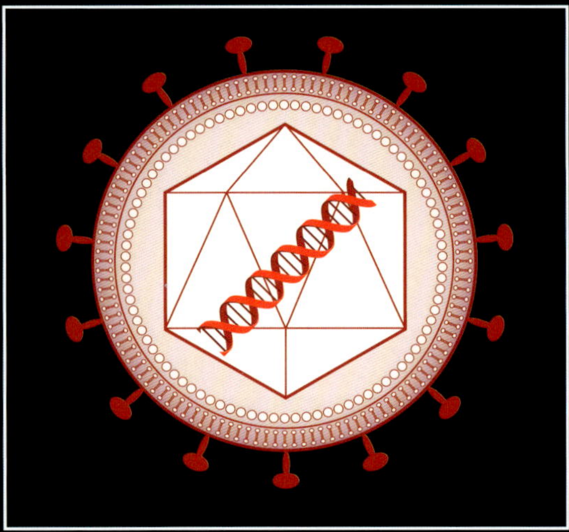

Most important features of the herpesviruses associated with their pathogenic ability:

- Establishment of lytic infection in the host cell.
- Induction of latency.
- Formation of inclusion bodies.
- Thermosensitivity: ability to multiply at temperatures below 37 °C.

Some surface glycoproteins of the virus, such as gB, induce an effective and protective immune response.

Herpesviruses are very sensitive to the action of the majority of disinfectants.

Canine herpesvirus type 1 infection in dogs is associated with reproductive disorders and mortality in pups under two or three weeks of age.

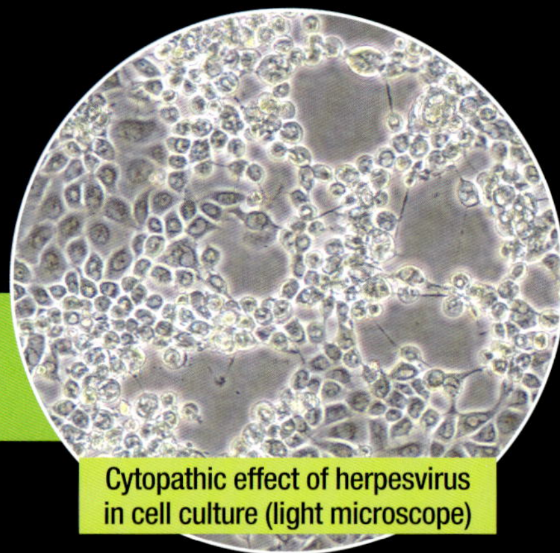

Cytopathic effect of herpesvirus in cell culture (light microscope)

EPIDEMIOLOGY

Seroprevalence in canine populations is highly variable and can range between 40 and 80 %, depending on the country.

SHEDDING

- Mainly through oronasal and genital secretions.
- Other: urine, feces, saliva and tears. Fetuses and fetal membranes contain large loads of virus (in abortions).
- The virus can be shed up to between two to three weeks post-infection.

Infection is restricted to dogs and wild canids.

TRANSMISSION

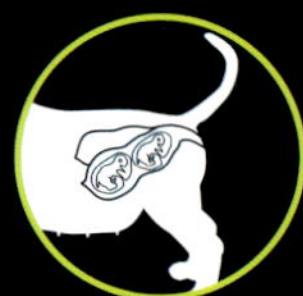

- Maternal-fetal (in uterus and through the birth canal).

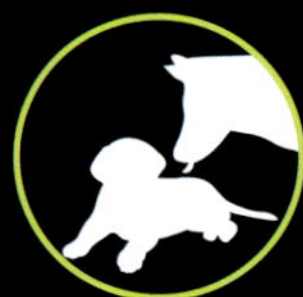

- Oronasal: by contact with oral or respiratory secretions of the mother (through licking) or of other infected animals.

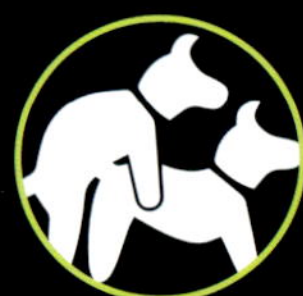

- Venereal.

CLINICAL FORMS

- Reproductive form.
- Neonatal form: systemic disease in puppies younger than three weeks old.
- Respiratory form: in young and adult animals.
- Venereal form: restricted to the genital area in adults.

FACTORS CRITICAL TO NEONATAL INFECTION

- Titer of maternal antibodies.
- Immunological maturity or immune competence of the puppy.
- Inability of the puppy to regulate its body temperature (the virus multiplies at 35 °C).

Over 80 % of the infected puppies less than one week old may die in two or three days.

Due to the reproductive problems and the high mortality in neonates, the infection by canine herpesvirus type 1 is a serious problem for breeders.

PATHOGENESIS

1 Contact with oronasal secretions. Early viral replication takes place in the nasal epithelium and mucosa, tonsils and pharynx.

2 Subsequently, an early viremia develops (2-4 days post-infection) associated with monocytes that can cause:

- **2a** A systemic infection (liver, spleen, kidney, lymphoid tissue, CNS, adrenals and heart) in less than three week old puppies.
- **2b** A localized infection in the respiratory tract of young and adult dogs.
- **2c** A persistent infection in the genital tract of adult animals.

In **systemic infections**, the multiplication of the virus induces multifocal cell death in different tissues and organs, such as the endothelium and the CNS, and can cause bleeding, thrombocytopenia and meningoencephalitis.

When the infection occurs in a **pregnant bitch**, cell-associated viruses enter the uterus and can produce from stillbirth to neonatal illness (systemic infection), depending on the stage of gestation.

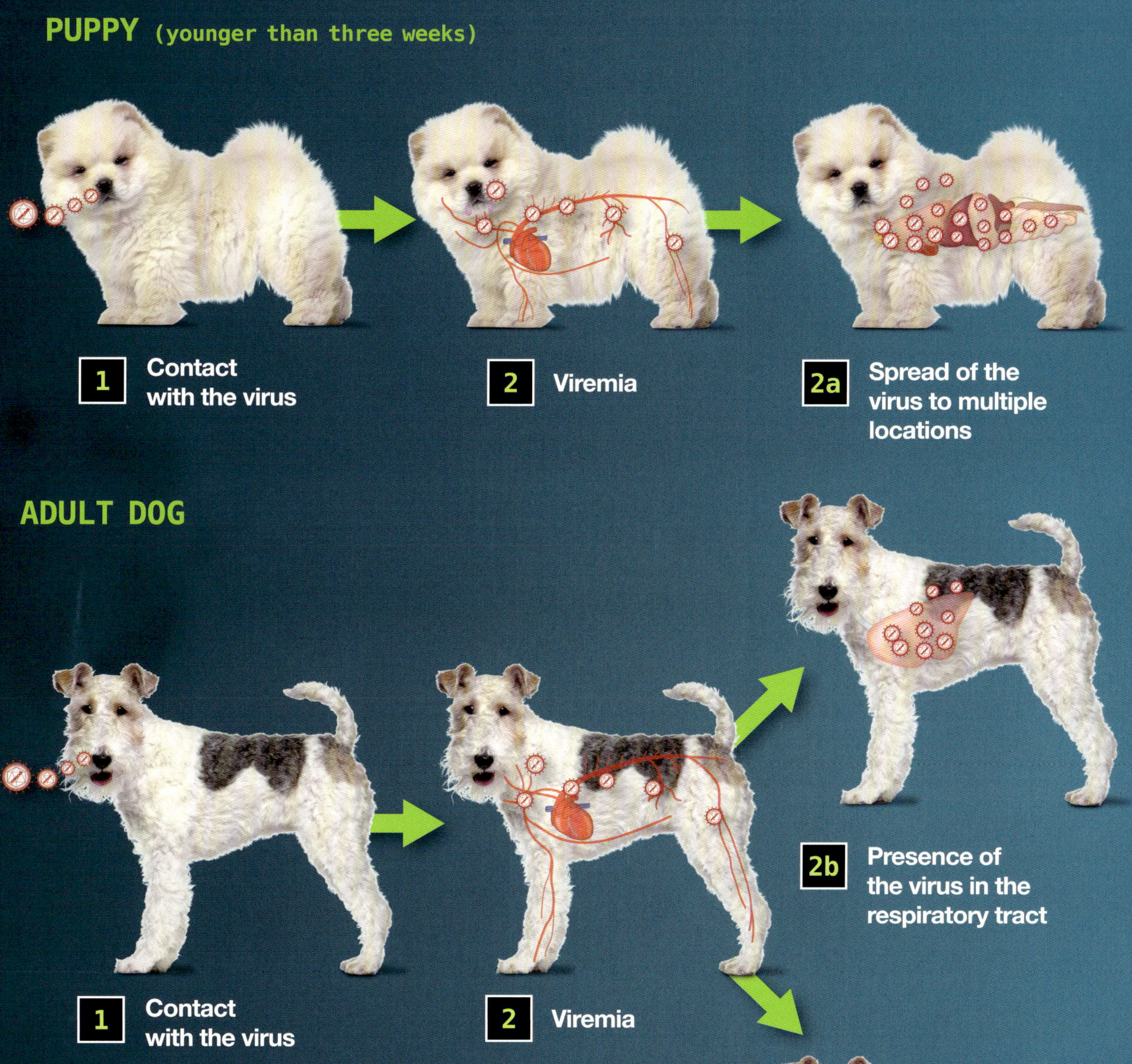

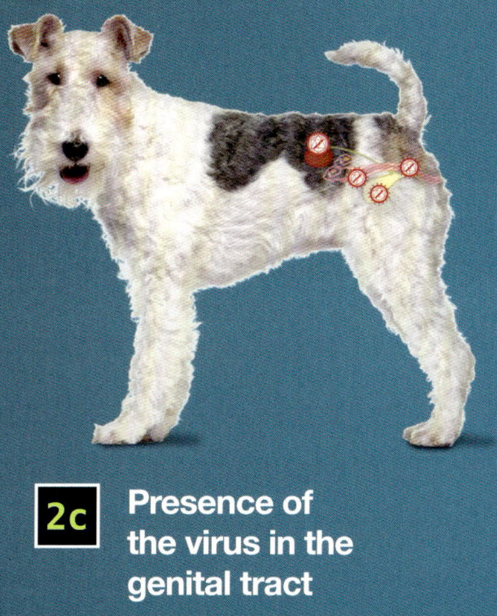

- The infection may be **subclinical** in puppies over three weeks of age and in adults.
- Canine herpesvirus type 1 produces **latent infections** in nerve cells, especially of the trigeminal and lumbosacral ganglions.
- Reactivation of a latent infection may be caused by stress, immune suppression or gestation. Reactivated viruses may be shed again through oronasal and genital secretions.

Animals can be persistently infected.

REPRODUCTIVE FORM

Abortion, stillbirths, premature births and infertility.

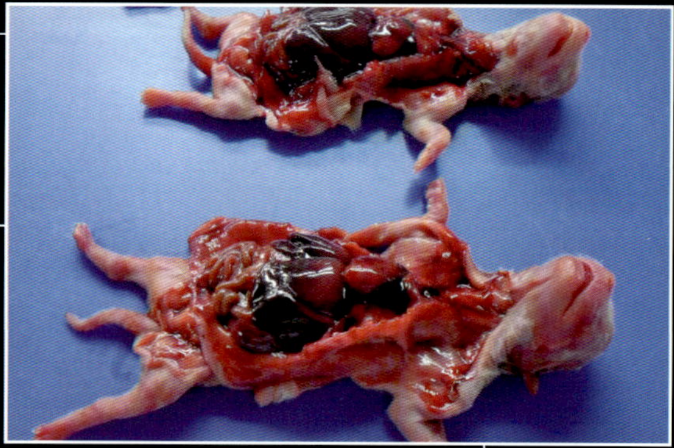

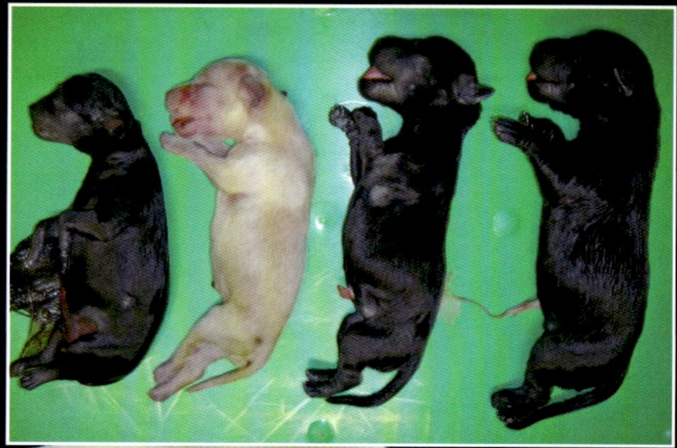

NEONATAL FORM

CLINICAL SIGNS

Puppies have anorexia, weakness, abdominal pain (whining), diarrhea, dyspnea, nasal discharge, loss of suckling reflex (they refuse to suck) and neurologic dysfunction (such as opisthotonos and seizures).

After recovery, some puppies may develop sequelae such as optic neuritis and uveitis with keratitis.

LESIONS

- Renal ecchymosis and discoloration ("speckled kidney").
- Splenomegaly.
- Effusion in cavities.
- Necrotic foci and haemorrhages in various tissues and organs (liver, lung and digestive tract).

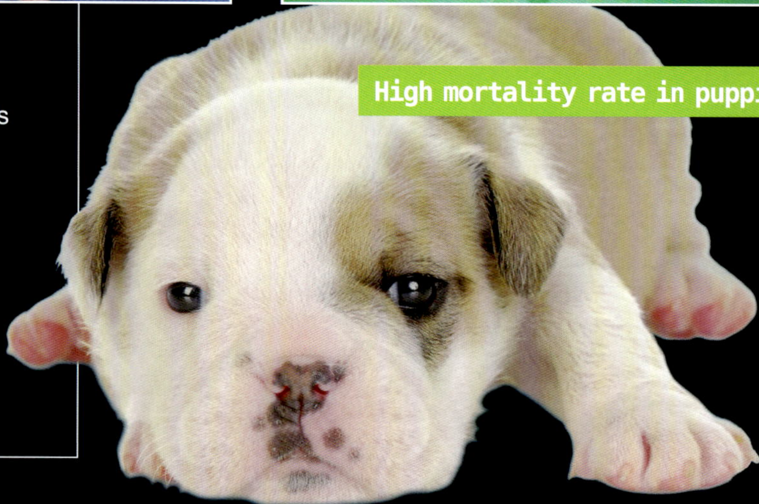

High mortality rate in puppies.

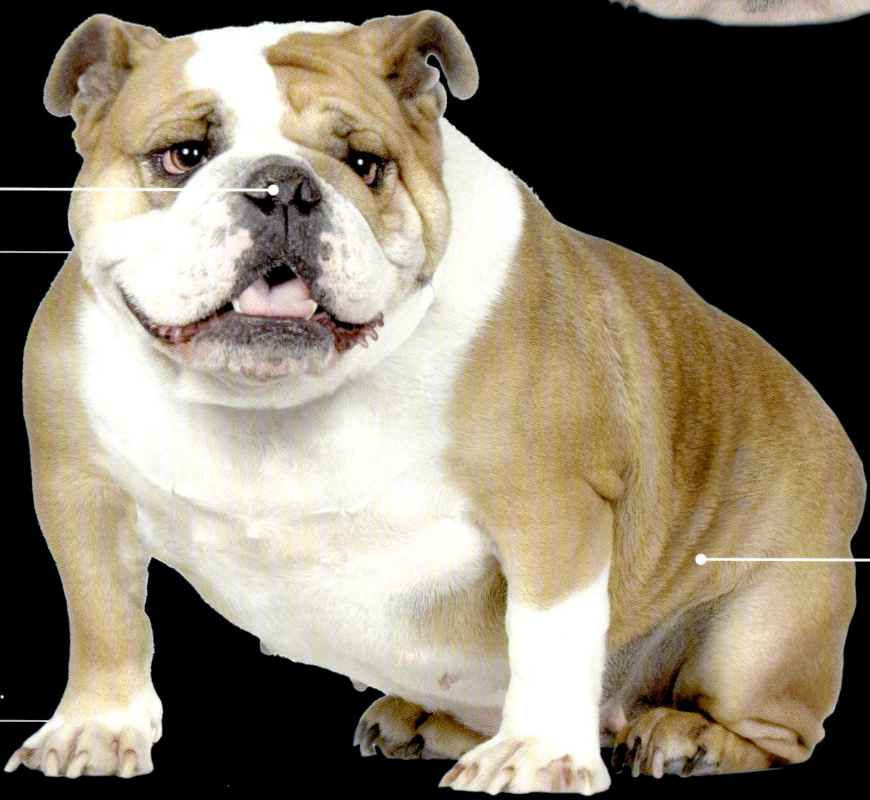

RESPIRATORY FORM

Transient mild respiratory and ocular manifestations may be observed in young and adult dogs.

CLINICAL SIGNS

- Cough.
- Conjunctivitis.
- Keratitis.
- Ocular and nasal discharges.

VENEREAL FORM

In adults the virus may accumulate in the genital tract and produce vesicular vaginitis or posthitis.

DIAGNOSIS

CLINICAL AND DIFFERENTIAL DIAGNOSIS

The age, physiological state and genetic value (breeders) of the animal should be taken into account. In addition, it should be considered whether the disease affects an individual dog or a population.

In populations, if there are respiratory clinical signs in young animals, it may be necessary to resort to a differential diagnosis with canine distemper, canine infectious respiratory disease or infectious canine hepatitis.

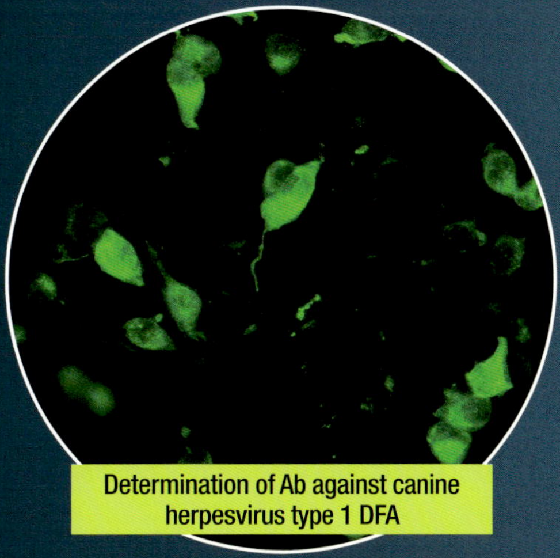

Determination of Ab against canine herpesvirus type 1 DFA

LABORATORY DIAGNOSIS

Techniques	Samples	Observations
Viral detection (DFA and PCR) and histology	• *In vivo:* respiratory and genital secretions. • *Post-mortem:* lung, lymphoid tissue, spleen, liver, adrenal glands, kidney and CNS.	• Observation of fluorescent cells and the presence of intranuclear inclusion bodies (DFA). • Control of frozen semen. • The most widely used.
Serology (ELISA, IFA and neutralization)	Serum (two extractions: days 0 and 21).	It is necessary to assess seroconversión.

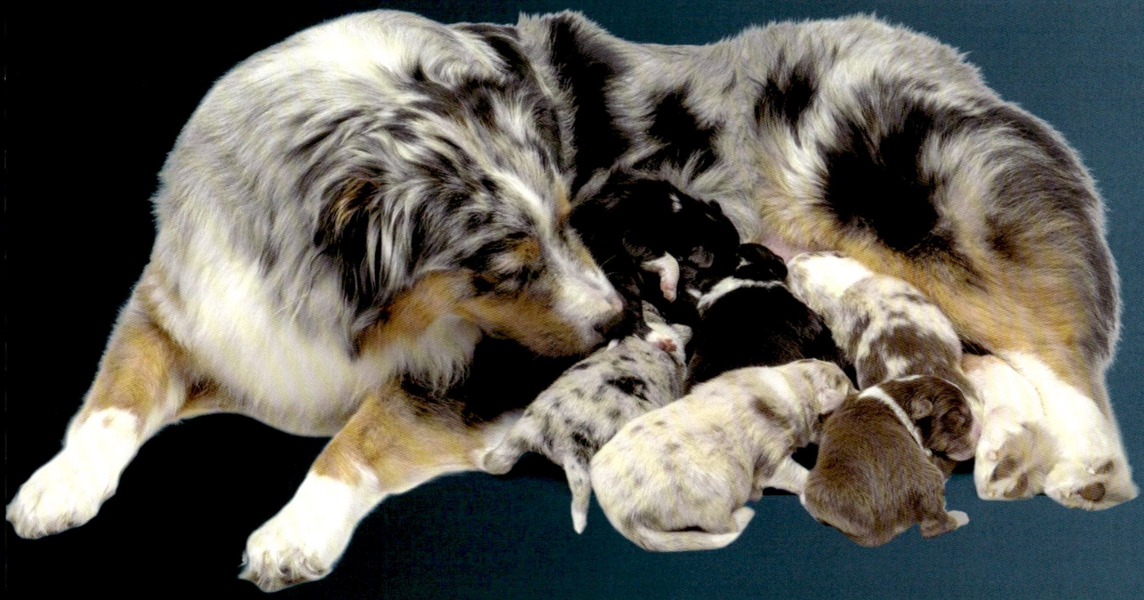

The presence of abortion of a single pup in the litter is not usually indicative of infection by herpesvirus.

TREATMENT

- **Glucocorticoids and vitamin complexes** to treat respiratory, ocular or neurological manifestations.
- **Antibiotics**, administered parenterally or in ophthalmic solution to prevent secondary bacterial infections.
- **Interferon** to limit viral replication.

PREVENTION AND CONTROL

VACCINATION

The vaccine against canine herpesvirus 1 is monovalent and is composed of subunits (containing gB). It is used in Europe.

Since puppies may become infected *in utero* or early after birth, immunization programs are designed to immunize mothers (two doses of the vaccine: 1st, one or two weeks after mating; 2nd, around two weeks before whelping).

Vaccination reduces the clinical incidence of reproductive disorders, but does not prevent the emergence of carriers.

CONTROL MEASURES IN POPULATIONS

For **control of the infection in breeding kennels** with a history of reproductive disease it is necessary to:

- Implement quarantine and control measures when replacing breeder dogs and during transportation.
- Isolate pregnant females from about three weeks before the expected date of whelping up to three weeks post-partum.
- Install heat lamps in the maternity ward to keep the body temperature of the puppies at 38 to 39 °C.

Removal of infected breeding animals should be considered.

CANINE BABESIOSIS

ETIOLOGY

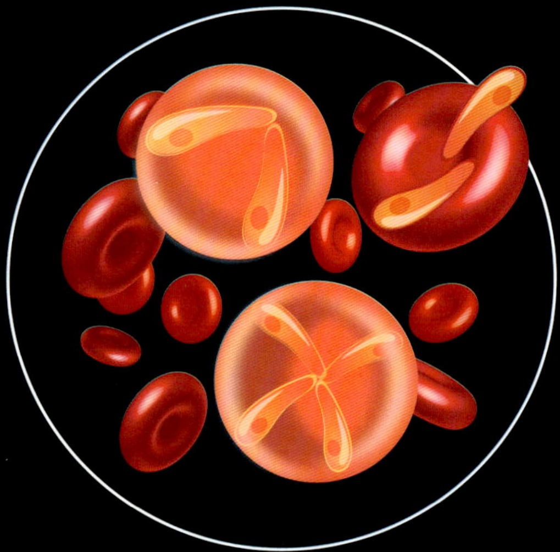

The two types of *Babesia* known to infect dogs are:

- *Babesia canis* and *Babesia vogeli*, also known as "large babesias".
- *Babesia gibsoni* and *Babesia microti*-like or *Theileria annae* (pending classification), called "small babesias".

Babesias infect red blood cells, where merozoites may be observed. These are pyriform, sub-spherical, or rounded forms of the parasite, which may occur in pairs or alone.

PATHOGENESIS

It depends on several factors:

- **The parasite:** virulence of the isolate, primary infection or re-infection, infecting dose.
- **The host:** young animals or those with concomitant diseases, and those who have had no prior contact with the parasite and are introduced in endemic areas are more susceptible to the infection and the disease is more severe.

The pathogenesis is similar for the different species of *Babesia*:

- Mechanical action: there is a destruction of the red blood cells due to the multiplication of the zoites inside these cells. This causes severe anemia (intravascular hemolysis) which persists throughout the parasitemia.
- The increase in vascular permeability produces edema, vasodilation, hypotension and blood stasis, leading to metabolic acidosis which aggravates the disease.
- Red blood cells stick to the endothelium of blood vessels with the risk of thrombosis. The process is made worse by the formation of immune complexes that are deposited on the membrane of parasitized erythrocytes and in certain tissues (see Chart 21). Different clinical outcomes will occur according to the affected organ (liver, kidneys, lungs, skeletal muscle or heart, CNS).

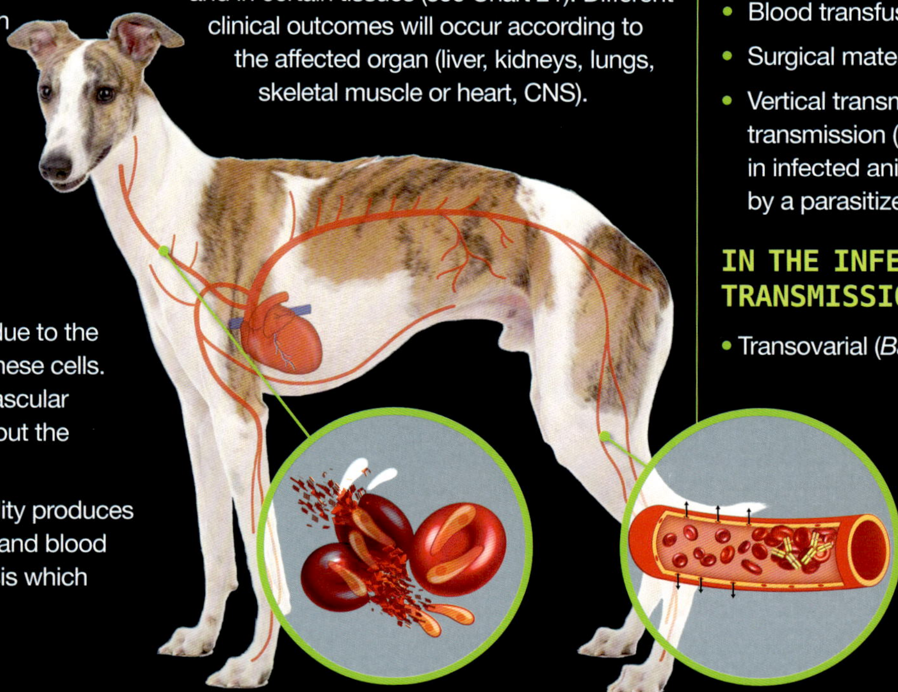

EPIDEMIOLOGY

Seasonal disease (summer), linked to the climate needs of its vector, the *Ixodidae* or hard ticks.

Several species of *Babesia* have been described in different European countries: *B. canis*, *B. vogeli*, *Theileria annae* (syn. *B. microti-like*) and *B. gibsoni*.

TRANSMISSION

MAIN SOURCES OF INFECTION

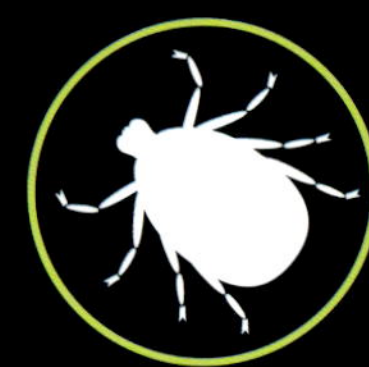

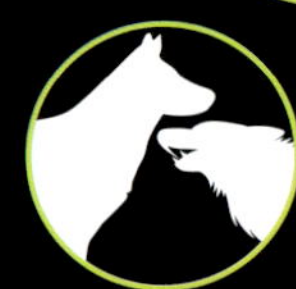

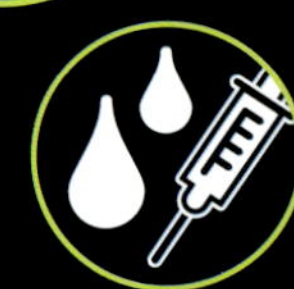

- Infected ticks.
- Sick animals.
- Clinically healthy carriers, common in endemic areas.

OTHER LESS FREQUENT ROUTES OF INFECTION

- Blood transfusions.
- Surgical material.
- Vertical transmission and dog-to-dog transmission (described for *B. gibsoni* in infected animals after being bitten by a parasitized dog).

IN THE INFECTED TICK, TRANSMISSION MAY BE:

- Transovarial (*Babesia* spp.).
- Transestadial (*Theileria* spp.), *i.e.*, the tick is infected in a stage of evolution and maintains the protozoan in the following stage.

CLINICAL SIGNS AND LESIONS

CLINICAL EVOLUTION

It depends on the species of parasite, age of the animal, hygiene and diet conditions.

The prepatent period is short, ranging from 4 to 20 days, and occasionally it can be even 1 or 2 days.

- In young animals, *Babesia* infections are usually acute, with a prepatent period of 4-6 days, and a patent period ranging between 7-10 days. In this age group, babesiosis can be fatal.
- In adults, in general, a flare-up of a chronic form in the case of immune compromise is more frequent.

CLINICAL SIGNS

- Hyperthermia (up to 41°C).
- Asthenia, anorexia, weight loss.
- Dehydration.
- Digestive disorders (vomiting, diarrhea).
- Hepatosplenomegaly, edema, ascites, jaundice, hemorrhages in skin and mucous membranes, dyspnea, pallor, muscle pain, paresis, ataxia (see figures).
- **Clinico-pathological abnormalities** include: normochromic, normocytic, non-regenerative anemia, neutropenia, thrombocytopenia and hemoglobinuria.

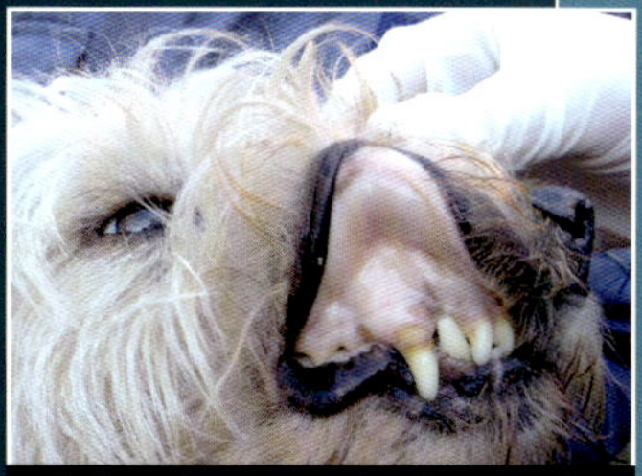

Pallor of mucosa due to anemia

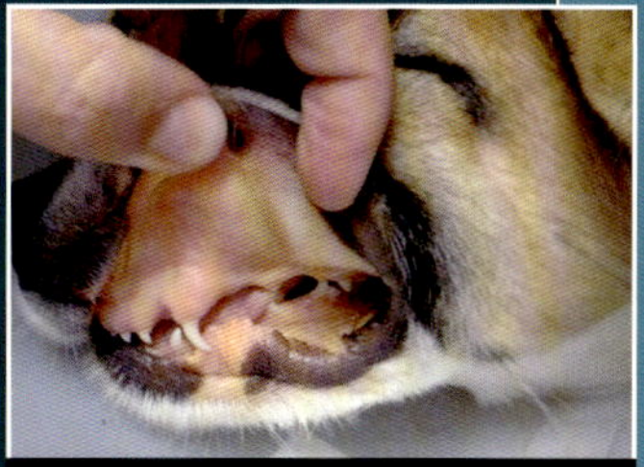

Jaundice

DIAGNOSIS

CLINICAL DIAGNOSIS

Based on physical examination and laboratory abnormalities.

SPECIFIC DIAGNOSIS

Blood smear, molecular diagnosis, and serology.

- **Stained blood smears:** it is difficult to **detect parasites** in blood due to the limited period of parasitemia. Thin layer smears are prepared using peripheral blood (tip of the ear, toenail capillary beds) (see figures).
- **Molecular diagnosis:** PCR, especially in cases of low parasitemia and to differentiate species of *Babesia*. It can be done using blood and/or spleen samples.
- **Serology** is not considered the method of choice due to cross-reactivity between *B. canis* and *B. gibsoni* mainly, but also cross-reactions may occur between the remaining species, hampering interpretation. In addition, it is not possible to differentiate between a past and a present infection. In any case, it is convenient to analyze samples during convalescence and repeat a second sample 3-4 weeks later to assess seroconversion.

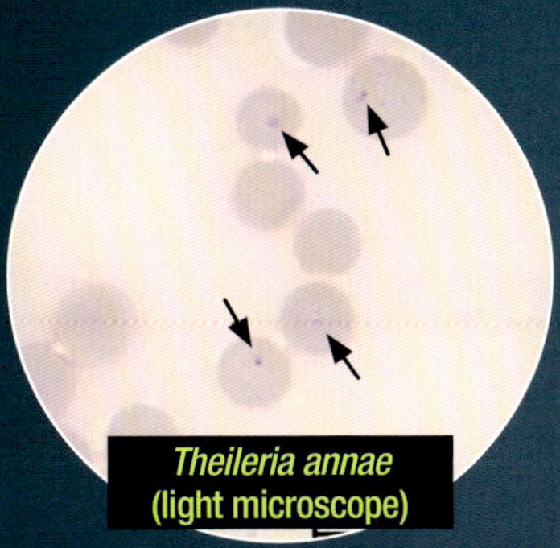

Theileria annae (light microscope)

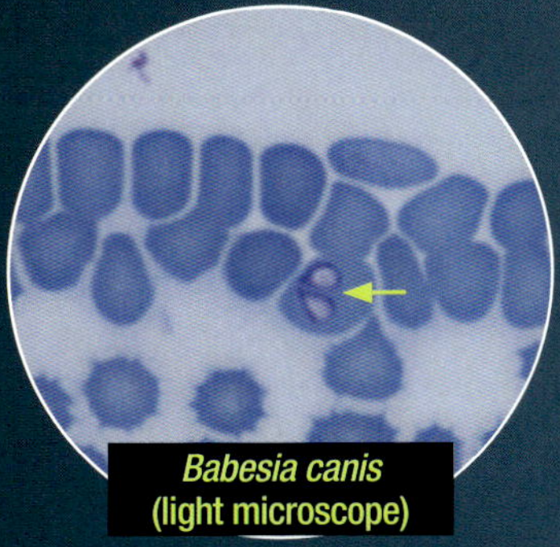

Babesia canis (light microscope)

TREATMENT

- **Babesicides:** imidocarb dipropionate. Effective in the treatment of infections due to *Babesia canis* and *Babesia vogeli*.
- **Theilericides:** atovaquone and buparvaquone.
- **Supportive treatment:** according to clinical and laboratory alterations.
- Other drugs can be used, such as the phenamidine, pentamidines or diminazene, but they present a greater toxicity and reduced efficacy.
- Doxycycline and clindamycin are indicated in some cases.

Dogs may remain infected for life.

PREVENTION AND CONTROL

Two vaccines against *B. canis* based on soluble parasite antigens grown in specific cultures are commercially available. Both induce only a partial protection, but can reduce the severity of the clinical outcome, parasitemia, and/or the duration of the disease.

These vaccines are mainly indicated in endemic areas and for splenectomized animals.

Puppies may be vaccinated from 5 months of age, with a reboost 3-6 weeks later.

Routine application of topical acaricides and daily checks for ticks and their early removal is essential for preventing infection by *Babesia* spp.

LEISHMANIOSIS

ETIOLOGY

In Europe canine leishmaniosis is a zoonotic disease produced exclusively by the protozoan *Leishmania infantum*.

The zymodeme MON-1 is responsible for most infections in dogs and other hosts. Its differentiation and characterization is important in establishing the influence that intraspecific variation can have on the epidemiology of this infection.

EPIDEMIOLOGY

- **Vector-borne transmission:** *Leishmania*'s life cycle involves two hosts: an arthropod vector (in the Mediterranean basin species of sandflies, genus *Phlebotomus*), where the flagellated form of *Leishmania* **(promastigote)** resides in the gut; and a vertebrate host, mainly inside macrophages, in its non-flagellated form **(amastigote)**.
- **Other routes of transmission:** vertical (MON-1), venereal and blood transfusion.
- **Domestic cycle of the infection by *L. infantum*:** the dog is the main reservoir.
  The infection is not always synonymous with clinical disease, since in endemic areas there is a high percentage of clinically healthy infected dogs (50 %) and a much lower rate of sick dogs (5 %).
- **Sylvatic cycle of the infection by *L. infantum*:** maintained by wild canids (wolf and jackal, but mainly fox). Foxes act as a link between both cycles for their tendency to live near human populations (dumps), and able to act as a secondary reservoir.
- **Prevalence:** canine leishmaniosis extends in 50 of the 88 countries where human leishmaniosis is present. It is more prevalent in Brazil, China and the Mediterranean basin.
- **Incidence:** some breeds (Boxer, Cocker Spaniel, Rottweiler and German shepherd) seem to be more susceptible to the disease. The distribution of the disease follows a bimodal pattern with respect to age, with the highest prevalence reported in dogs < 2-3 years old and > 8 years old.
- **Other receptive hosts:** *L. infantum* has been detected in wolves, rodents, horses, cats and recently in hares (producing a major outbreak of human leishmaniosis in Madrid (Spain) since 2010

BIOLOGICAL CYCLE OF *LEISHMANIA INFANTUM*

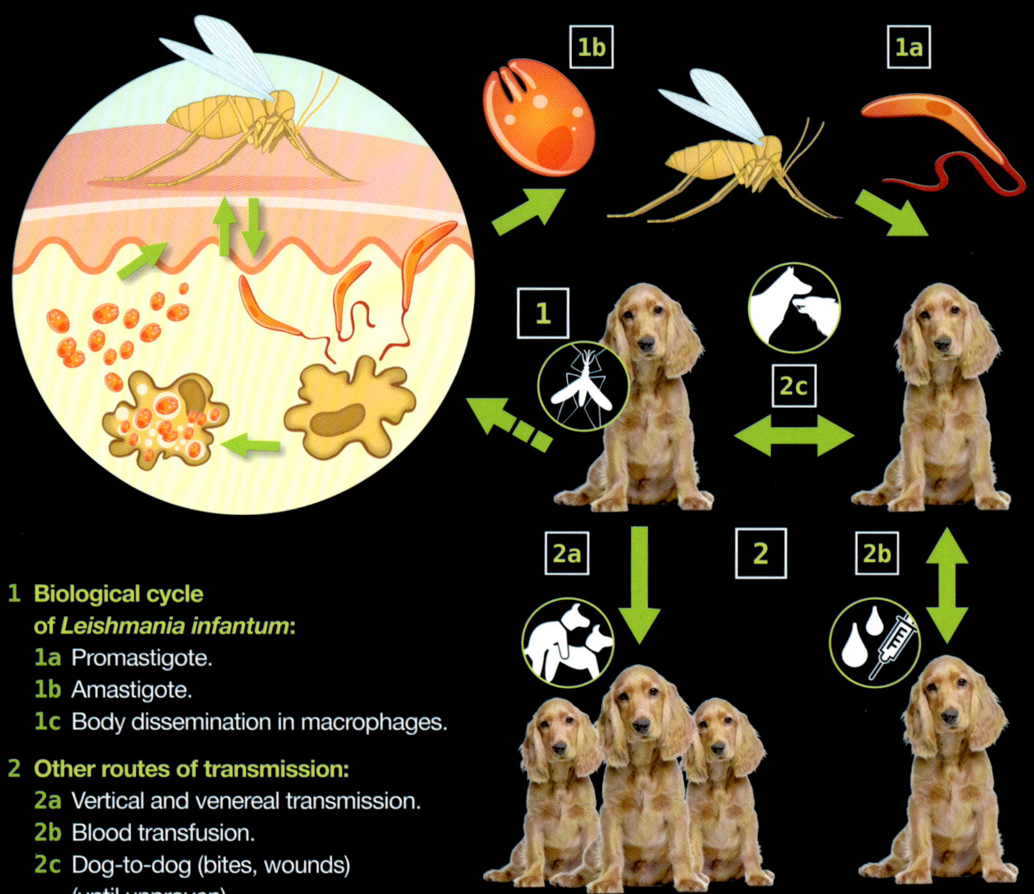

1 Biological cycle of *Leishmania infantum*:
- **1a** Promastigote.
- **1b** Amastigote.
- **1c** Body dissemination in macrophages.

2 Other routes of transmission:
- **2a** Vertical and venereal transmission.
- **2b** Blood transfusion.
- **2c** Dog-to-dog (bites, wounds) (until unproven).

PATHOGENESIS

The pathogenesis is a consequence of the strong humoral immune response of the host to the parasite. Due to the continuous antigenic stimulation caused by the high parasite load and exaggerated production of non-protective antibodies, the deposition of immune complexes can produce severe consequences: glomerulonephritis, vasculitis, polyarthritis, uveitis and meningitis.

IMMUNOPATHOLOGY

There are **two types of response to the infection** by *L. infantum* in the dog (see Chart 16):

- Clinically healthy infected dogs that develop a mild humoral immune response (low antibody titers) and a predominant protective specific cell-mediated immunity against the parasite, which allows for control of the infection **(Th1 response)**.
- Sick infected dogs that develop an exaggerated humoral response and reduced/absent non-protective specific cell-mediated immune response that allows multiplication and dissemination of the parasite **(Th2 response)**.

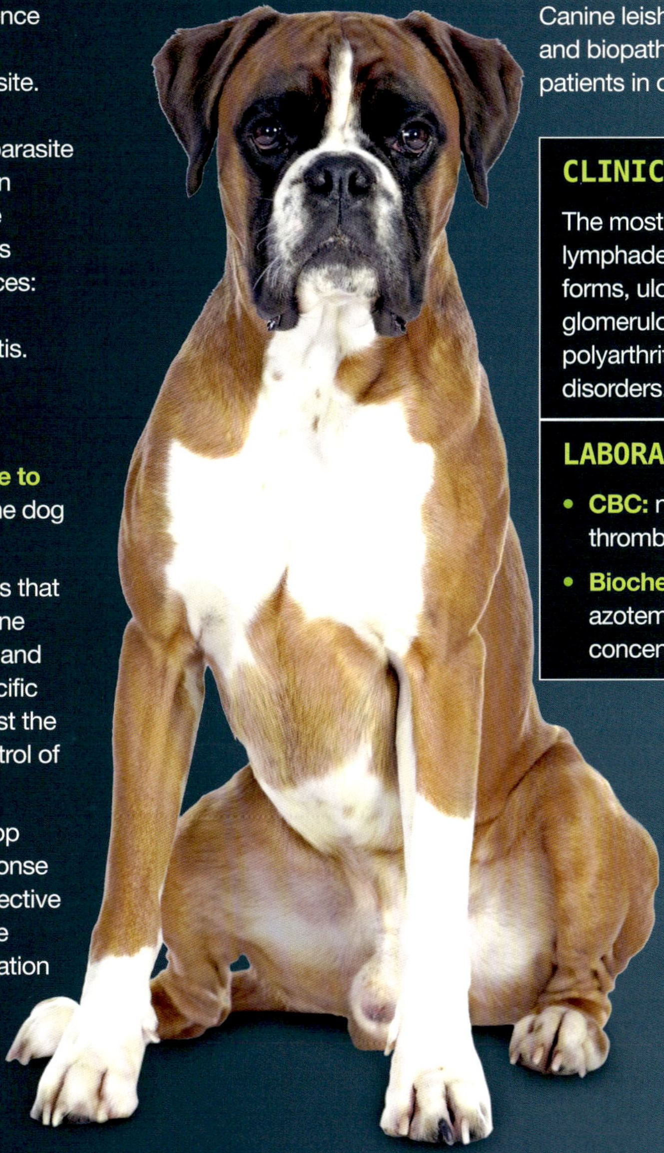

CLINICAL SIGNS AND LESIONS

Canine leishmaniosis is characterized by a wide range of clinical signs and biopathological alterations that should always be evaluated in patients in order to establish appropriate treatment and prognosis.

CLINICAL SIGNS

The most frequent systemic signs are weight loss, asthenia, lymphadenomegaly and cutaneous lesions (keratoseborrheic forms, ulcerative forms and nodular forms). Less frequent are glomerulonephritis and associated signs, such as vasculitis, polyarthritis, cardiorespiratory, digestive and neurological disorders.

LABORATORY ABNORMALITIES

- **CBC:** non-regenerative anemia, leukocytosis or leukopenia, thrombocytopathy.
- **Biochemical profile:** Hyper beta-gammaglobulinemia, azotemia, proteinuria, hypoalbuminemia and increased concentration of liver enzymes.

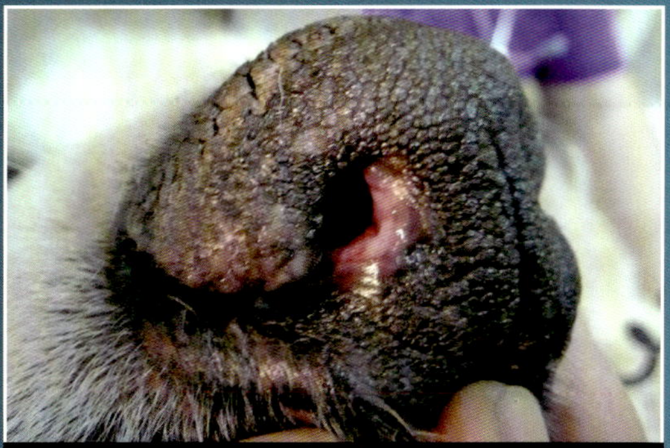

Nose hyperkeratosis with depigmentation of the mucocutaneous boundary

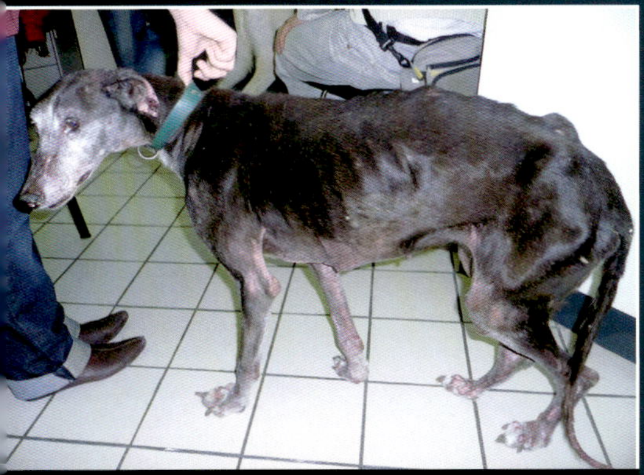

Chronic wasting

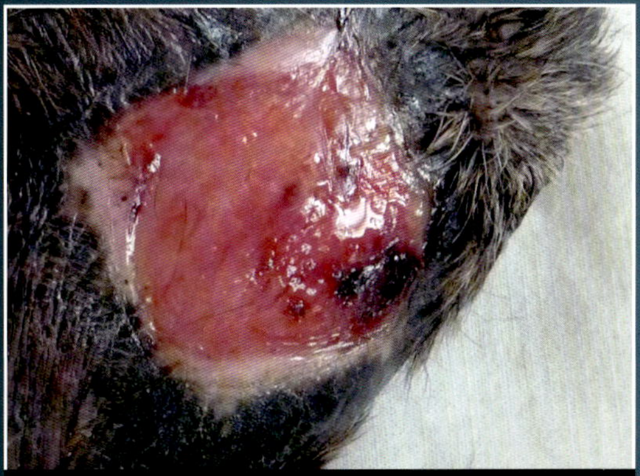

Ulcerative form

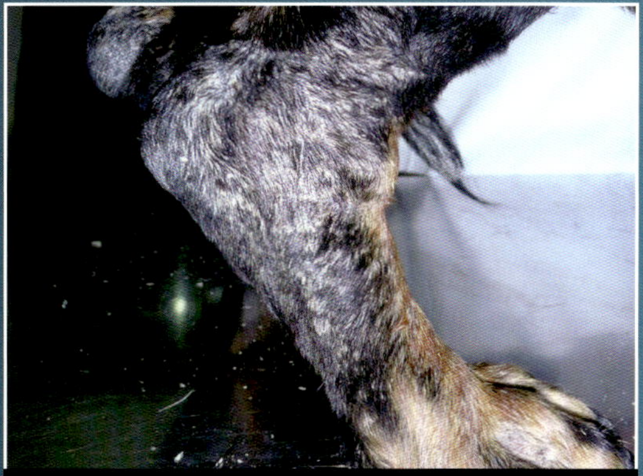

Exfoliative dermatitis and onychogryphosis

DIAGNOSIS

CLINICAL DIAGNOSIS

Clinically healthy infected dogs are those who after a physical examination and routine laboratory tests do NOT show any clinical sign or laboratory abnormalities, but in which infection is confirmed.

Sick dogs are those that present clinical signs or compatible laboratory abnormalities and in which infection is confirmed.

LABORATORY DIAGNOSIS

- Observation of amastigotes in cytological tests of skin lesions or aspirates from lymph nodes or bone marrow (see figure).
- Evaluation of biopsies of skin or other organs by immunohistochemistry (IHC).

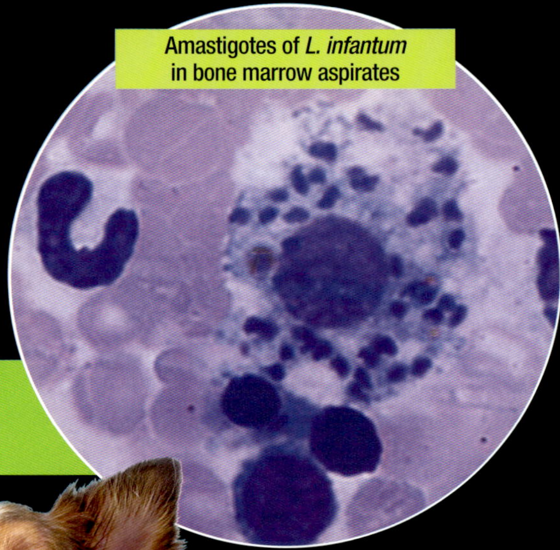

Amastigotes of *L. infantum* in bone marrow aspirates

A serologic diagnosis should be based on quantitative techniques (IFA or ELISA): high levels of antibodies are associated with high parasite load and disease.

In dogs with low levels of antibodies, other complementary tests are necessary to confirm or rule out clinical leishmaniosis: cytology, histopathology, or PCR.

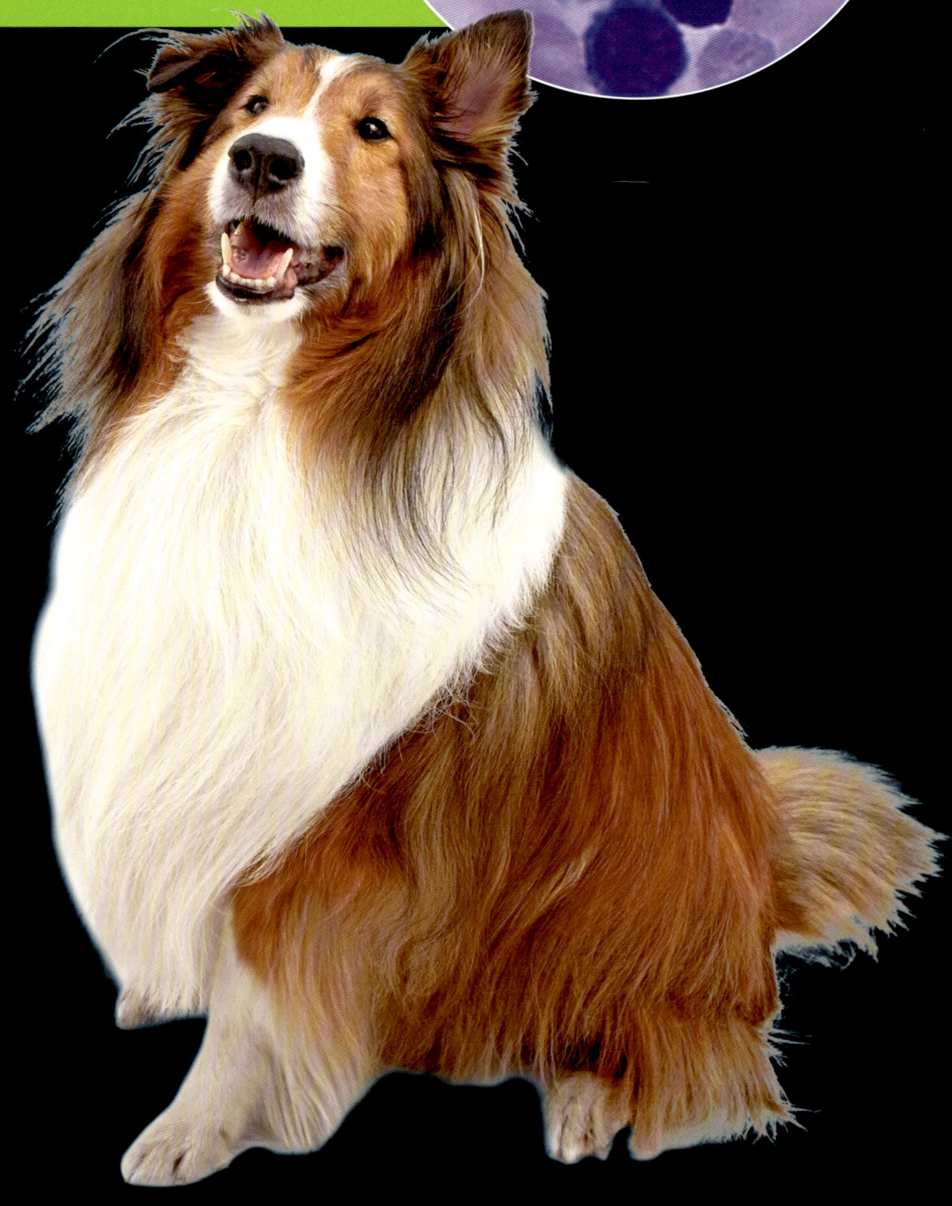

TREATMENT

To date no drug has proven to be consistently curative for canine leishmaniosis.

In most dogs, clinical signs improve after treatment, but there is no "parasitological cure" and in many cases there may be relapses.

ANTI-LEISHMANIAL DRUGS

- **Pentavalent antimonials:** a cycle for 4-6 weeks at conventional doses or
- **Miltefosine:** a cycle of 4 weeks per os, given with food.

These leishmanicides are always combined with allopurinol which, due to its safety and effectiveness, is the best leishmaniostatic drug. The allopurinol must be administered for a minimum of 6-12 months depending on the clinical evolution of the patient. These long therapies may produce adverse effects, such as urolithiasis or nefrolithiasis by xanthine, which need to be monitored.

PREVENTION AND CONTROL

- Topical use of **repellents or insecticides** based on synthetic pyrethroids to prevent sandflies biting and, therefore, the transmission of *L. infantum*.
  - Collars: they require 7-14 days to be effective:
    - Deltamethrin.
  - Pipettes: they require 24-48 hours to be effective:
    - Permethrin.
    - Permethrin + imidacloprid.
- Install **mosquito screens** of 0.3-0.4 mm² fine mesh on windows and doors of houses and doghouses.
- **Immunoprophylaxis:** a vaccine is available based on a purified antigen excreted by cultured promastigotes of *L. infantum*. It includes MDP (muramyl dipeptide) as an adjunvant. Healthy seronegative animals can be vaccinated from 6 months of age. It is recommended to administer 3 doses at 3 week intervals and to reboost annually with a single dose.

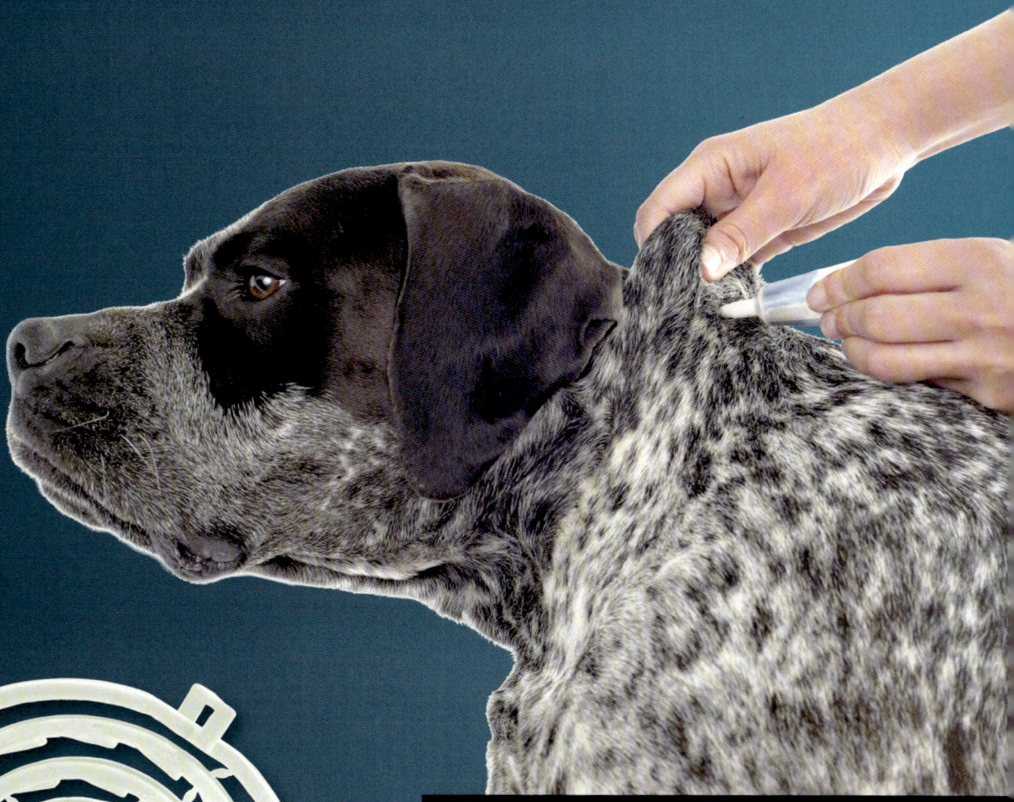

Topical prophylaxis against *L. infantum*: use of pipettes

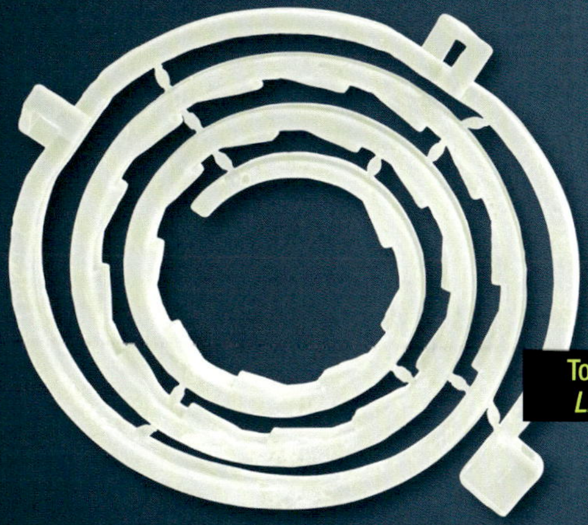

Topical prophylaxis against *L. infantum*: use of collars

FELINE LEISHMANIOSIS

Feline leishmaniosis, caused by *Leishmania infantum*, has been described in the same endemic areas as canine leishmaniosis.

Subclinical infection is more common than the patent disease. When present, the clinical signs include skin lesions on the face and ears, with nodular or ulcerative forms. Systemic illness is rarely observed.

The infection is diagnosed by the same methods as used for dogs.

Information on treatment is limited although **allopurinol** is commonly used, which produces good clinical response.

To date, there are no preventive measures that avoid infection in cats.

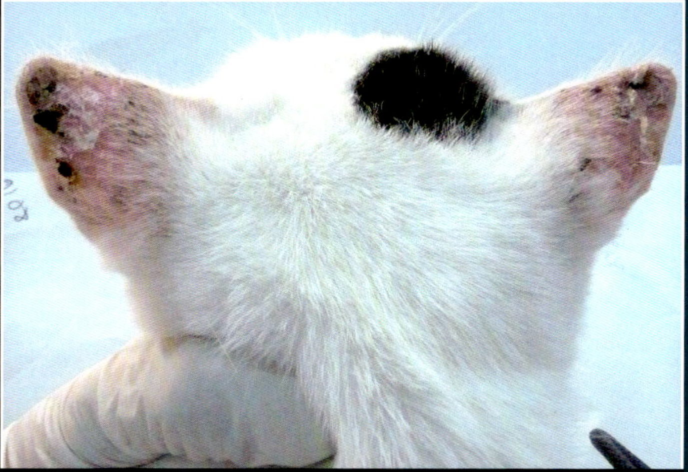

Alopecia and exfoliative dermatitis on the pinna in a cat with leishmaniosis

RABIES

ETIOLOGY

Rabies virus belongs to the family *Rhabdoviridae* (enveloped RNA viruses), genus *Lyssavirus*. Virions have a characteristic bullet shape.

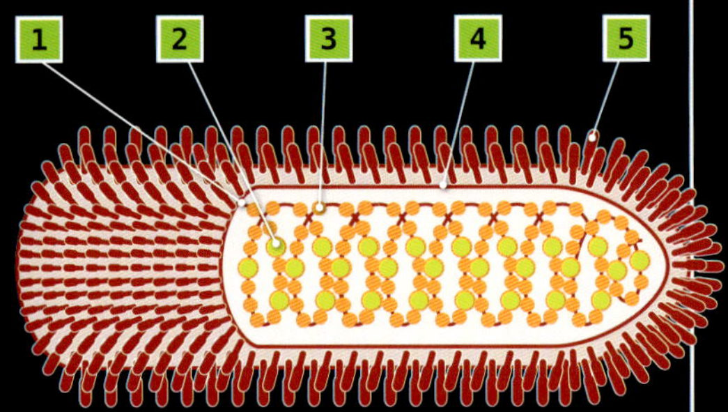

1 Nucleoprotein
2 Polymerase
3 Phosphoprotein
4 Matrix protein
5 Glycoprotein G

PROTEINS OF INTEREST

- **Nucleoprotein:** most abundant protein, it is associated with the genomic RNA, is resistant to RNAses and is highly conserved among the different rhabdoviruses.
- **Glycoprotein G:** contains a large extracellular domain and forms spikes (trimers) which protrude from the envelope, and which play a key role in the pathogenesis (binding to the cell receptor, entry into the cell and collaboration in viral assembly).

Glycoprotein G is the only responsible protein for the induction of protective neutralizing antibodies.

DIVERSITY OF THE GENUS *LYSSAVIRUS*

Seven genotypes have been described so far. They are grouped into three phylogroups (I to III) on the basis of their genetic, pathogenic and immunogenic characteristics.

Rabies virus belongs to genotype 1, its original hosts are carnivores, and it has a worldwide distribution.

European bat lyssaviruses types 1 and 2 (EBLV-1 and EBLV-2) belong to genotypes 5 and 6, respectively; they are present in Europe, are isolated from insectivorous bats and can occasionally be transmitted to man ("splashes" of saliva).

The rabies virus can remain viable at 20 °C for several days in carcasses or tissues.

EPIDEMIOLOGY

TYPES OF EPIDEMIOLOGICAL CYCLES

- **Air-borne cycle**, maintained by **bats**.
- **Terrestrial**, maintained by **carnivores**. It has two types of distribution:
  - **Urban** rabies, whose main reservoir is the dog.
  - **Sylvatic** wildlife rabies, whose reservoirs are other animal species.

Dogs are the source of infection in the majority of cases of human rabies.

One or more "air-borne" infection cycles in bats and one or more "terrestrial" cycles in carnivores can coexist in the same geographic area. In Europe two cycles of bat rabies by EBLV-1 and EBLV-2 coexist with the cycle associated with the common fox.

The degree of susceptibility among various animal species varies considerably.

SHEDDING

Rabies virus is shed mainly with saliva even before the first clinical signs of the disease appear.

FORMS OF TRANSMISSION

- Contact with the infected saliva after being bitten or scratched by an infected animal (most frequent form).
- Air-borne route.

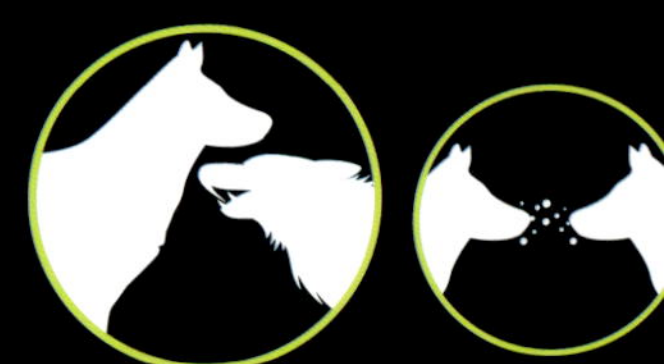

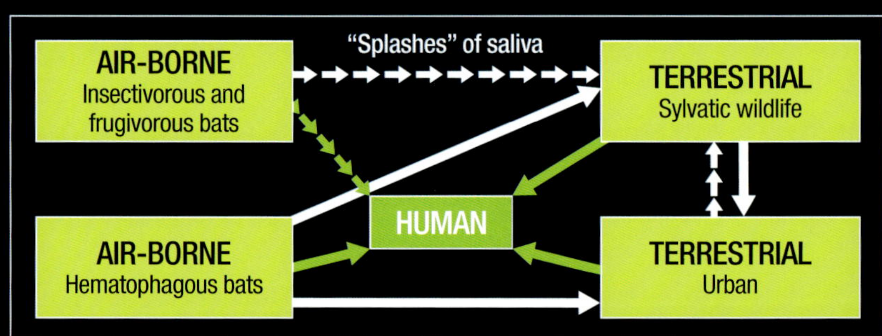

PATHOGENESIS

PATHOGENIC MECHANISM

1 Rabies virus, once inoculated through the infected saliva, binds to the cell receptors and can replicate either in the cells of the striated muscle or directly infect nerve cells.

2 The virus then travels via retrograde axoplasmatic transport mechanisms to the CNS. Both motor and sensory fibers may be involved.

3 Once in the CNS, the virus multiplies rapidly in the gray matter (Ammon's horn, medulla oblongata, and cerebellum), giving rise to the onset of encephalitic symptoms.

4 The virus can be transported later from the CNS along the peripheral nerves to multiple locations, including the salivary glands (crucial for transmission).

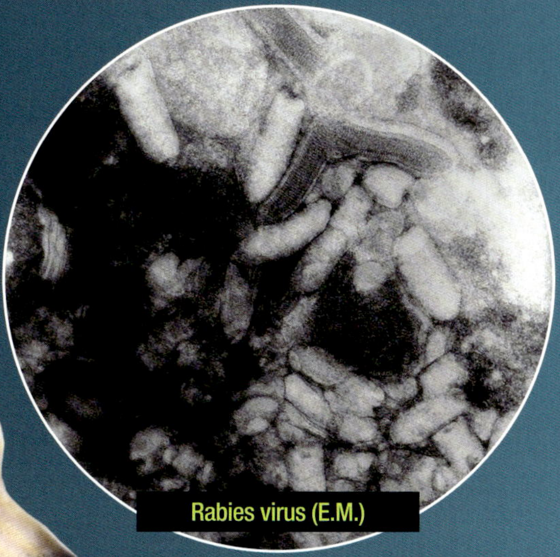

Rabies virus (E.M.)

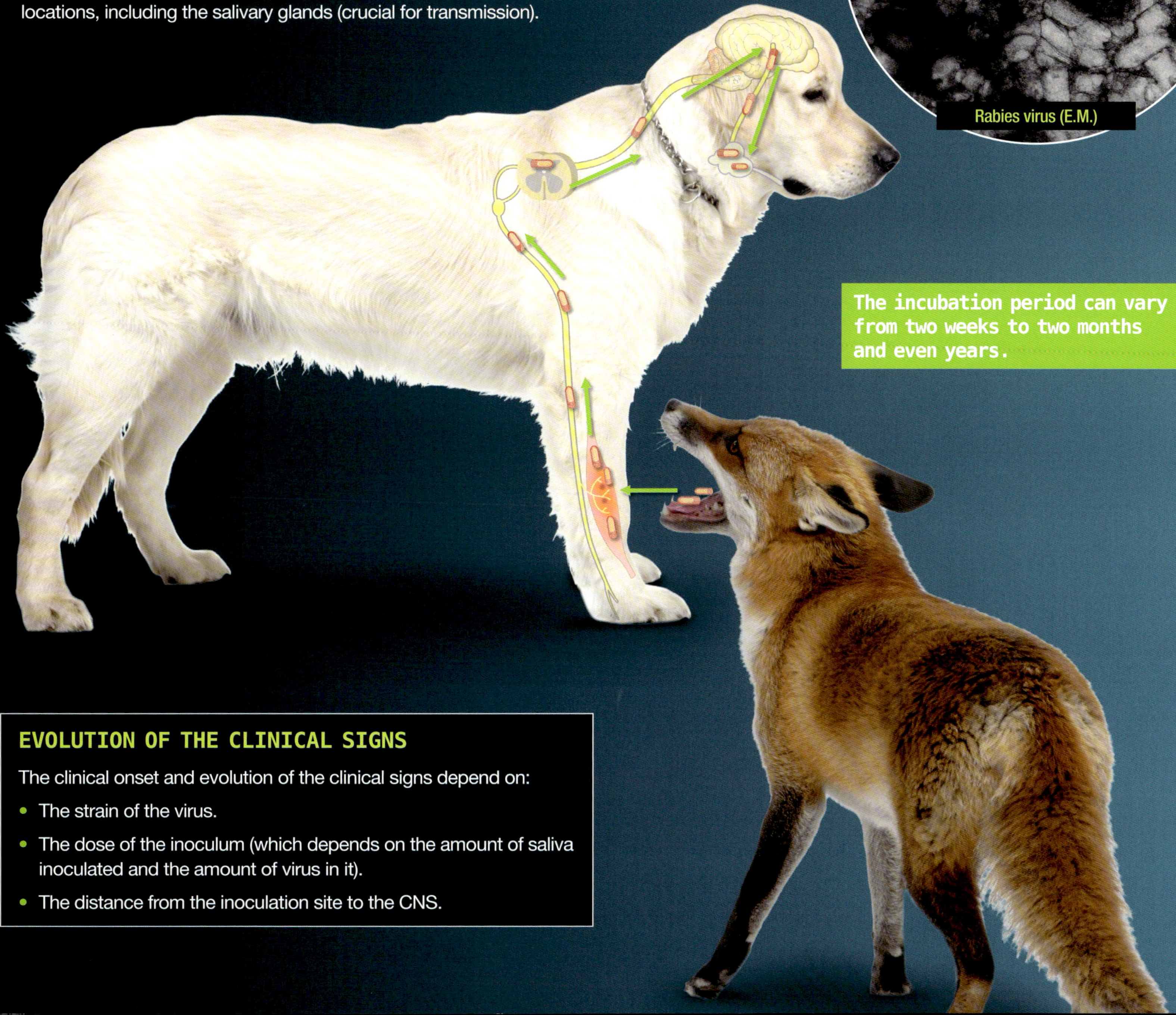

The incubation period can vary from two weeks to two months and even years.

EVOLUTION OF THE CLINICAL SIGNS

The clinical onset and evolution of the clinical signs depend on:

- The strain of the virus.
- The dose of the inoculum (which depends on the amount of saliva inoculated and the amount of virus in it).
- The distance from the inoculation site to the CNS.

CLINICAL SIGNS AND LESIONS

Three stages of rabies are recognized from the clinical point of view:

1 PRODROMAL STAGE

It usually lasts from 1 to 3 days and is characterized by behavioral changes, aggressiveness, irritability, and appetite disorders. There may be itching in the inoculation area, which the animal bites itself and it gets ulcerated.

2 FURIOUS RABIES

It is manifested by intense excitation, alternating with depression. The animal is highly aggressive, bites at anything near and utters a characteristic bark (high and furious). It can die during this stage even without exhibiting paralysis.

3 PARALYTIC OR "DUMB" STAGE

It is defined by an inability to swallow (typical sign of drooling) and the development of a flaccid, progressive, generalized and ascending paralysis. Death occurs due to cardiorespiratory arrest.

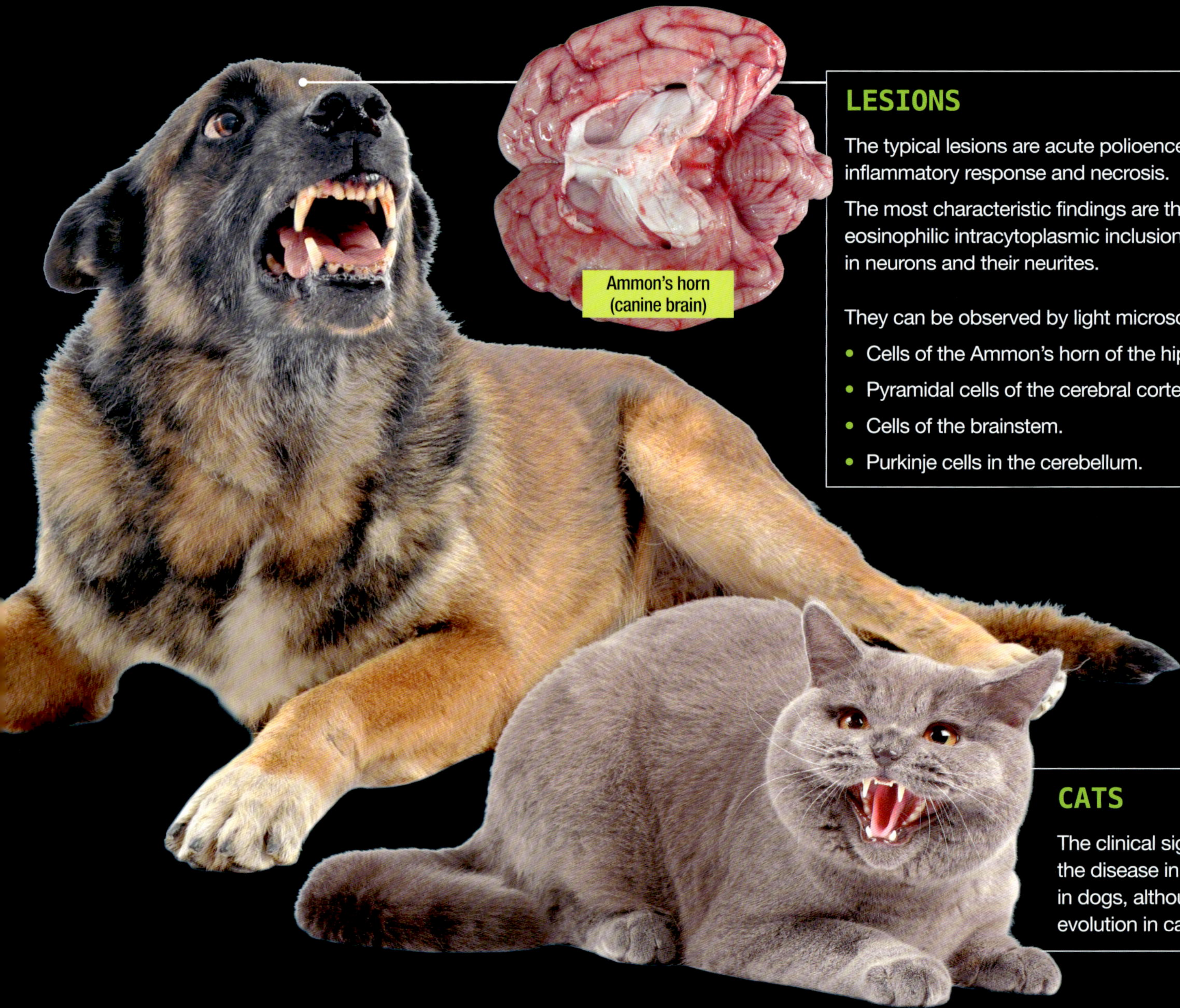

LESIONS

The typical lesions are acute polioencephalomyelitis with low inflammatory response and necrosis.

The most characteristic findings are the **Negri bodies**: eosinophilic intracytoplasmic inclusions which are formed in neurons and their neurites.

They can be observed by light microscopy in:

- Cells of the Ammon's horn of the hippocampus (mainly).
- Pyramidal cells of the cerebral cortex.
- Cells of the brainstem.
- Purkinje cells in the cerebellum.

CATS

The clinical signs and evolution of the disease in cats is similar to those in dogs, although in general the evolution in cats can be faster.

DIAGNOSIS

CLINICAL AND DIFFERENTIAL DIAGNOSIS

Rabies is a notifiable disease.

An animal should be "suspected" as nfected by rabies when it exhibits any abnormal neurological disorder along with aggression to people.

Dogs and cats suspected of suffering from rabies will be placed under observation.

f the animal dies during the observation period, an official diagnosis in a reference aboratory is mandatory.

LABORATORY DIAGNOSIS

Techniques	Samples	Observations
DFA	Nervous tissue (spinal cord, cerebellum and hippocampus).	• OIE and WHO criteria must be followed. • Reference technique applied in official laboratories.
Biological techniques: • **Mouse inoculation** • **Cell culture**	Nervous tissue and salivary glands.	Complementary reference tecniques also applied in official laboratories.
Viral detection (PCR)	Nervous tissue and saliva.	They are complementary techniques to the reference one, they do not substitute it.

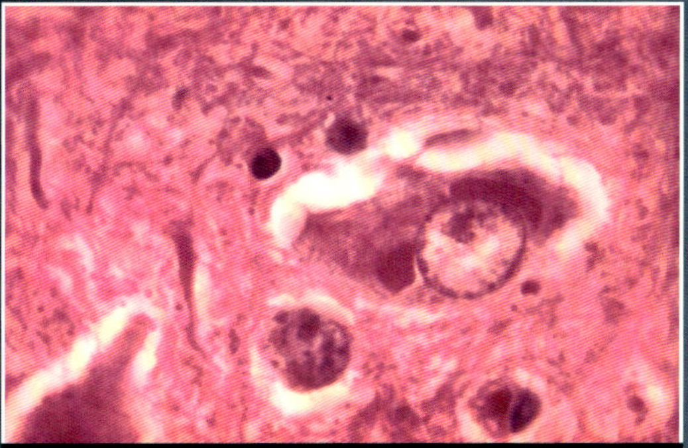

Negri bodies within the neuronal cytoplasm, characteristic finding of rabies. H&E stain

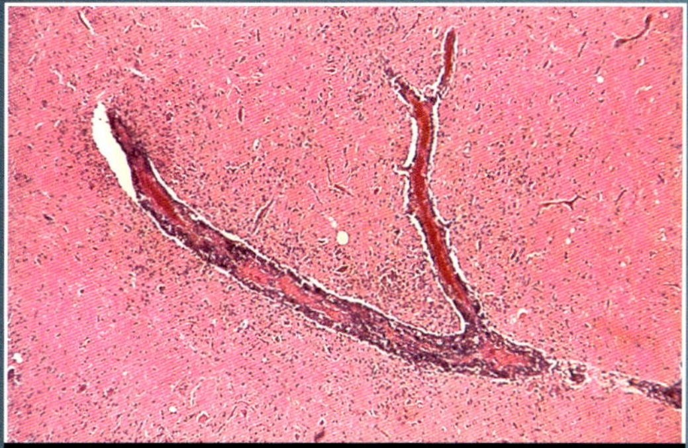

Perivascular cuffing asociated to encephalitis produced by rabies virus. The figure depicts the accumulation of inflammatory cell infiltrates around the cerebral blood vessel. H&E stain

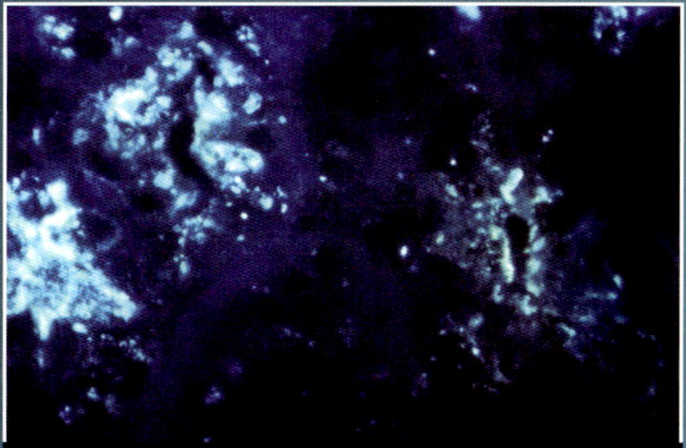

DFA, reference technique which reveals rabies viral antigen in infected tissues

TREATMENT

No treatment is applied.

PREVENTION AND CONTROL

Vaccines used for the control of rabies in dogs and cats (some licensed also for mustelids –ferrets and mink– and different livestock) are inactivated (the majority) or prepared by recombinant vector techniques (only for cats) and can be mono or multivalent (for dogs only).

From the epidemiological point of view, the control of rabies in Europe is aimed at eliminating or reducing the disease in foxes by placing baits containing live vaccines.

Compulsory vaccination of pets varies according to the areas or countries.

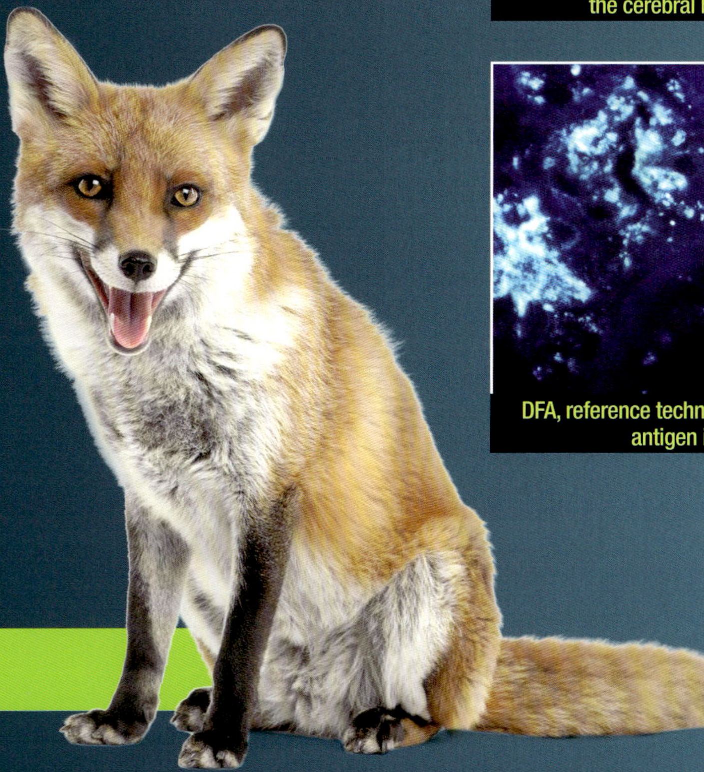

FELINE LEUKEMIA

ETIOLOGY

Feline leukemia virus (FeLV) is a retrovirus of the family *Retroviridae*, genus *Gammaretrovirus*, which causes neoplastic and non-neoplastic diseases in the cat.

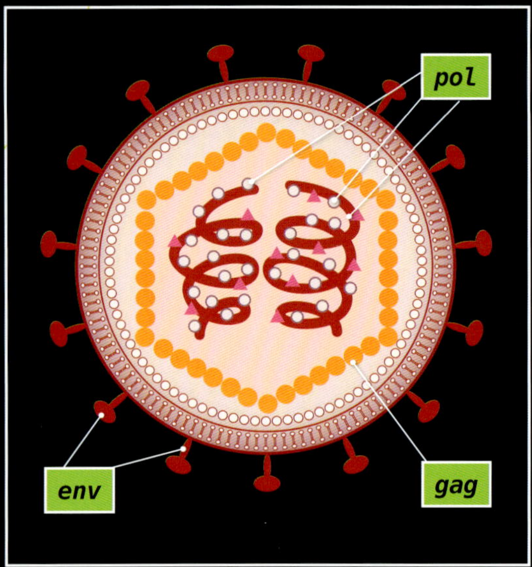

Retroviruses are RNA viruses that replicate through a DNA intermediate thanks to the enzyme reverse transcriptase, which transcribes the genetic information from RNA to DNA. This viral DNA binds to the DNA of the host cell to form the provirus, which remains generally integrated into the cellular genome for life.

The retroviral virion consists of: envelope, capsid and RNA.

RETROVIRAL RNA CONTAINS THE FOLLOWING GENES:

- *gag*: encodes the capsid proteins.
- *pol*: encodes reverse transcriptase.
- *env*: encodes the envelope proteins.

There are three **genotypes** of FeLV: I, II, and III.

FeLV can be also classified into **sub-groups** according to their interaction with the host and to differences in the envelope region (caused by recombination between different variants of FeLV or with endogenous retroviruses), which have been linked to different processes: FeLV-A, FeLV-B, FeLV-C, FeLV-D and FeLV-T.

PROTEINS OF INTEREST

- p27/CA (capsid): protein detected by different commercial diagnostic tests for screening.
- gp70/SU (surface): glycoprotein which binds to receptors on target cells. It induces neutralizing antibodies.

Different FeLV subgroups are recognized by different cell receptors.

Only FeLV-A are transmitted cat-to-cat.

EPIDEMIOLOGY

FeLV only causes disease in felines.

CLINICAL FORMS

Neoplastic and non-neoplastic forms.

INCIDENCE

Higher in stray cats with increased risk of concomitant diseases and in cats around 2 years of age. In recent years, the incidence has dropped, probably due to routine diagnosis and population control measures.

SHEDDING

Saliva, blood, tears, feces, urine and milk.

TRANSMISSION

Direct, through contact with saliva and grooming habits between animals, but also through bites and, occasionally, orally, venereal, transplacental and calostral.

The infection of new animals requires close and prolonged contact with infected animals.

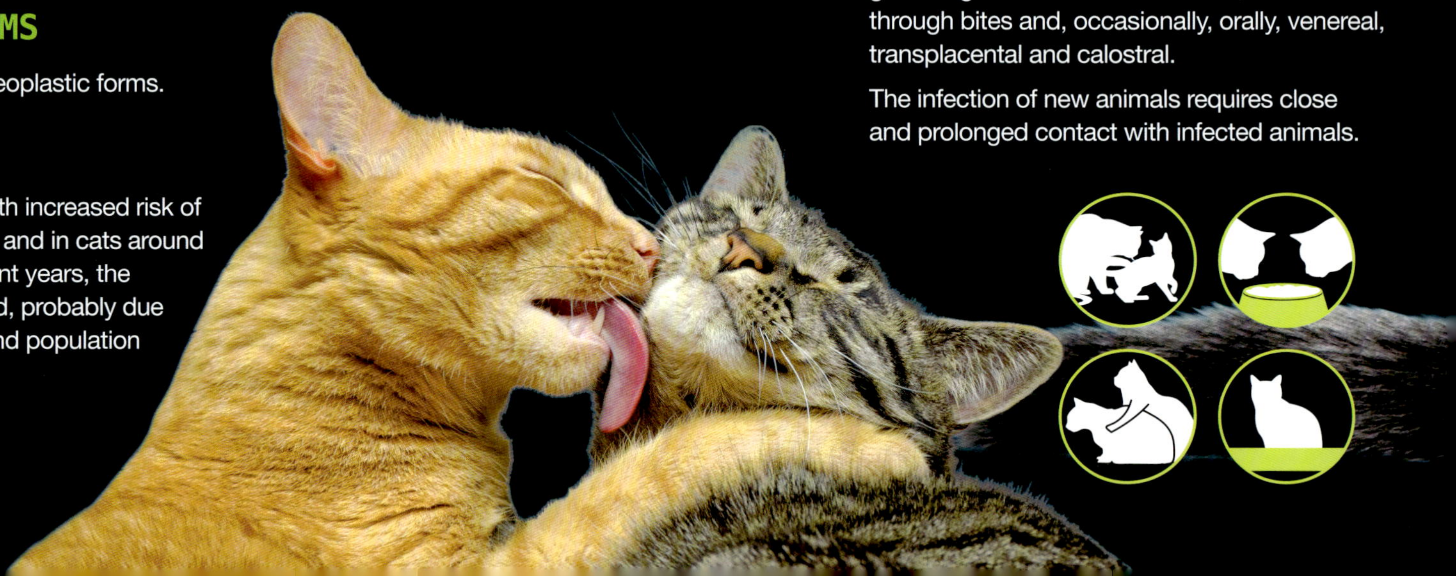

PATHOGENESIS

FeLV enters the host and replicates in the lymphoid tissue of the oropharynx. Subsequently, the infection can evolve in different ways:

1. **Abortive infection:** an effective immune response develops in a small number of animals. It is characterized by high neutralizing antibody titers that remove the virus from all cells before it originates viremia. These animals are negative to p27 Ag, viral RNA and proviral DNA.
2. **Regressive infection:**
   - FeLV produces a transient viremia associated to monocytes which allows, in some cases, the entry of the virus in the bone marrow and the development of a latent infection. Cats are positive to p27 Ag and shed virus through saliva (usually from 3-6 weeks) only during the initial phase. Some cats can eliminate the latent infection within several months post-infection.
   - In latent infections, the viral genomes are present in the host cells although the viruses do not replicate (these animals, after the initial phase, are negative to the usual diagnostic tests). Occasionally, latent infections may reactivate and evolve to progressive infections.
   - Although the majority of cats with latent infections show no clinical signs, some may develop tumors or immune suppression (these cats are negative to p27 Ag and to viral RNA, but are proviral DNA positive).

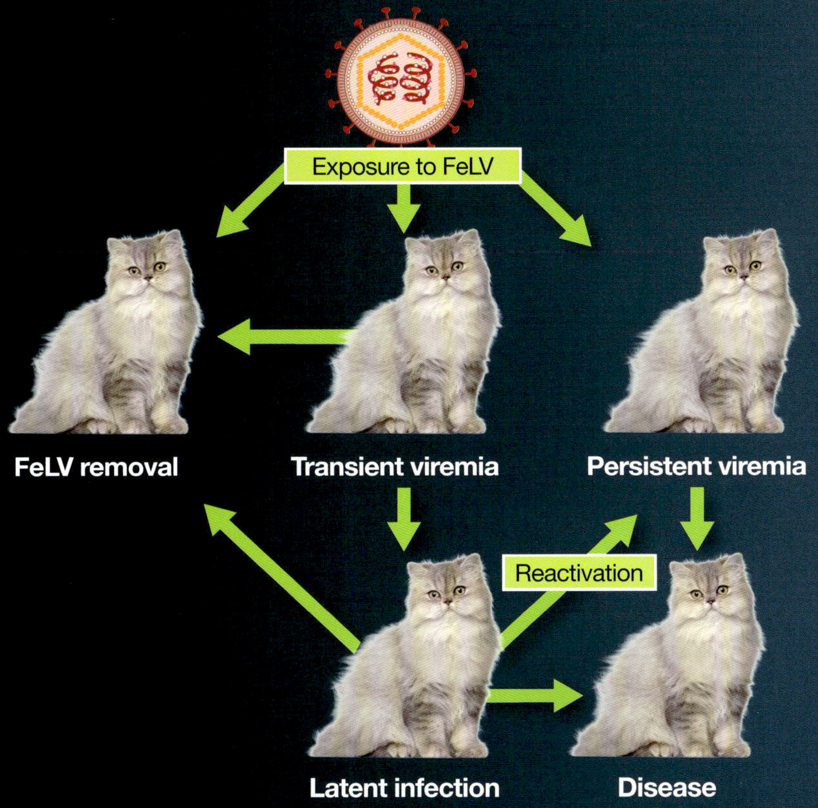

3. **Progressive infection:** FeLV replicates extensively, first in the oropharynx, later in the bone marrow and, lastly, in mucous membranes and epithelia. These cats develop a persistent viremia, shed viruses and are positive to all diagnostic tests. In most, the prognosis is unfavorable and their average life expectancy is short, even with proper treatment.
4. **Atypical or focal infection:** it is rare. FeLV replicates in locations different from the bone marrow (mammary glands, bladder, eyes, etc.) and the evolution of the disease is variable.

Immune response

The production of antibodies, mainly against gp70 (SU), and the development of cell-mediated immunity shortly after infection, protect the cat from developing clinical signs.

FeLV CAN CAUSE MANY ALTERATIONS THROUGH DIFFERENT MECHANISMS:

- **Tumors:** certain FeLV strains cause tumors because they encode oncogenes, while the rest of the strains induce tumors by an unknown mechanism (activation of cellular oncogenes?).
- **Immunodeficiency:** most of the strains of FeLV originate immunodeficiency by an unknown mechanism, although it has been associated with alterations in neutrophils. FeLV-T strains, in combination with FeLV-A, originate an intense immune deficiency caused by a decrease in T cells, sometimes both CD4+ and CD8+ cells, and at other times only the CD4+ T cells.
- **Anemia:** FeLV originates regenerative and non-regenerative anemia. The first may be due to secondary infections (usually by mycoplasmas), immune-mediated hemolytic anemia and bleeding because of platelet disorders. Most of the non-regenerative anemias combine with other alterations. They may be caused by disease or by chronic inflammation or replacement of the precursor cells of erythrocytes by infectious agents or neoplastic cells. Only in co-infections by FeLV-A and -C (< 1 % of infections by FeLV) a pure red cell aplasia develops. FeLV-C interferes with a protein which transports the heme group.
- **Other hematological alterations:** FeLV can cause pure platelet disorders (thrombocytopenia and thrombopathies) and non-regenerative pancytopenia (when all precursors of blood cells in the bone marrow are affected).
- **Neurological alterations:** during viremia, FeLV can cross the blood-brain barrier and cause a neurotoxic effect.

DIAGNOSIS

DIFFERENTIAL DIAGNOSIS

Other illnesses that involve tumors, immune deficiency and anemia.

LABORATORY DIAGNOSIS

Type of infection by FeLV	Detection of p27 in blood (ELISA, IC and DFA) and bone marrow (DFA)	Detection of viral RNA in blood (PCR)	Detection of proviral DNA in blood (PCR)
Abortive	−	−	−
Regressive (transient viremia)	+	+	+
Regressive (latent)	−	−	+
Progressive	+	+	+
Atypical	+ −	+ −	+ −

The most commonly used diagnostic tests are the detection of the p27 Ag using commercial in-office ELISA and IC, which can be exclusive for FeLV or combined with the detection of feline immunodeficiency virus (see figure).

To differentiate a progressive infection from a regressive or atypical infection it is necessary to analyze two tests separated by between 6 to 10 weeks.

Serology is not useful since it can be positive in non-viremic cats and negative in cats with progressive infection.

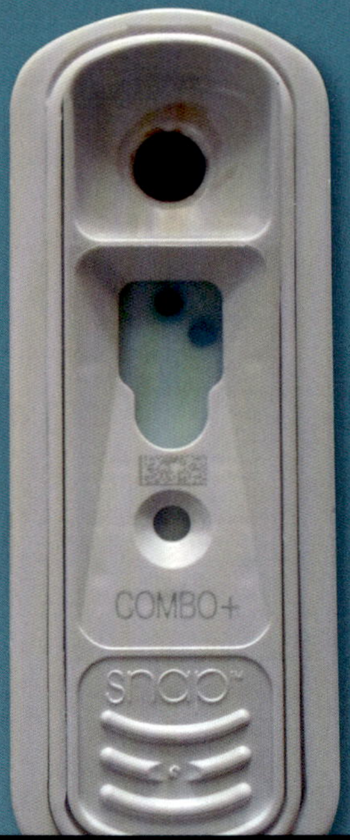

Commercial IC for the combined detection of p27 Ag of FeLV and Ab against feline immunodeficiency virus

TREATMENT

1 SYMPTOMATIC TREATMENT

Antibiotics: to combat secondary bacterial infections, as well as the appropriate drugs according to the concurrent problems that arise.

2 CYCLES OF INTERFERON

Cycles of interferon (alpha, of human origin, or omega, of feline origin) can be used to limit viral replication.

Although antiviral treatment cannot eliminate the latent infections or reverse the persistent viremia, it often significantly improves the clinical outcome and increases life expectancy.

PREVENTION AND CONTROL

A test to detect p27 Ag (usually combined with the detection of feline immunodeficiency virus) is recommended prior to vaccination.

There are inactivated, subunit and recombinant vector vaccines available. They may be monovalent or polyvalent.

Although vaccines are not fully efficacious, it is advisable to vaccinate cats.

As a general control measure, positive and negative animals should not live together. In communities, and for stable populations, animals should be routinely checked and vaccinated periodically. To prevent the spread of the infection, it is possible to consider sanitation measures and euthanasia of positive animals.

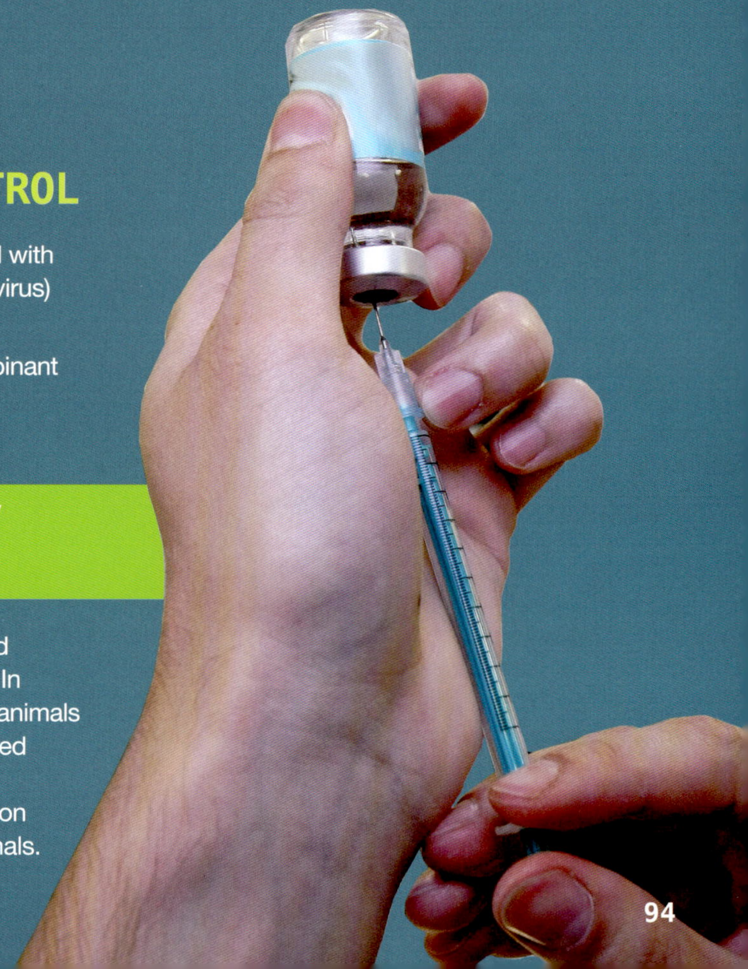

CLINICAL SIGNS AND LESIONS

NEOPLASTIC FORM

- **Lymphomas (lymphosarcomas):** is the most frequent tumor produced by FeLV. They are usually mediastinal or multicentric and, less frequently, digestive (see figures).
- **Lymphoid or myeloid leukemias:** can be either acute or chronic. The most common is acute myeloid leukemia.

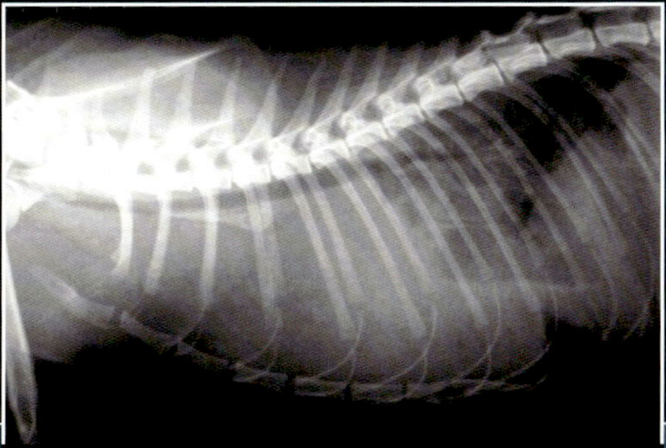

Mediastinal lymphoma: X-ray of the thorax in which increased density in the tracheal mediastinum, elevation of the trachea and pleural effusion are observed

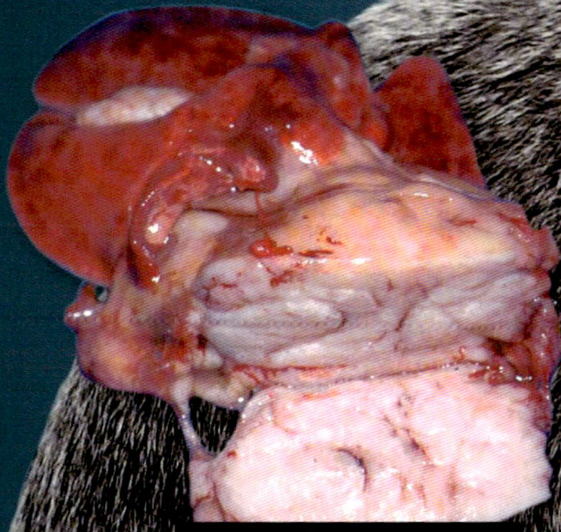

Mediastinal lymphoma

NON-NEOPLASTIC FORM

- **Immune deficiency:** secondary and opportunistic infections.
- **Anemia:** usually non-regenerative and combined with other alterations.
- **Other outcomes:** immune-mediated diseases (glomerulonephritis, uveitis and polyarthritis), reproductive alterations (infertility, miscarriages and neonatal mortality), neurological disorders (anisocoria, blindness, locomotive disorders, paresis, paralysis and incontinence) and myeloblastopenia-enteritis syndrome (occurs with panleukopenia and enteritis with diarrhea).

FELINE IMMUNODEFICIENCY

ETIOLOGY

Feline immunodeficiency virus (FIV) is a retrovirus (family *Retroviridae*, enveloped RNA virus) included in the genus *Lentivirus*.

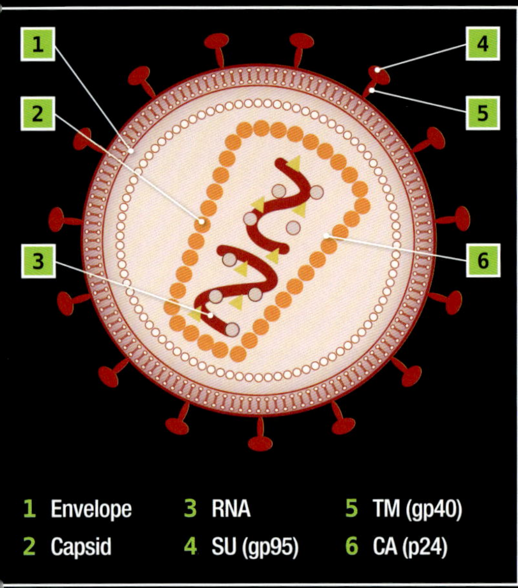

FIV infects initially CD4+ T cells and macrophages, later CD8+ T cells and B cells and, from the beginning of the immunodeficiency syndrome, also other cell types (dendritic cells, monocytes, microglia, astrocytes and neurons).

Six subtypes of FIV (A-F) have been identified on the basis of differences in the env gene (envelope).

FIV strains differ in their pathogenicity.

PROTEINS OF INTEREST

- p24/CA (capsid): it induces antibodies which are used for routine diagnosis.
- gp40/TM (transmembrane).
- gp95/SU (surface): located in the envelope. It is recognized by cell receptors for viral adherence.

EPIDEMIOLOGY

FIV only produces disease in domestic cats and in some wild felids (panther, puma).

Incidence: higher in males > 3 years, stray cats, cats with greater exposure to multiple pathogens and closed populations.

The prevalence of the disease varies between countries.

SHEDDING

Saliva, blood, tears and milk.

TRANSMISSION

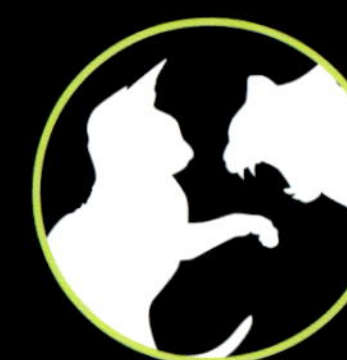

- **Mainly bites**, but also direct contact with infected saliva or through mucous membranes.

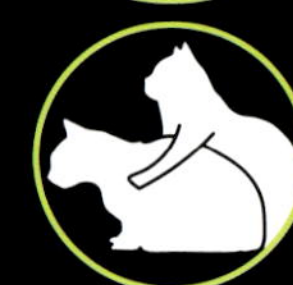

- **Other routes:** venereal, trasplacental and calostral.

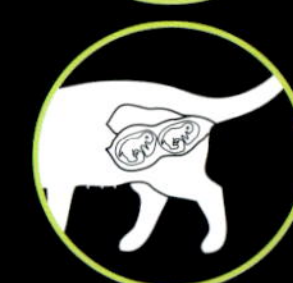

Infected cats remain infected for life. Many never develop immunodeficiency, although they represent a source of virus.

PATHOGENESIS

Upon entering the host, FIV replicates in the local lymphoid tissue and viremia develops quickly. This disseminates the virus to the thymus, spleen and lymph nodes. The replication of the virus stimulates the synthesis of proinflammatory lymphokines and activates the production of B cells. When the infection becomes established (digestive system, kidneys and CNS), the constant activation of the immune system originates lymphocytic hyperplasia.

Antibodies may be detected from the 2nd-4th week post-infection and they modulate, along with the cell-mediated immune response, the maintenance of a persistent viremia from 4-6 weeks post-infection).

The control of the infection depends on the ability of the host to remove the virus from the bloodstream and to reduce the viral load in different tissues.

In animals with persistent viremia unable to control the infection, FIV crosses the blood-brain barrier and infects microglia, astrocytes and neurons, and can develop various neurological signs. Cats with persistent viremia also have a higher incidence of tumors.

Infected animals generally do not develop clinical signs.

IMMUNODEFICIENCY SYNDROME

Its development is related to a high level of viral replication and to lymphoid depletion with drastic decrease of CD4+ T cell counts and the resulting increase in susceptibility to secondary and opportunistic infections.

FIV causes immunodeficiency through various mechanisms; the most important is that it induces cell death and apoptosis of lymphocytes.

CLINICAL SIGNS AND LESIONS

he progression of the disease is highly variable (many nfected cats remain at a stage of clinical latency hroughout their lives).

CLINICAL SIGNS

Clinical signs are usually observed the first two years post-infection and can include:

- Fever, lymphadenopathy, leukopenia, anemia, and disorders of the skin, eye, respiratory, oral cavity (stomatitis, gingivitis), etc. They are caused by secondary and opportunistic infections. These animals can suffer a wasting syndrome.
- Tumors: occasionally, mostly lymphomas.
- Neurological and behavioral disorders (5 % of the sick cats): ataxia, seizures, tremors, changes in behavior and dementia.

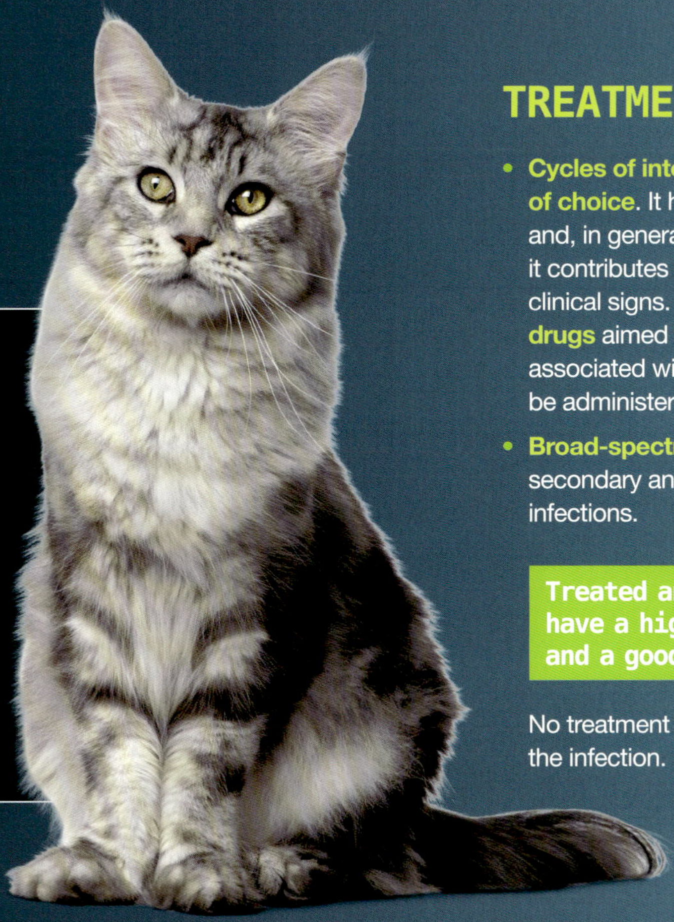

TREATMENT

- **Cycles of interferon:** it is the **treatment of choice.** It helps limit viral replication and, in general, if it is administered early, it contributes to the rapid remission of the clinical signs. **Immunomodulators and drugs** aimed to alleviate the clinical signs associated with secondary pathogens may be administered simultaneously.
- **Broad-spectrum antibiotics** to treat secondary and opportunistic bacterial infections.

Treated and well cared for cats have a high rate of survival and a good quality of life.

No treatment completely eliminates the infection.

DIAGNOSIS

PRESUMPTIVE CLINICAL DIAGNOSIS

t is based on epidemiological data, clinical signs and age group. Biopathological analyses are useful and suggestive of immunodeficiency.

LABORATORY DIAGNOSIS

Techniques	Samples	Observations
Serology (ELISA, IC)	Serum.	• Commercial ELISA and IC available, exclusive for FIV or combined with feline leukemia virus (the most widely used for screening). • A positive diagnosis needs to be confirmed by PCR.
Viral detection (PCR and ELISA)	Blood, bone marrow and several tissues.	

n countries, where vaccine is not available commercially, the presence of specific antibodies to FIV is considered as a positive infection.

A positive serological diagnosis can be confirmed by PCR.

PREVENTION AND CONTROL

VACCINATION

In certain countries, such us U.S.A., inactivated vaccines are used with only limited succes.

CONTROL MEASURES

The infection by FIV usually does not produce very severe clinical signs or an elevated impact that reduces the population in shelters.

MEASURES RECOMMENDED IN POPULATIONS

- Separation of animals.
- Neutering of males (to reduce the aggressiveness and, hence, the dissemination of the infection).
- Sacrifice of the positive or aggressive animals.

All new animals should be quarantined and tested for the infection.

FELINE PANLEUKOPENIA

ETIOLOGY

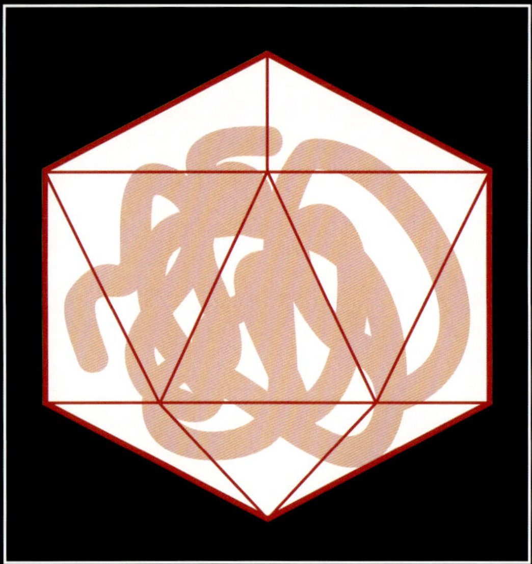

Feline panleukopenia (also known as feline infectious enteritis or feline distemper) is produced by a virus of the family *Parvoviridae*, genus *Parvovirus* (non-enveloped small size DNA viruses, with icosahedral symmetry). It is considered the type species of this Genus.

It is one of the most conserved viruses of the group and has been known for over 100 years.

It shares 98 % homology with canine parvovirus type 2 (CPV-2, see Chart 29).

Parvoviruses need cellular factors expressed during the S phase of the cell cycle to complete their replication cycle. This determines the type of target cells, which are preferably located in tissues with high mitotic index (rapidly dividing), such as the intestine and the lymphoid tissue.

The virus is able to cross the placental barrier.

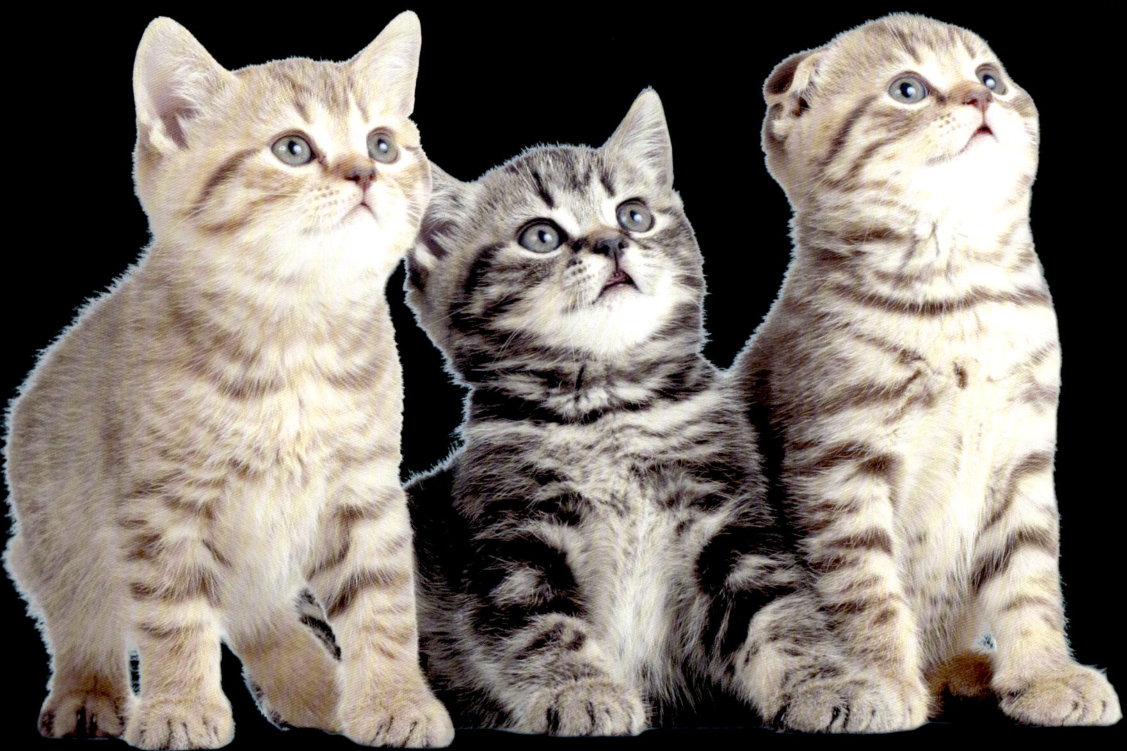

EPIDEMIOLOGY

TRANSMISSION

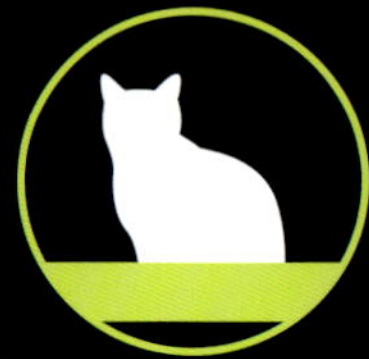

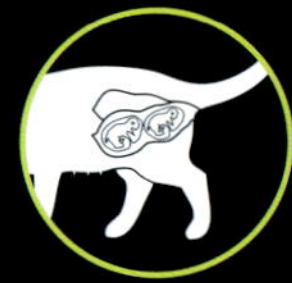

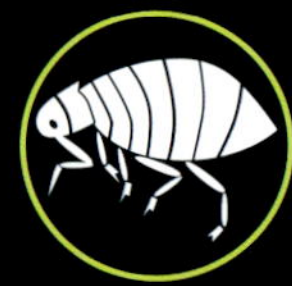

- **Mainly** through the **oral route** (direct contact with contaminated feces, urine, etc.).
- **Other routes:** the infection may also be acquired in utero and by flea bites (vectors of the virus).

SUSCEPTIBLE SPECIES

- Domestic cat and some wild carnivores.
- The dog can become infected, but does not develop disease. However, some variants of canine parvovirus (CPV-2a and CPV-2b) can infect and cause disease in cats.

INCIDENCE

Mainly in kittens 2-4 months of age with low immune profile.

In adults, the infection may go unnoticed.

CLINICAL PRESENTATION

The clinical outcome depends to a great extent on:

- Age.
- Immune status.
- Physiological stage (pregnancy, stage of development of the fetus).

Young animals suffer from an enteric syndrome, whereas pregnant queens can experience a reproductive disorder.

In recent years, regular vaccination of the population has reduced the occurrence of the disease.

PATHOGENESIS

ENTERIC FORM

- The virus enters the host **orally** and during the first 18-24 hours post-infection replicates in the nasopharynx-associated lymphoid tissue (NALT, see Chart 11).
- Subsequently, a short **viremia** (2-5 days post-infection) develops.
- **The virus disseminates to various tissues and organs with rapidly dividing cells** (thymus, bone marrow and lymph nodes, among others). Initially, the multiplication of the virus produces transient leukopenia, mostly by a drop in the neutrophil counts, and transient immunosuppression.
- The virus also **multiplies in the cells of the crypts of the intestinal villi** in the jejunum and ileum, producing cell death. This precipitates shortening of the intestinal villi, triggering acute diarrhea.

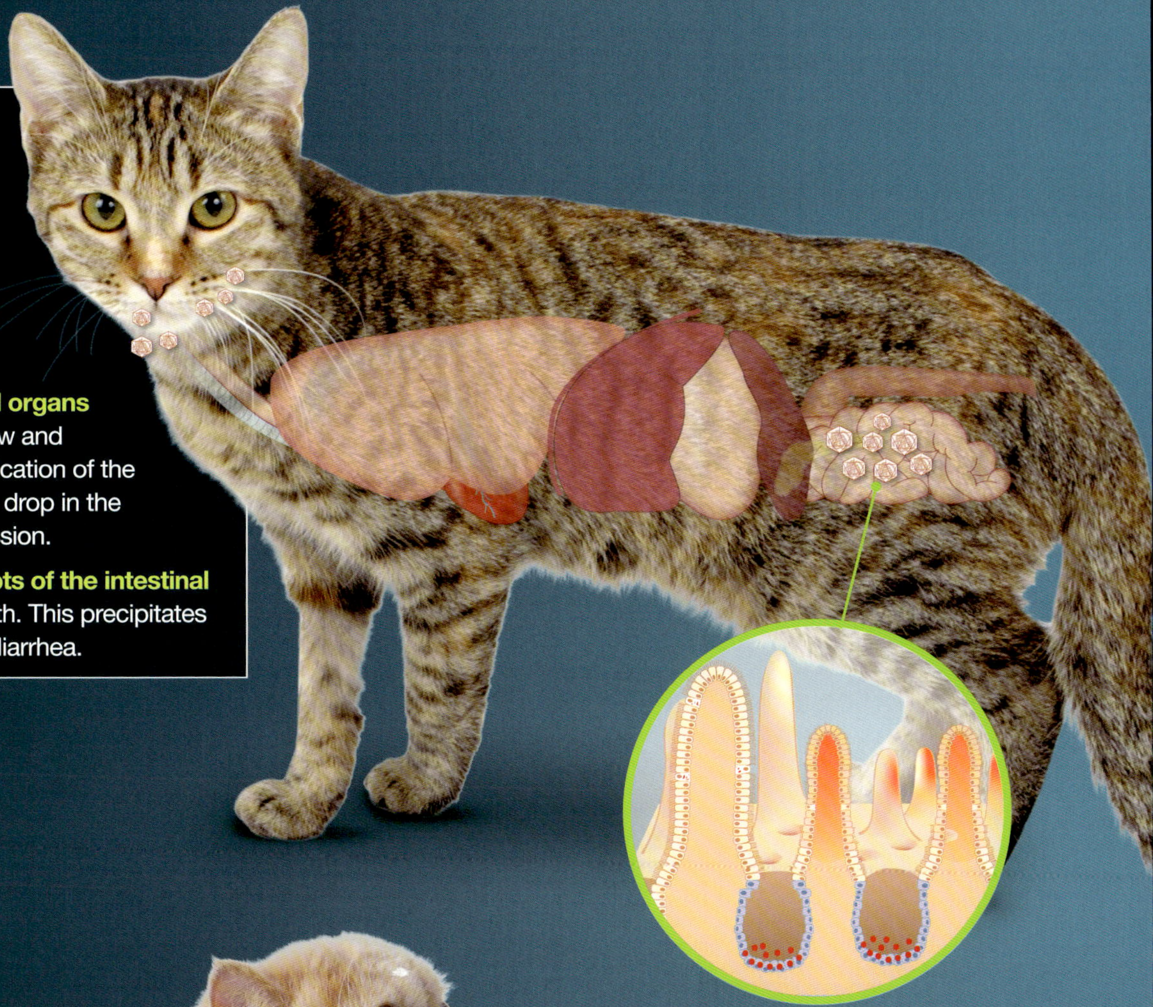

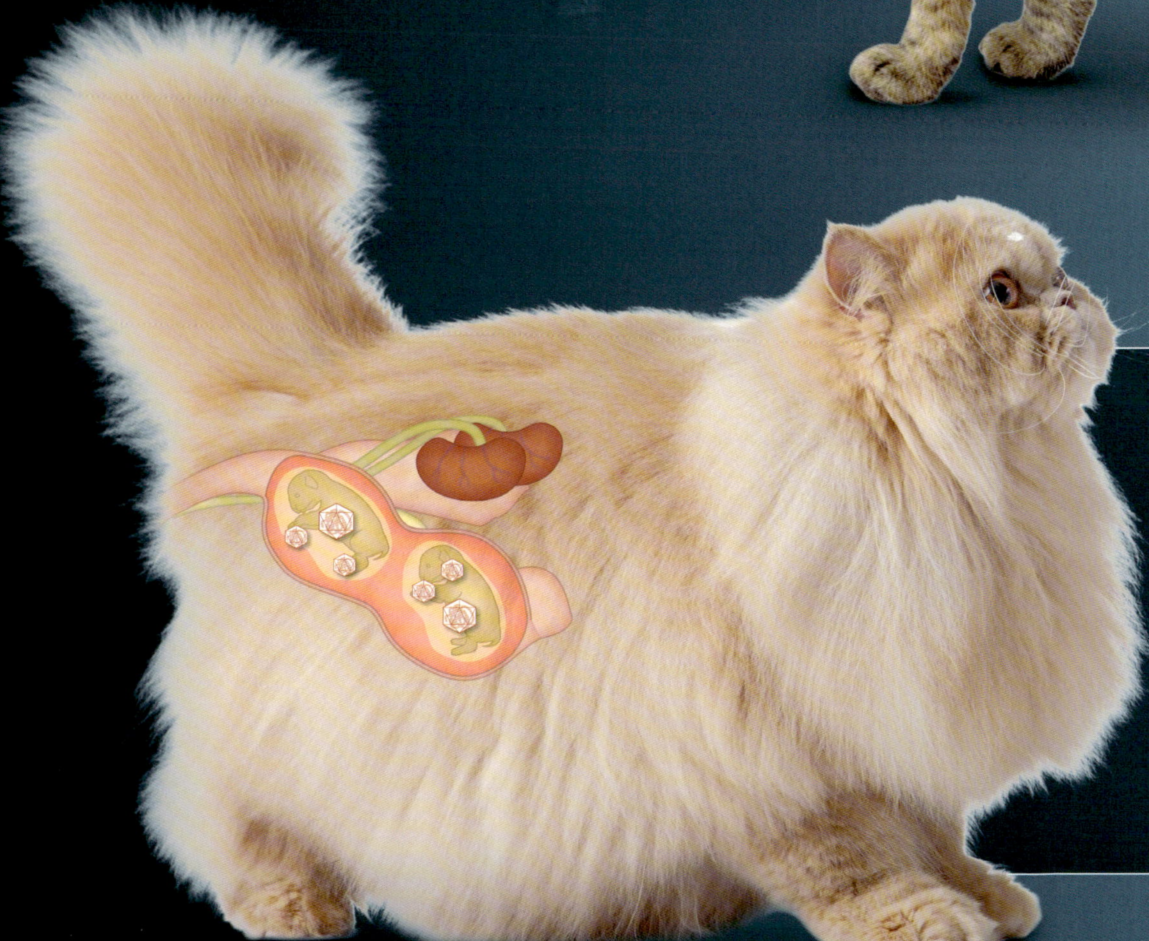

REPRODUCTIVE DISORDERS

If the **infection** occurs in a **pregnant queen** that lacks immunity, the virus crosses the placenta and infects the fetus; it may cause different disorders depending on the stage of gestation:

- **Early:** fetal death and resorption.
- **Medium:** abortions, and mummified fetuses.
- **Late:** teratogenic abnormalities. Kittens are born alive but with low viability. Similar alterations can be observed in **neonatal infections** (2-3 weeks of life).

CLINICAL SIGNS AND LESIONS

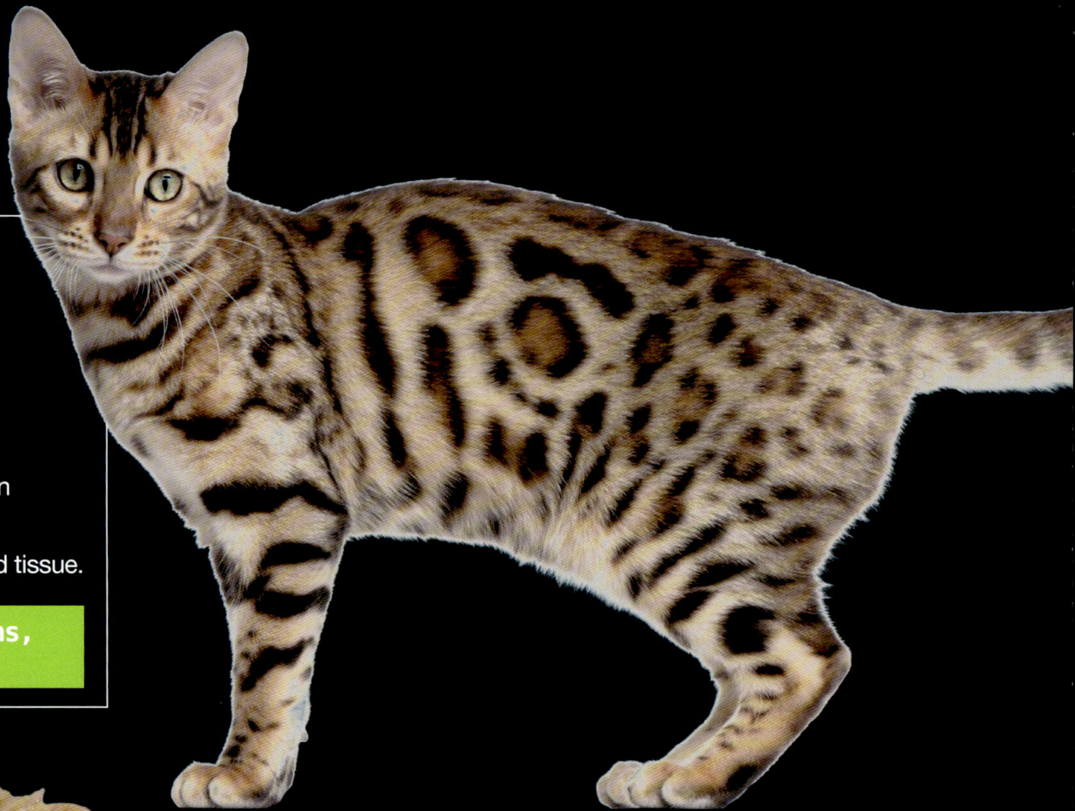

ENTERIC FORM

Young kittens 2-4 months of age: vomiting, profuse watery diarrhea which is often blood-tinged, and rapid dehydration. Sick cats may sit for long periods of time in front of their water bowls but not drink much water.

The alteration of the lymphoid tissue (panleukopenia) can cause severe immunosuppression and will condition the outcome of the disease.

Lesions concentrate in the jejunum, ileum, and lymphoid tissue.

Death is often due to concurrent infections, lack of treatment, and shock.

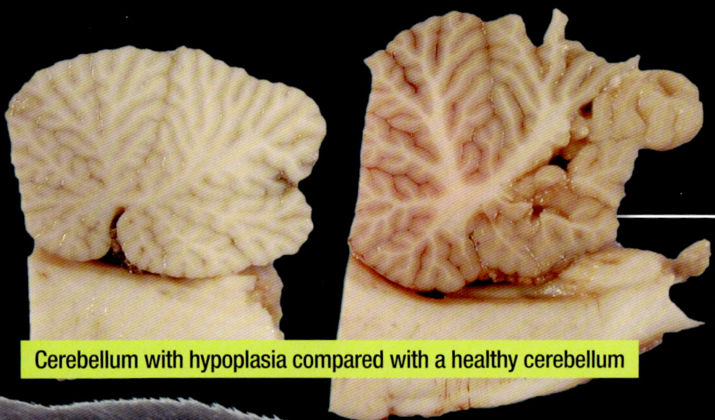

Cerebellum with hypoplasia compared with a healthy cerebellum

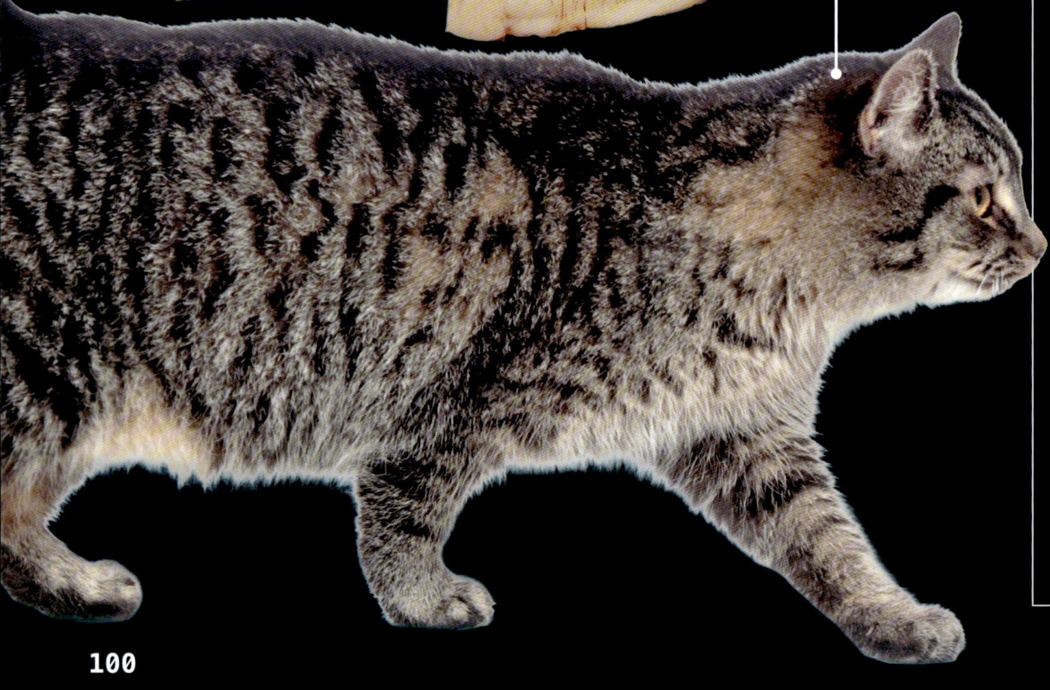

REPRODUCTIVE DISORDERS

Infection in the uterus has different consequences depending on the stage of pregnancy:

- **Early:** infertility (return to estrus due to fetal mortality and subsequent fetal resorption).
- **Medium:** abortions and birth of mummified fetuses.
- **Late:** viral multiplication in lymphoid tissues, eyes and CNS of the fetus, causing hydrocephalus, ocular abnormalities and, above all, cerebellar hypoplasia (see figure). These animals are born alive but have short viability. They will present severe neurological disorders associated with control of movement, and various neuropathies (such as atrophy of the optic nerve) or retinal dysplasia.

The clinical signs in animals that have been infected **shortly after birth** (2nd-3rd week) are similar to those seen in late infection in the uterus.

Postnatal infection in kittens a few weeks old, which have ingested insufficient colostrum and have a lactation deficit, occurs with viral replication in lymphoid tissues and intestine. This infection can go clinically unnoticed or present mild digestive alterations.

DIAGNOSIS

PRESUMPTIVE DIAGNOSIS

Factors to be considered in presumptive diagnosis:

- Age.
- Previous history.
- Whether it is an individual cat or it belongs to a population.

Circumstances which are suggestive of feline panleukopenia are: a young unvaccinated kitten, with acute digestive alterations, and compatible blood cell counts. When reproductive failure is present, feline panleukopenia should always be considered.

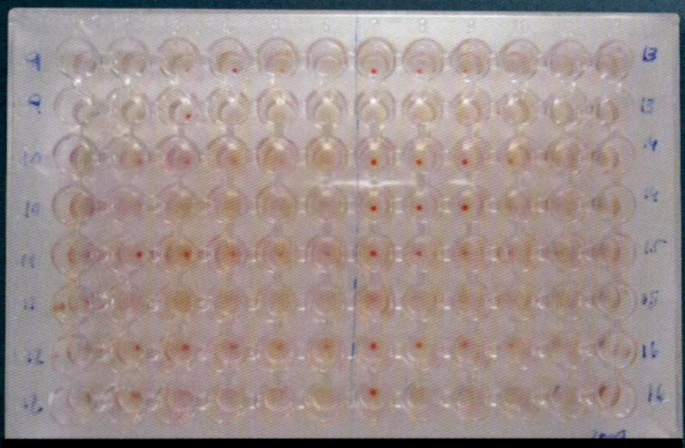

HAI for detecting Ab against the feline panleukopenia virus.

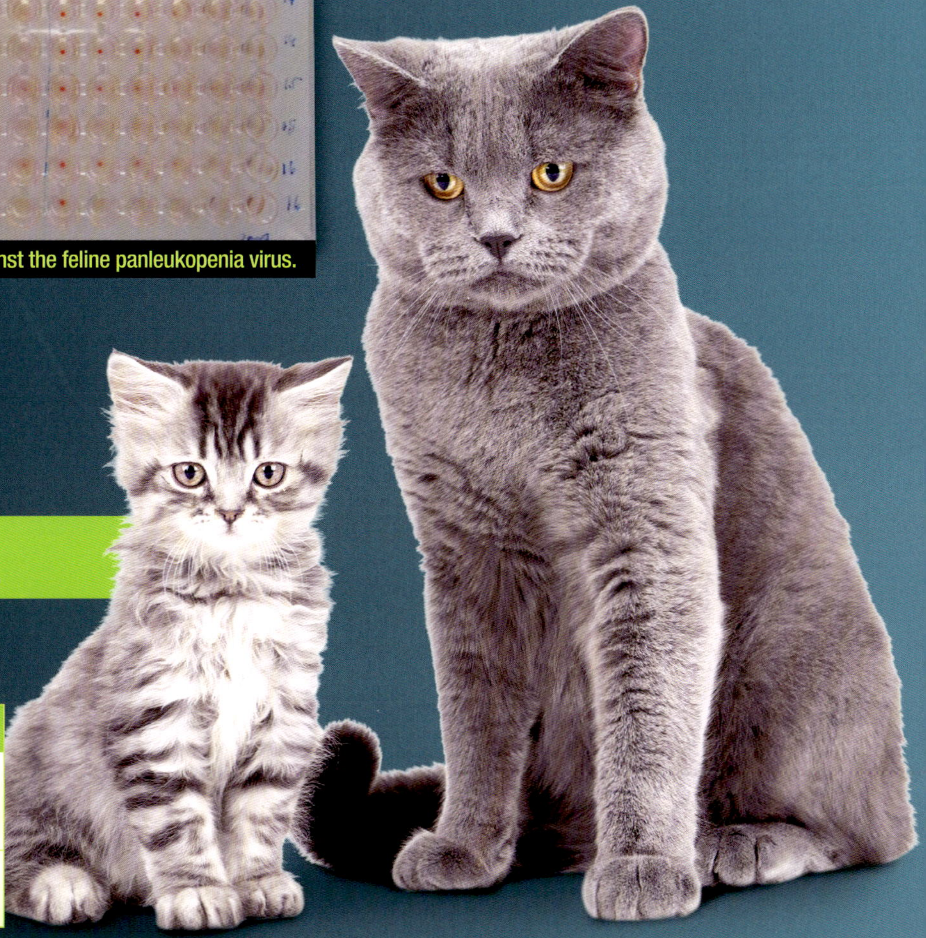

Usually, there is a direct relationship between the intensity of leukopenia and the severity of the disease.

LABORATORY DIAGNOSIS

Techniques	Samples	Observations
Viral detection (IC, HA and PCR)	Stools.	Commercial IC available (the most widely used; they can be specific for feline panleukopenia or broadly-reactive for canine parvoviruses).
Serology (ELISA and HAI)	Serum (two extractions: days 0 and 21).	• It is necessary to assess seroconversion. • Commercial in-office ELISA available.

TREATMENT

- **Fluid therapy:** this type of treatment is crucial to correct dehydration and avoid hypovolemic shock. Crystalloid isotonics and colloids, which can be combined with plasma or whole blood transfusions, are administered initially, to continue with supportive fluid therapy.
- **Antibiotics and antiemetic and antisecretory drugs:** are indicated according to the characteristics of the patient and the presence or absence of fever.

There is no clear data on the effectiveness of IFN-ω in the treatment of this disease.

There is no treatment for cerebellar hypoplasia.

VACCINES

Vaccines for feline panleukopenia are attenuated and multivalent.

Pregnant queens or kittens < 4 weeks old should not be vaccinated.

Vaccines induce a strong and lasting immunity. They are included in all core vaccination protocols.

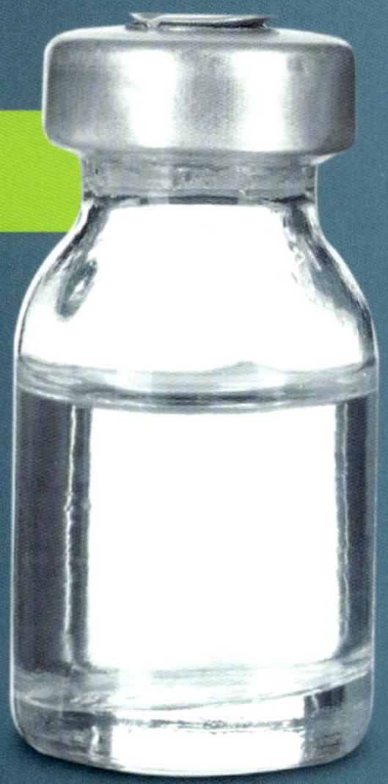

FELINE INFECTIOUS PERITONITIS

ETIOLOGY

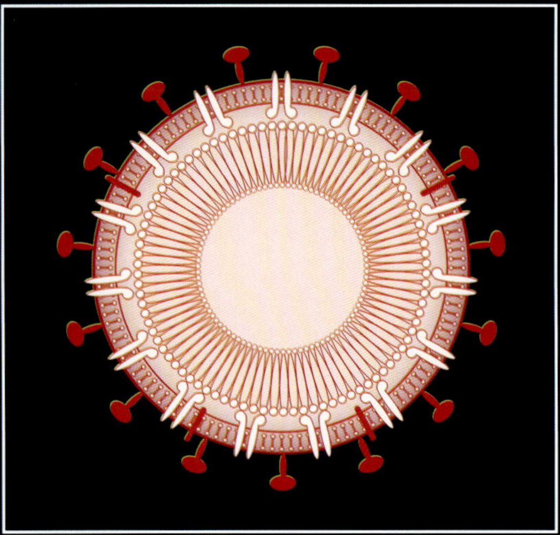

Feline Infectious peritonitis (FIP) is produced by feline coronaviruses (FCoV), which belong to the family *Coronaviridae*, genus *Alphacoronavirus*. They are enveloped RNA viruses with spikes on their surface (peplomers) resembling a crown.

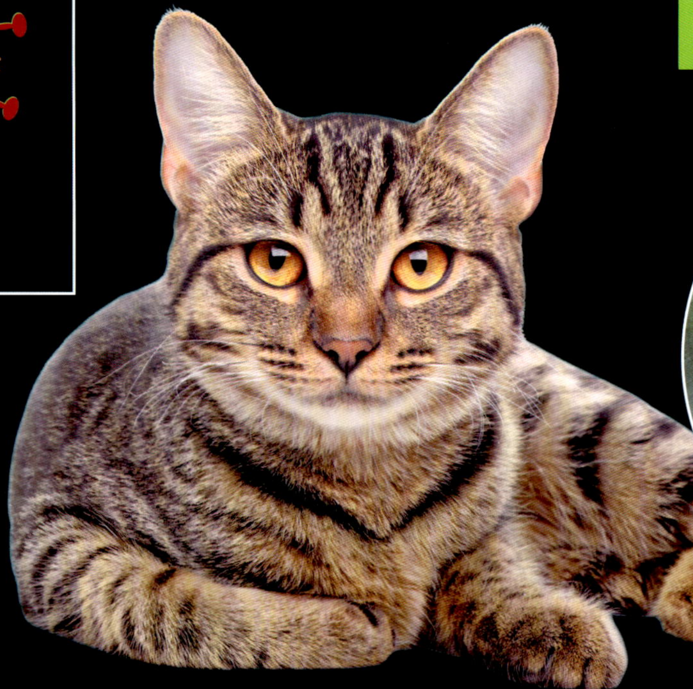

FCoV strains are classified into two types: I and II, related to the canine coronavirus I and II, respectively. Both can cause FIP.

Coronaviruses are sensitive to temperature and to the action of common detergents and disinfectants.

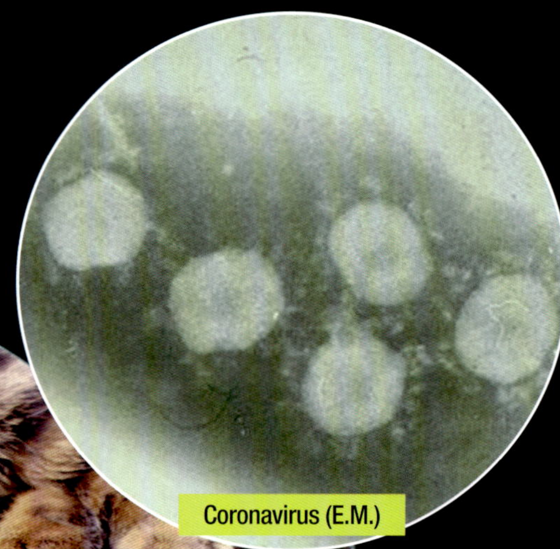

Coronavirus (E.M.)

EPIDEMIOLOGY

SUSCEPTIBLE SPECIES

Domestic cats and wild felids.

INCIDENCE

More common in young cats (< 12 months old).

Over 70 % of the cases of FIP occur in cats < 1 year old.

Higher incidence in catteries and in some breeds (Persian).

The percentage of seropositive cats is highly variable among different countries, since feline coronaviruses are present in many cats that live in populations with more than 6 animals. However, <10 % of those infected develop FIP.

SOURCE OF INFECTION

Cats with subclinical infections.

TRANSMISSION

Viruses are shed mainly by feces, but also by nasal secretions, saliva, etc. Normally, entry occurs orally and, occasionally, by inhalation, either directly or indirectly.

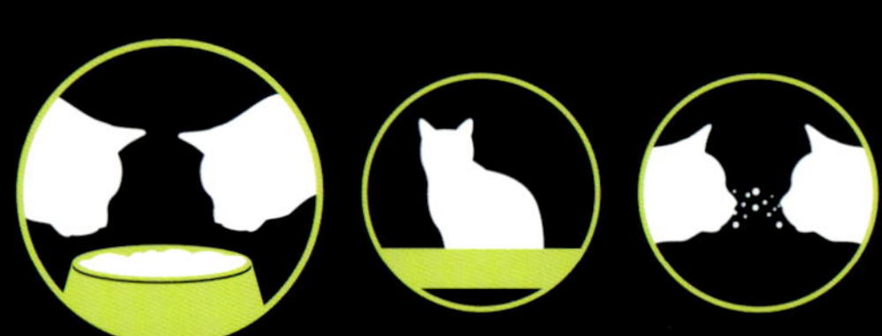

The incidence of FIP in developed countries has increased in recent years.

THE CLINICAL OUTCOME DEPENDS TO A GREAT EXTENT ON:

Ethological characteristics of cats, shedding period of the virus through feces (a few weeks for type II, 2-3 months for type I), entry route and strain of the virus, age, immune status and genetics, density and average age of the population, management measures (especially of reproduction) and quarantine, prevalence of concurrent diseases, mean antibody titer and breed.

PATHOGENESIS

- After ingestion or inhalation, **FCoV replicate in the tonsils and oropharynx** and quickly reach the intestine (ileum and colon; 2nd day post-infection).
- **Target cells** for FIP virus ("peritonitis" virus) are **monocytes /macrophages and endothelial cells of small vessels**. This tropism is essential for the "conversion" of the "enteric" virus (which replicates in enterocytes and whose infection is restricted to the digestive tract without crossing the mucosal membrane) into the "peritonitis" virus.

Cytokines and other inflammatory mediators determine the intensity and severity of the clinical manifestations.

- **Replication** of the FCoV **in macrophages** occurs slowly during the first two weeks post-infection, during which specific antibodies are raised. During this period many infected felines can eliminate the infection without developing the disease.
- In those who develop disease, the **presence of antibodies** enhances its development. Specific antibodies against the peplomers facilitate the entry of the virus in macrophages through the Fc receptors (see Chart 14), which favors replication and increases budding from the infected macrophages.

- Later, the **infection spreads** rapidly through the gut, spleen, liver, pancreas, kidney, pleura, peritoneum, CNS, and eyes, with successive cycles of phagocytosis → replication → release of the virus. Infection is accompanied with a highly inflammatory component which originates the development of pyogranulomatous lesions in multiple organs. The degree in which effusion is present in the body cavities characterizes the form of presentation of the disease: effusive or dry. The effusion is the accumulation of clear amber liquid with a high concentration of protein and a low concentration of cells (neutrophils, lymphocytes and plasma cells).

Some researchers believe that the clinical outcome depends on the intensity of the cell-mediated immune response and on the development of hypersensitivity reactions. If the cell-mediated immune response is strong, cats neutralize the virus, whereas if it is insufficient (no viral neutralization) and there is a prior coronavirus infection, Type III (effusive form) or IV (dry form) hypersensitivity may develop (see Chart 21).

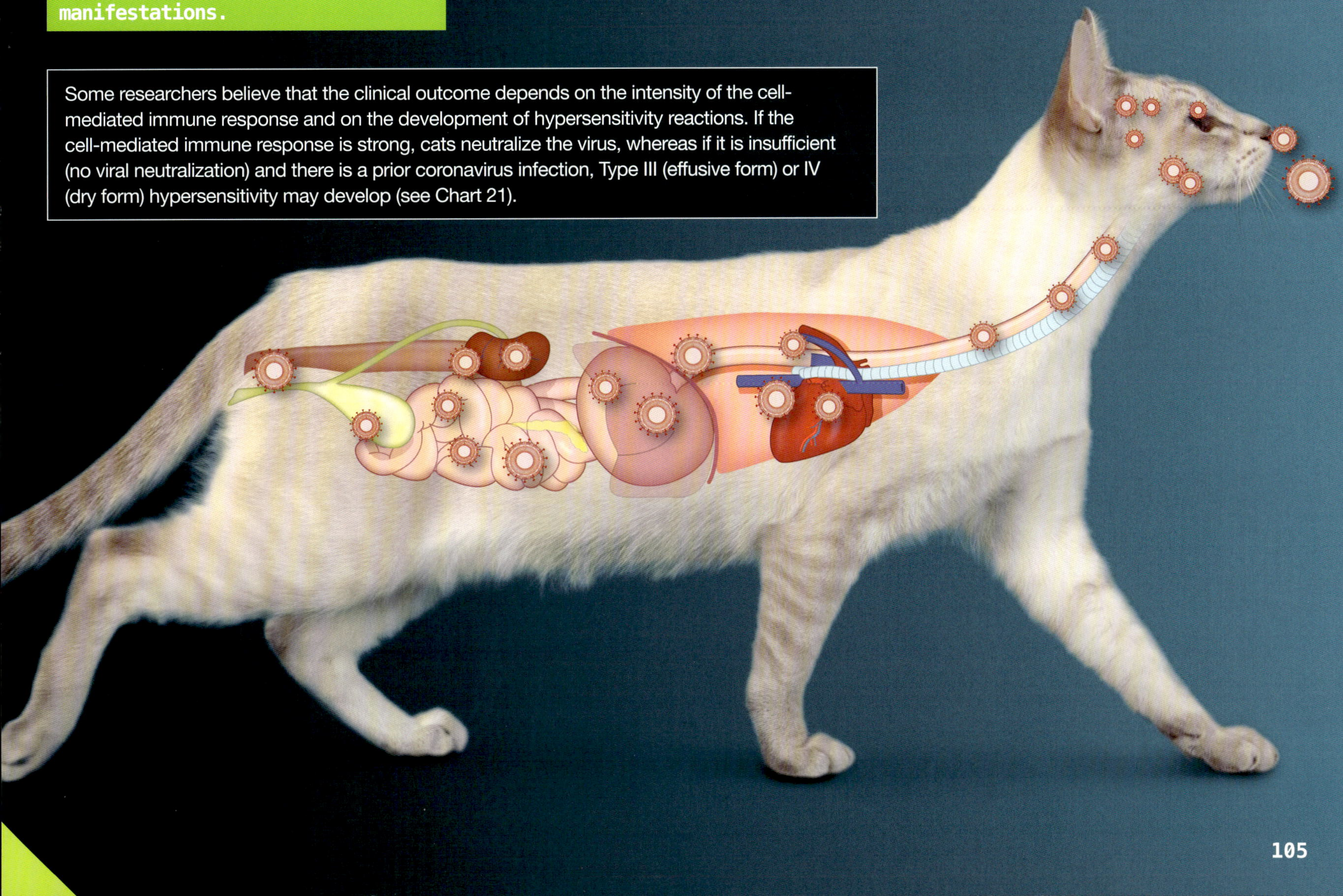

DIAGNOSIS

DIFFERENTIAL DIAGNOSIS

It is based on the clinical history and on the epidemiological data.

In the effusive form, *in vivo* diagnosis is mainly based on analysis of ascitic fluid. The altered proteinogram of ascitic fluid is indicative of FIP, but the presence of coronaviruses or specific antibodies against them must be confirmed.

The *post-mortem* gross pathology and histopathological diagnoses are definitive.

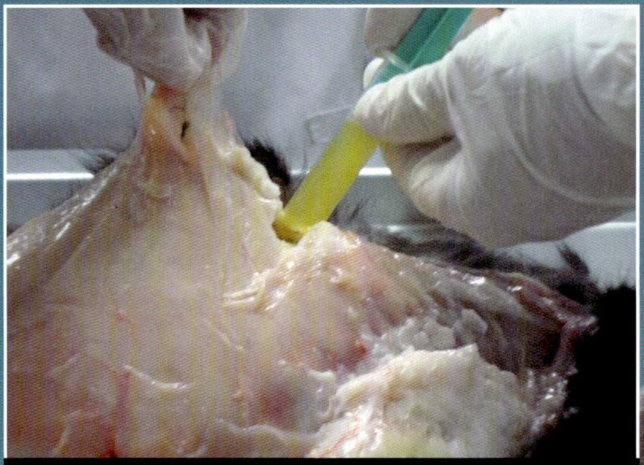
Effusive form of FIP: ascitic fluid

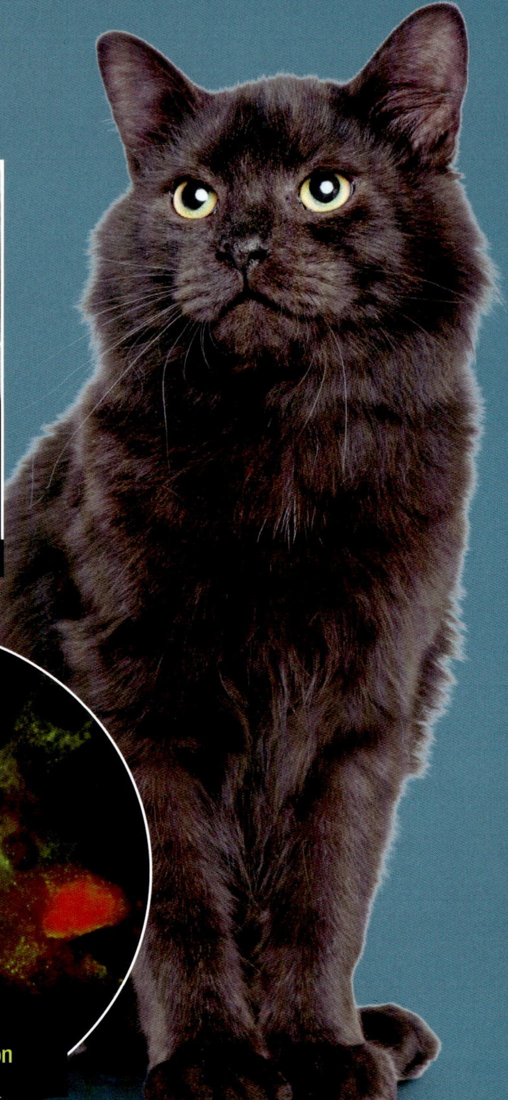

LABORATORY DIAGNOSIS

Techniques	Samples	Observations
Histopathology	Liver, spleen, kidney, lymph nodes, peritoneal and pleural exudates and pyogranulomas.	The most widely used.
Detection of viral antigens (DFA and IP)	Peritoneal and pleural exudates and pyogranulomas.	Reliable but not always possible (it detects virus in macrophages).
Detection of viral nucleic acids (PCR)	Blood and stools.	It does not differentiate pathogenic from non-pathogenic strains.
Serology (ELISA and IFA)	Serum.	• High titers are only suggestive of FIP. • Commercial ELISA available.

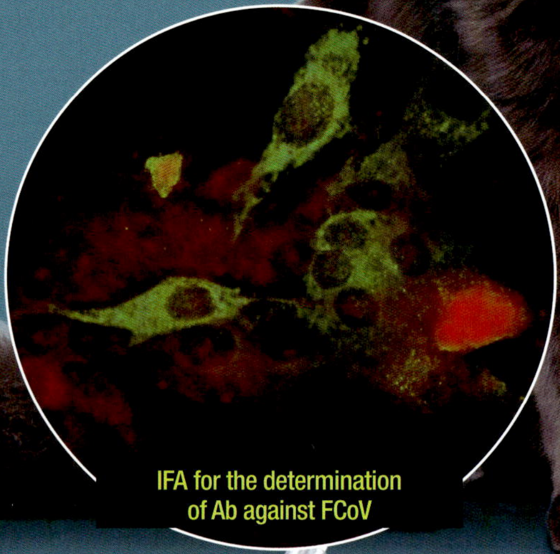
IFA for the determination of Ab against FCoV

TREATMENT

Therapy only delays the progression of the disease. It includes:

- **Corticosteroids and immunosuppressive drugs** (especially in the effusive form) to avoid inflammatory and immune-mediated responses.
- **Broad-spectrum antibiotics** to prevent secondary bacterial infections.
- **Fluid therapy** to prevent dehydration.

It is advisable to consider euthanasia of those cats that do not improve within a few days of starting treatment.

The prognosis is usually unfavorable.

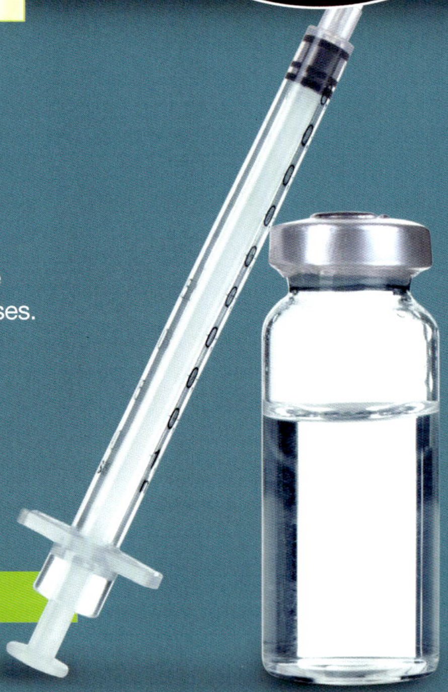

VACCINES

A temperature-sensitive vaccine is commercially available, whose effectiveness and security is controversial. It is administered intranasally.

This vaccine is not currently recommended for most animals.

CLINICAL SIGNS AND LESIONS

CLINICAL FORMS

1 EFFUSIVE OR WET FORM

- **Presence of clear amber effusion** with a high protein concentration in body cavities, and **necrotic and pyogranulomatous lesions**. Presence of fibrin in peritoneum, pleura and the surface of various organs.
- It usually starts as an **insidious disease** with progressive weight loss, depression, anorexia, fever, pleural effusion and discrete appearance of edema which settles in lower regions.
- Some cats develop **jaundice** and **pericarditis**.
- **Death** usually occurs **3-6 months after** the clinical signs begin. For humanitarian reasons, cats are usually euthanized earlier than this.

In the effusive form, 90 % of the cats suffer peritonitis and 25-40 % pleuritis.

2 NON-EFFUSIVE OR DRY FORM

- **Pyogranulomatous lesions** identical to those of the effusive form but with reduced exudation.
- The **progression** is **slow** (months or years) due to the location of pyogranulomas in one or more organs, mainly kidneys, liver, pancreas, mesenteric lymph nodes, CNS and eyes.
- Cats develop **hepatic or renal insufficiency**, pancreatic disease and disorders of the CNS.
- **Nervous signs,** appearing in 10-30 % of cases, include paresis of hind legs, paralysis, tremors, ataxia and muscle stiffness.
- A high number of cats develop **ocular disorders**, such as keratitis, uveitis, alterations of the retina and panophtalmitis.

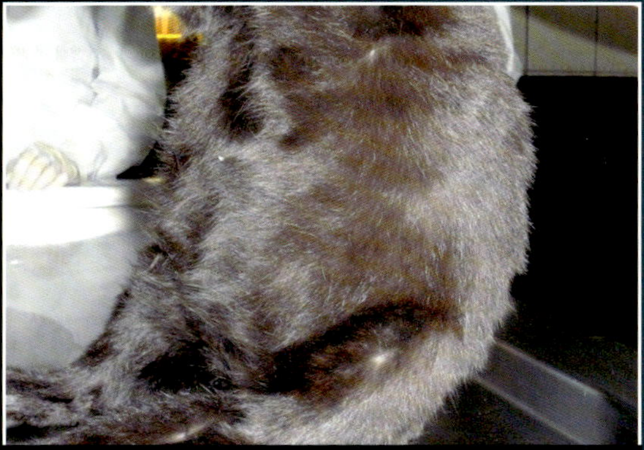

Effusive form of FIP: distention of abdomen

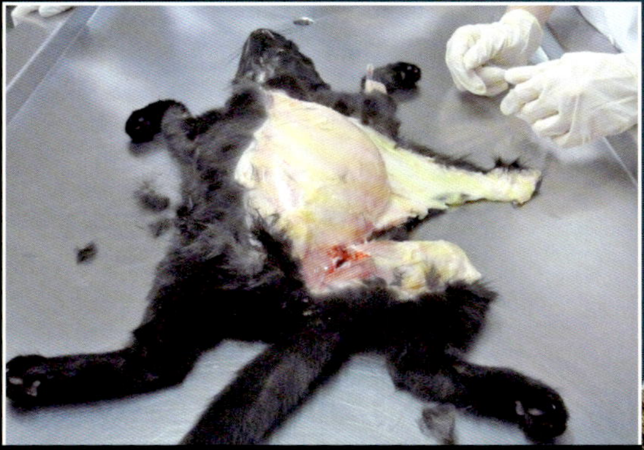

Effusive form of FIP: ascites

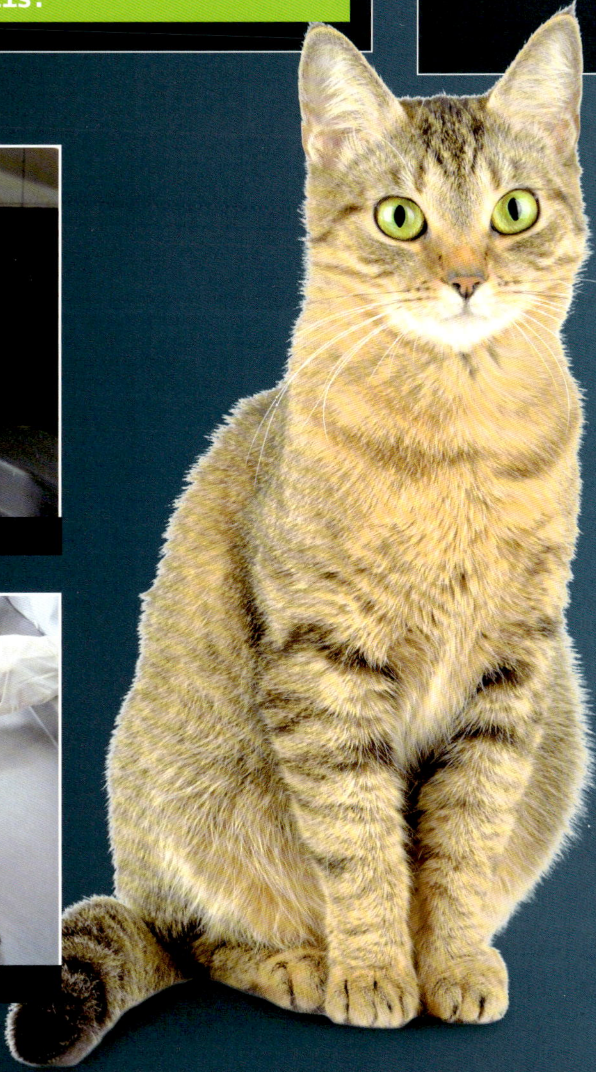

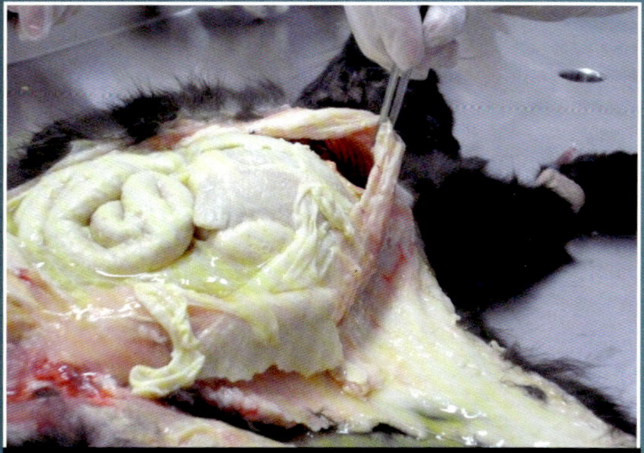

Effusive form of FIP: abdominal cavity with fibrin

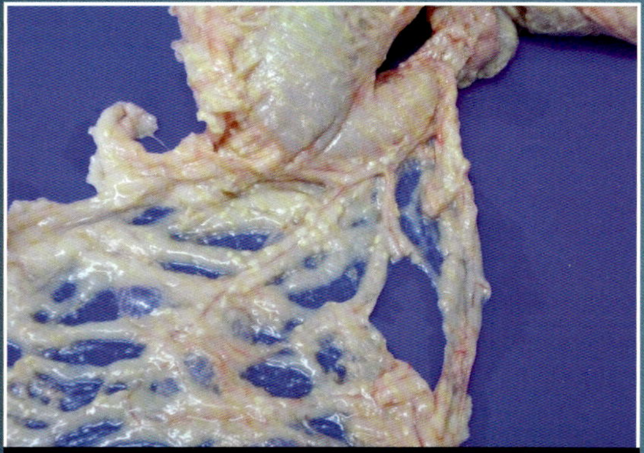

FIP: pyogranulomas in the mesentery

FELINE RESPIRATORY DISEASE

Infections by feline rhinotracheitis virus, feline calicivirus, *Bordetella bronchiseptica* and *Chlamydophila felis*.

ETIOLOGY

Main agents responsible for feline respiratory disease:

1 **Feline rhinotracheitis virus** (feline herpesvirus-1): it belongs to the family *Herpesviridae* (enveloped DNA virus), genus *Varicellovirus*. It can induce latent infections and colonize the upper respiratory tract.

2 **Feline caliciviruses:** classified in the family *Caliciviridae* (non-enveloped RNA viruses), genus *Vesivirus*. They present genetic, antigenic and clinical variability. They are often associated with oral ulcers, and with disorders of the upper respiratory tract ("feline coryza"). In recent years, highly virulent strains capable of producing a systemic disease have been described.

3 ***Bordetella bronchiseptica*:** a gram-negative coccobacillus, mobile by flagella, with fimbriae and which produces toxins. It colonizes the ciliated epithelium of the respiratory tract and is capable of inducing chronic infections.

4 ***Chlamydophila felis*** (formerly *Chlamydia psitacci*): is a chlamydia (a gram-negative microorganism that requires cells in which to multiply and, therefore, does not survive outside the host). Its primary multiplication site is the conjunctiva.

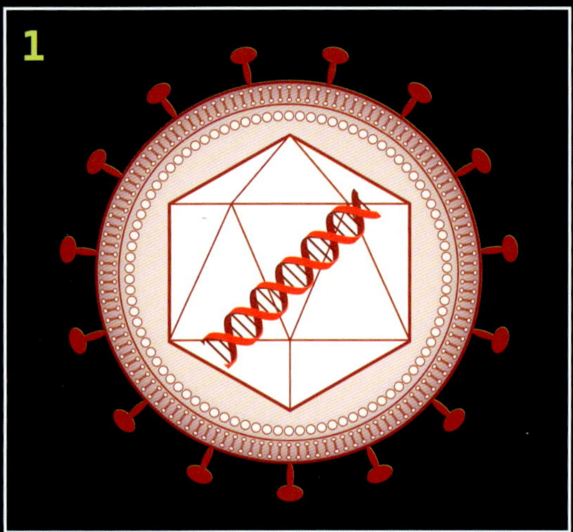

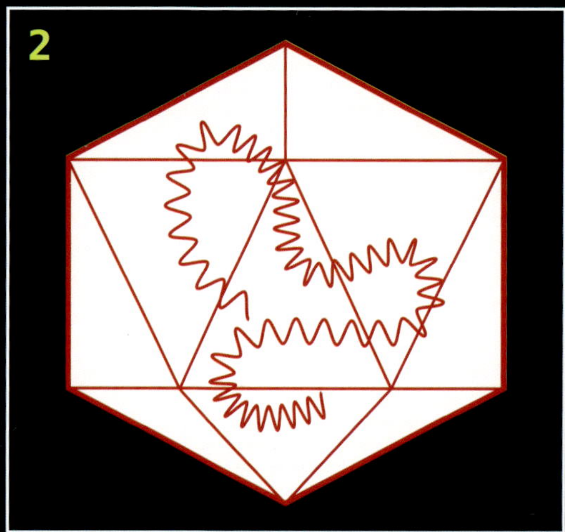

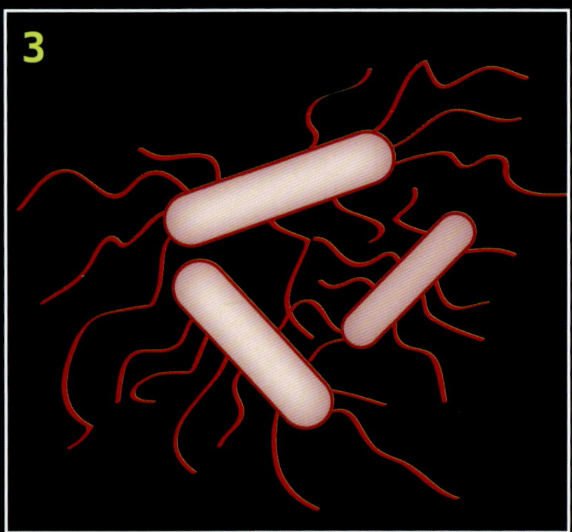

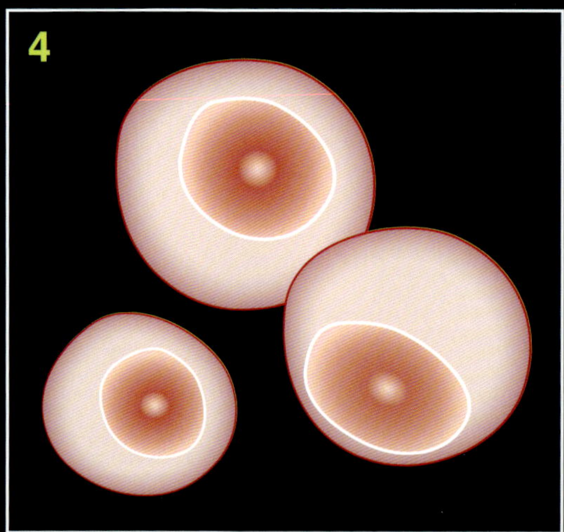

B. bronchiseptica (light microscope)

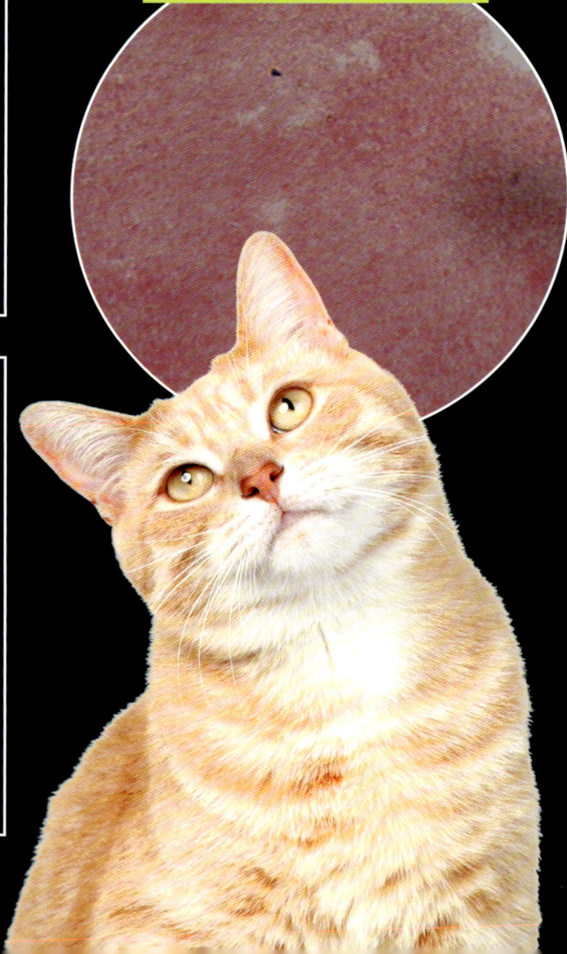

EPIDEMIOLOGY

The incidence of feline respiratory disease is higher in young animals (a few weeks old) and in populations (catteries).

Factors associated with the clinical development: number of different pathogens involved, virulence of strains, type of habitat, age, immune status and stress.

n populations, morbidity is usually high and mortality low. n recent years, outbreaks of the disease involving systemic nfection have been described. They are caused by strains of highly virulent calicivirus, which produce high mortality in young and adult cats.

The presence of carrier cats assures the permanence and circulation of these pathogens and that the situation becomes endemic, mainly in populations.

TRANSMISSION

Routes of transmission	Feline rhinotracheitis virus	Feline calicivirus	*B. bronchiseptica*	*C. felis*
Oral	+	+	+	
Nasal	+	+	+	
Conjunctival	+	+		+

Transmission of *C. felis* requires close contact between animals.

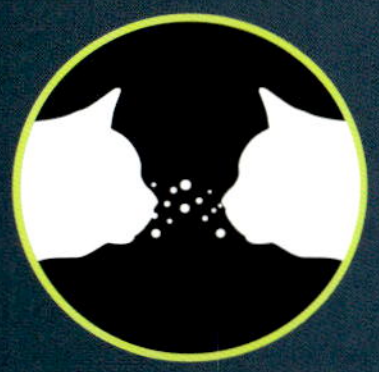

SHEDDING

- **Feline rhinotracheitis virus:** oronasal and conjunctival secretions for at least two weeks post-infection (it can stay latent after clinical recovery).
- **Calicivirus:** oronasal and conjunctival secretions.
- ***B. bronchiseptica:*** oral and nasal secretions.
- ***C. felis:*** conjunctival secretions.

PATHOGENESIS

- **Feline rhinotracheitis virus** multiplies in the conjunctiva, nasal turbinates and nasopharynx, and rarely produces viremia. It causes latent infections in various locations, mostly in the trigeminal ganglion.
- **Feline caliciviruses** replicate in the tongue, oropharynx, bronchi, lungs, digestive tract and, occasionally, in the joints.

  Highly virulent strains entering through aerosols may colonize pulmonary alveoli (acute exudative alveolitis) and other locations, producing systemic infections. Replication of these strains at the endothelium and the ensuing vasculitis are responsible for the development of skin lesions. In addition, highly virulent strains cause hemorrhagic disorders by DIC (disseminated intravascular coagulation) and alterations in various organs (such as liver and lung).

  They tend to persist in cats for 2-3 months, but a small percentage of infected cats may remain as carriers of the virus for years.
- ***B. bronchiseptica*** colonizes the ciliated epithelium of the respiratory tract and can cause chronic infections. It may produce toxins (dermonecrotic and tracheal) and stop the mucociliary escalator and denude the ciliary epithelium.
- ***C. felis*** mainly infects the conjunctiva, although it can also colonize the respiratory tract, especially the upper section.

The various agents involved in this syndrome can colonize different sections of the respiratory tract. In addition, some of them may even colonize other organs.

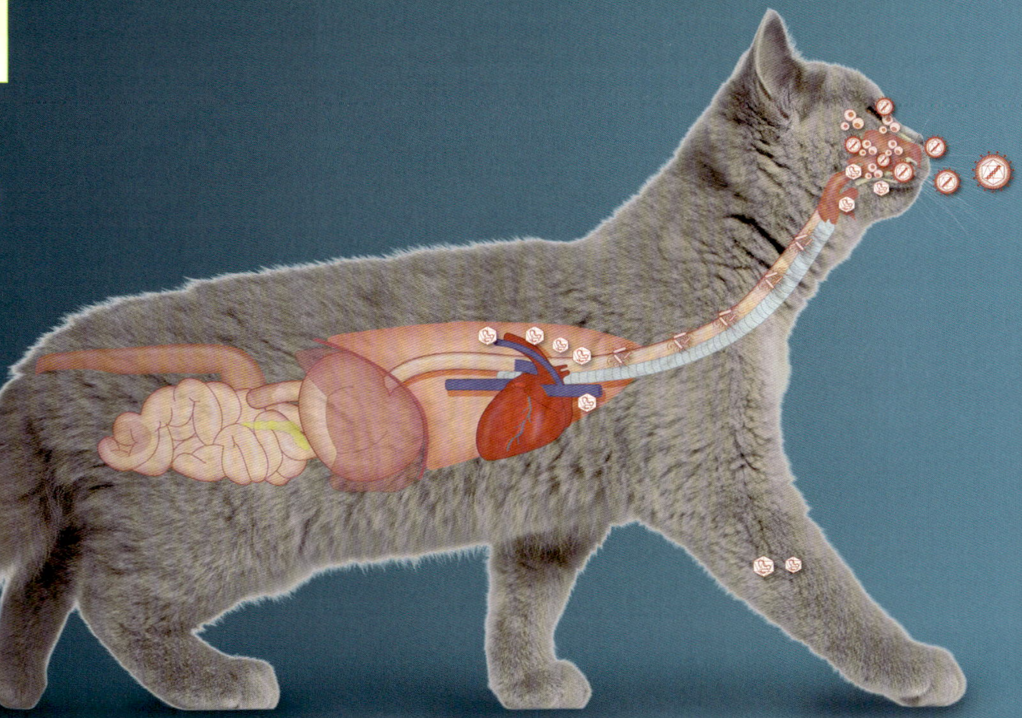

CLINICAL SIGNS AND LESIONS

Respiratory disorders range from mild to severe. They include shortness of breath and buildup of clear to mucous exudates that occlude the airway and prevent normal food ingestion. This results in rapid loss of body condition, dehydration, and anorexia (see figure).

Mortality occurs mostly in litters from queens which are allowed to roam, without veterinary care and intervention.

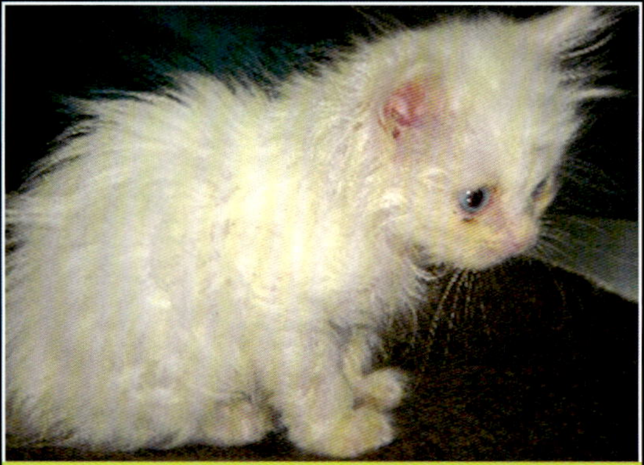

Kitten with feline respiratory disease

Each of the agents involved in this process can cause different clinical syndromes.

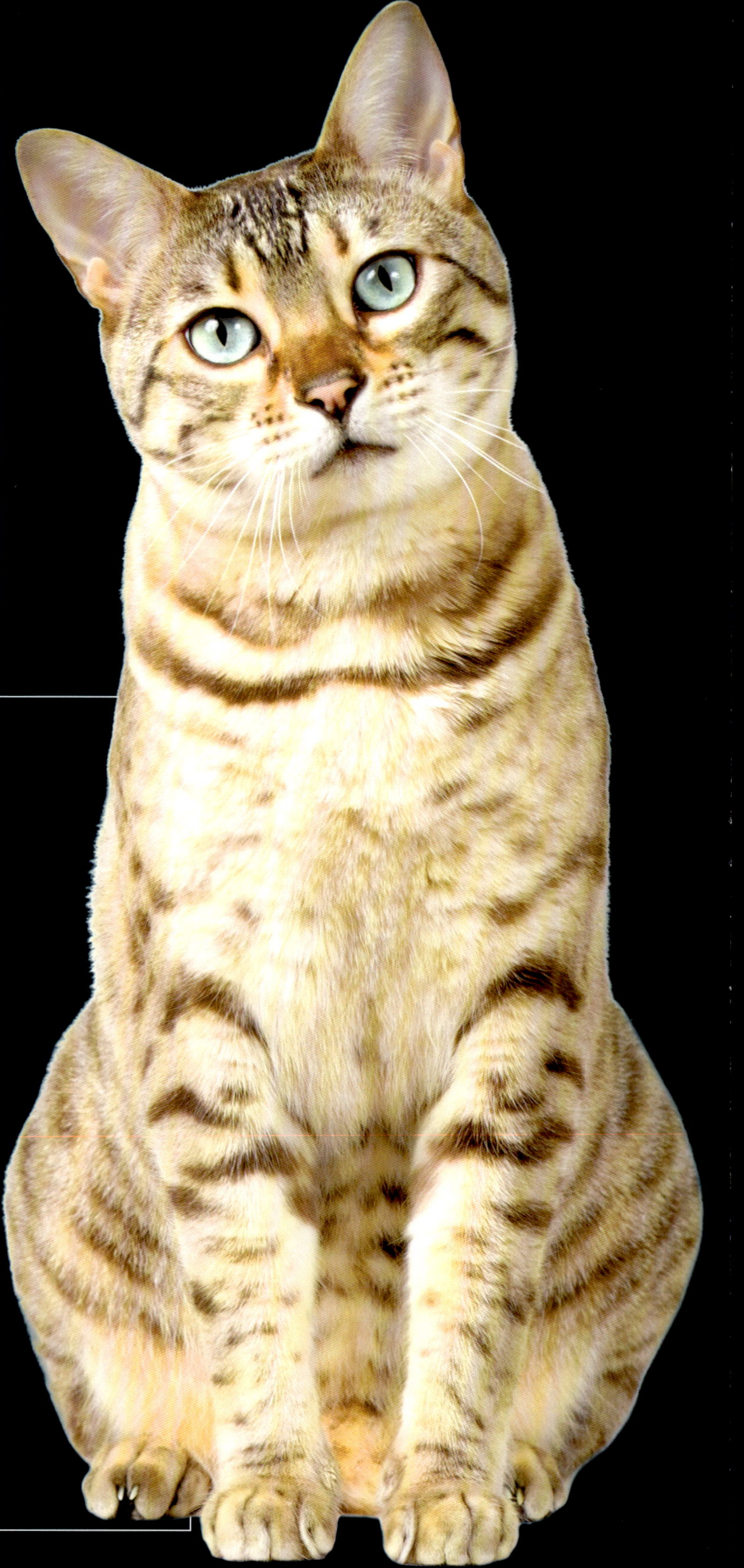

CLINICAL OUTCOMES

- **Feline rhinotracheitis virus** causes rhinitis, conjunctivitis, fever, depression and anorexia. The development of ulcerative keratitis is characteristic. Lesions include inflammation of the upper respiratory tract and, occasionally, osteolysis of the nasal turbinates.
- **Feline caliciviruses** can produce:
  1. **Typical disease:** acute, mild and self-limiting post-natal infection of the upper respiratory tract with presence of oral ulcers and vesicles. Occasionally, conjunctivitis, pneumonia, and intermittent claudication may be observed.
  2. **Systemic disease:** fever, severely affected lower respiratory tract, dyspnea, pneumonia, oral and footpad ulcerations, facial edema, enteritis, bleeding and jaundice. It can occur in kittens and adults, vaccinated or not, and is associated with high mortality (50-70 %), especially in adults.
  3. **Chronic stomatitis and gingivitis:** associated with persistent infections.
- ***B. bronchiseptica*** often causes mild hyperthermia, nasal catarrh, sneezing and conjunctivitis. Occasionally, other concurrent pathogens may complicate the disease and produce severe pneumonia and cyanosis.
- ***C. felis*** produces unilateral conjunctivitis, which can evolve to bilateral. Conjunctivitis is intense, with hyperemia of the nictitating membrane, blepharospasm and eye discomfort. It can be accompanied by transient fever, loss of appetite and weight loss.

DIAGNOSIS

Easy, in view of the clinical signs, age and background of the cat.

The involvement of multiple agents can complicate the etiologic diagnosis.

Frequently, diagnosis is limited to the isolation and identification of the bacteria present (*B. bronchiseptica* and secondary bacteria), complemented with the corresponding antibiogram (see figure).

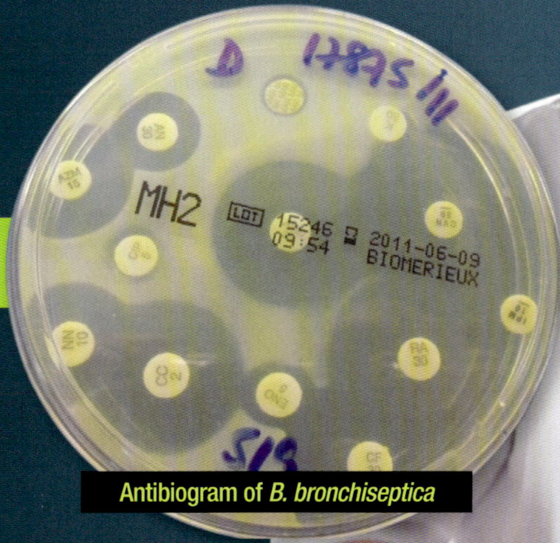

Antibiogram of *B. bronchiseptica*

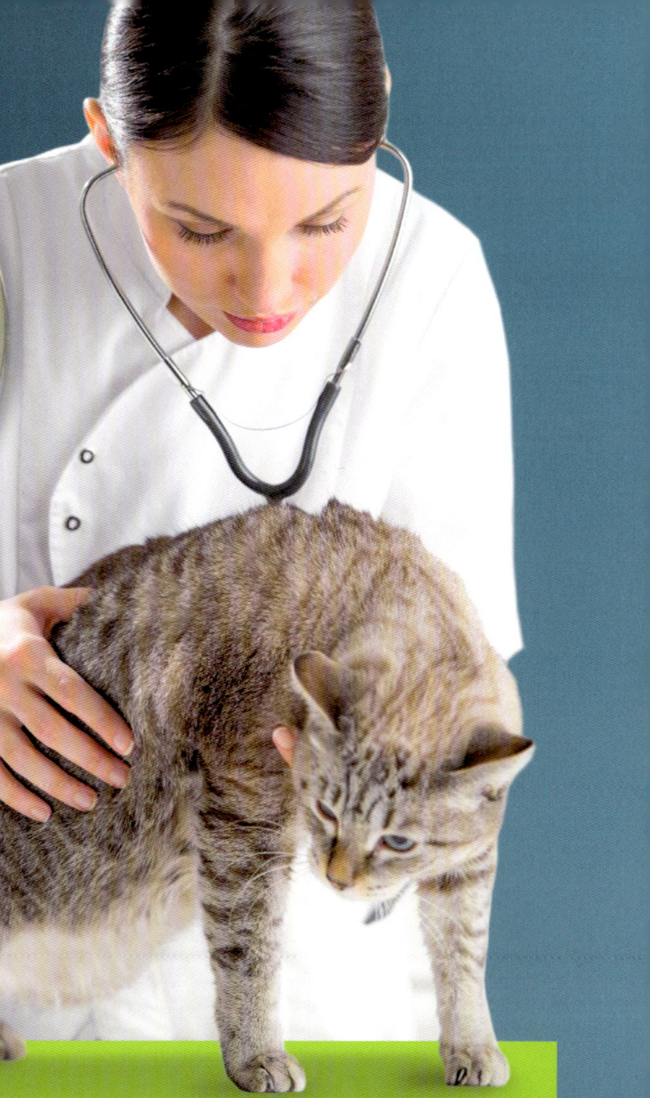

LABORATORY DIAGNOSIS

Techniques	Samples	Observations
Detection of viruses and bacteria (DFA and PCR)	Nasal and conjunctival secretions, and organs (tonsils, tongue, lung, GI tract, etc.).	PCR is more useful for detecting rhinotracheitis virus than caliciviruses.
Isolation of bacteria	Respiratory and conjunctival secretions.	Identification and antibiogram of *B. bronchiseptica* and secondary bacteria.
Serology	Serum (two extractions: days 0 and 21).	It is necessary to assess seroconversion.

Positive results of the diagnostic tests should be interpreted in the clinical context.

TREATMENT

The crucial elements are: support therapy, hygiene measures and neonatal care.

THERAPY CONSISTS OF:

- **Fluid therapy** to treat dehydration.
- **Mucolytics** to avoid the accumulation of exudates in the respiratory tract.
- **Antibiotics** to treat infections by *B. bronchiseptica* and secondary bacteria.
- **Topical antiviral drugs** or other medications to treat eye problems.
- **Very soft and palatable diet** in anorectic kittens due to the possible presence of oral ulcers.

VACCINES

Vaccines against feline rhinotracheitis virus, feline calicivirus, and *C. felis* can be attenuated, inactivated, or composed of subunits (the latter only for feline caliciviruses). All commercially available vaccines are multivalent.

Vaccines avoid or reduce the clinical signs, but do not prevent the infection in the cat, which eventually can become a carrier.

Protection against highly virulent feline calicivirus strains is very limited.

Routine vaccination of the population, especially in catteries, is highly recommended.

VACCINES AND VACCINATION

Vaccination or active immunization involves the administration of an antigen to the animal, so it responds effectively against it and develops a specific immune memory. Subsequent exposure to the same Ag will elicit a secondary response, faster and of greater intensity and duration than the primary.

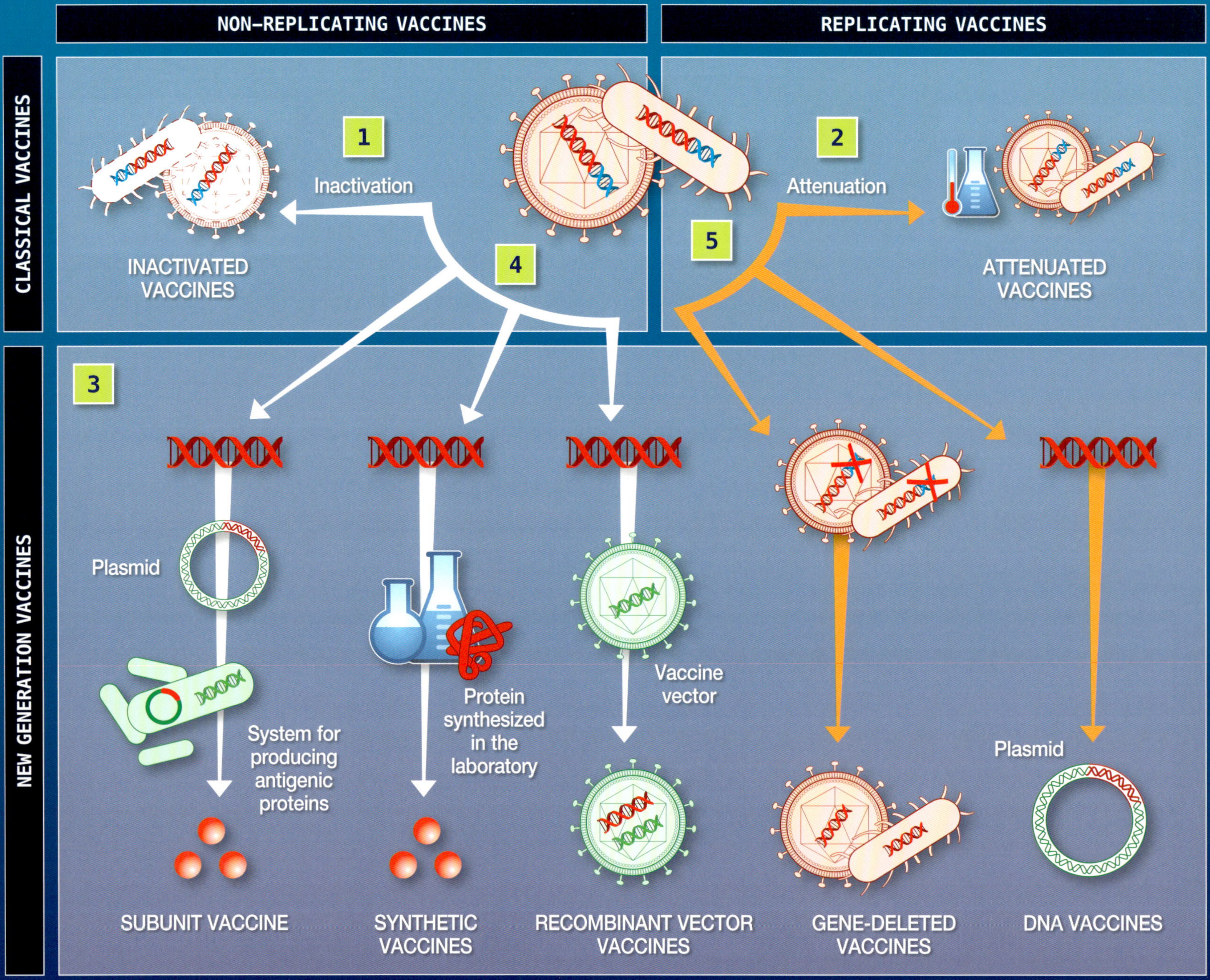

VACCINE ADMINISTRATION

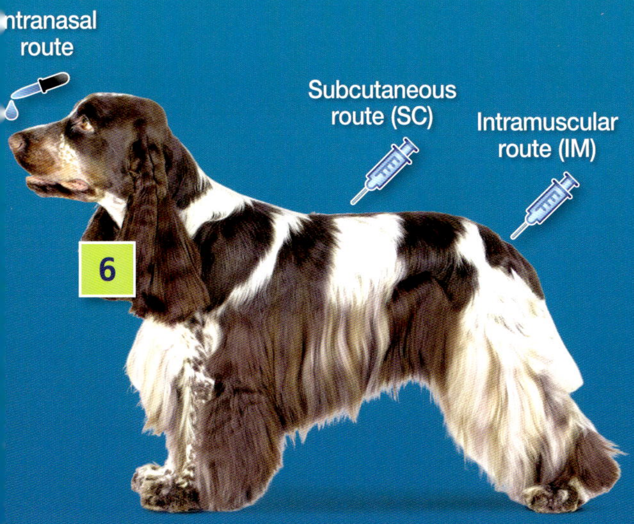

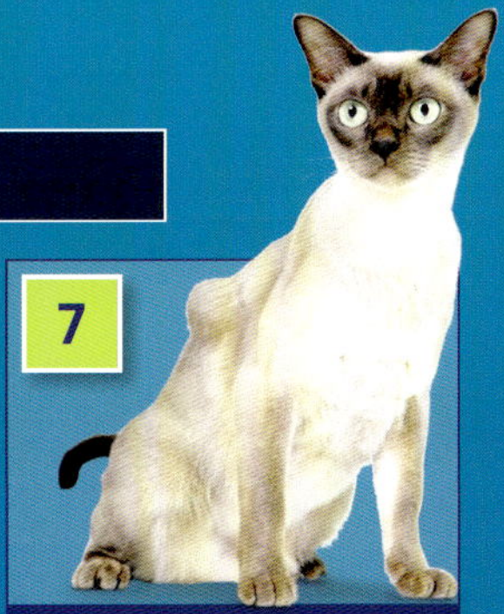

Sarcoma

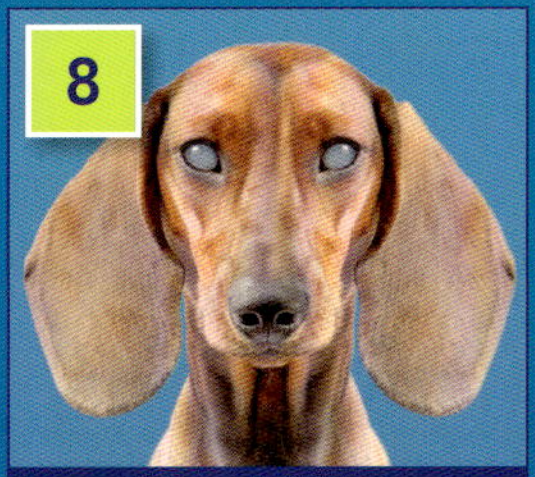

"Blue eye" due to Type III hypersensitivity

VACCINE FAILURES

9

		CAUSES
INADEQUATE ADMINISTRATION		• Inappropriate route of administration. • Inadequate moment for vaccinating. • Death of live vaccine.
ADEQUATE ADMINISTRATION	The animal responds but there is no protection	• Too late administration: the animal is already infected. • Wrong strain or organism used. • Non-protective Ab.
	The animal fails to respond	• Prior passive immunization. • Immunosuppressed animal. • Individual variability.

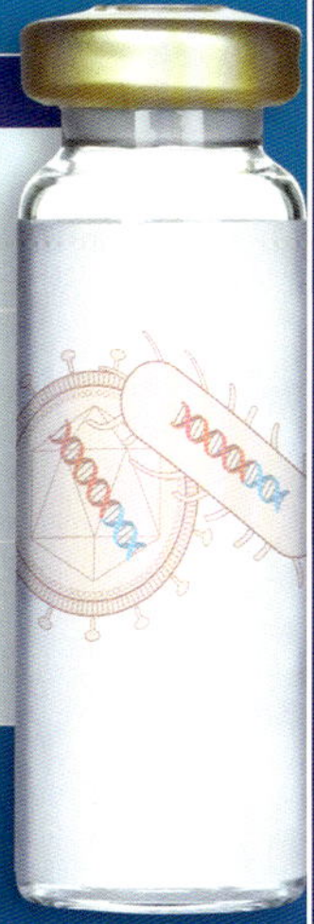

THE WINDOW OF SUSCEPTIBILITY

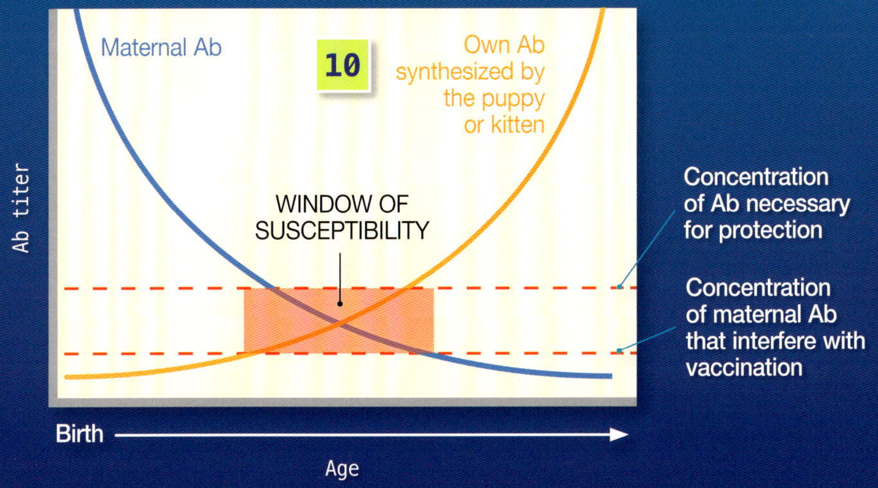

1 **Killed or inactivated vaccines** consist of complete but chemically- or physically-inactivated microorganisms, which retain their immunogenic properties. Inactivated bacterial exotoxins, called **toxoids**, are also considered killed vaccines (*e.g.*, tetanus toxoid).

2 **Attenuated vaccines** consist of **living non-virulent infectious agents**. Attenuation is achieved naturally (such as adaptation to a different host), by classic laboratory methods (*e.g.*, through passes or subcultures, adaptation to non-optimal temperatures), or through genetic manipulation. These vaccines usually provide a good level of protection, but are less safe than the inactivated ones (possible reversion to virulence).

3 **Modern vaccine technology** involves using genetic engineering to clone genes that encode immunogenic proteins of an infectious agent in different vectors, or to eliminate genes that encode proteins related to the virulence of a pathogen.

4 Inactivated organisms, synthetic and subunit vaccines act as exogenous antigens to induce a humoral immune response (Ab production and generation of memory B cells). In these cases, **adjuvants** are often included to enhance the immune response.

5 The living organisms in attenuated vaccines multiply in the host. Vector recombinant vaccines and DNA vaccines do not replicate in the animal, but lead to the synthesis of the antigenic proteins. In all these cases, the synthesis of these endogenous Ag stimulates a cell-mediated immune response (Th1) and the generation of memory Tc cells.

6 Vaccines in dogs and cats are usually administered by **subcutaneous** or **intramuscular** injection. Some live vaccines may also be administered intranasally. Amongst these are the vaccine against "kennel cough", and the temperature-sensitive vaccine against feline infectious peritonitis (FIP). In general, inactivated, synthetic and subunit vaccines often need several doses to provide adequate protection.

7 Vaccines normally elicit transient reactions at the point of inoculation, as effective protective immune responses require some degree of inflammation. Sometimes other **adverse side effects**, which are usually mild (pain, localized alopecia, abscesses), may be observed. Occasionally, side effects, such as the formation of sarcomas in cats, may be more serious.

8 Sometimes, **systemic adverse reactions** (such as fever or malaise) may develop after the administration of a vaccine. Less frequently, vaccines provoke other more serious problems such as abortions, reactions of hypersensitivity, autoimmunity or immunosuppression (see Charts 20 to 23).

9 Vaccines do not confer immediate protection after administration; it is necessary for the immune system to be activated and memory to develop. The effectiveness and duration of immune memory depends on various factors related to the vaccine, its administration and the characteristics of the vaccinated animal. **Vaccine failures** (when vaccination does not result in the animal being protected) sometimes occur for various reasons related to these factors.

10 The **window of susceptibility** is the period of time in which the level of maternal immunoglobulins acquired through colostrum is too low to provide protection against pathogens, but too high for the development of an effective response to the vaccination. Its duration varies between individuals, even within the same litter, and depends on the concentration of Ig in the colostrum, and on the amount of colostrum ingested and absorbed by the newborn (see Chart 12).

VACCINATION RECOMMENDATIONS FOR DOGS

Vaccination is one more tool of sanitary programs that may be used, both for individual dogs and for canine populations (kennels, shelters, etc.).

RECOMMENDATIONS FOR VACCINATION OF INDIVIDUALS

Vaccination protocols for individuals must be designed on the basis of various factors of the animal and its environment. Of special interest are:

- Age and breed.
- Immune and physiological status.
- Habits, activity, coexistence and fitness.
- Geographical area.

Immunization schedules must be flexible and prescribed by vets.

These factors will determine:

- Against which **diseases** dogs need to be protected. On the basis of its pathogenic category level and incidence in the geographical area where the animal lives.
- The choice of the **type of vaccine** (inactivated, subunit or attenuated). According to the characteristics of the individual to be protected.
- The **number of doses** and **administration interval**. Depending on the type of vaccine, age and health and physiological status of the dog.
- The use of **monovalent or polyvalent vaccines**. According to age and health and physiological status of the dog.
- The choice of the product with the **strain that is most appropriate for the area where the animal resides,** as there may be important differences between strains circulating in different geographical areas.
- The choice of the specific commercial product, once assessed the differences between equivalent vaccines, associated with the **titer or the concentration** of the microorganism or **the type of adjuvant**.

It is difficult to develop a single vaccination schedule, as it is not the same to design a program for a puppy, an adult or a pregnant bitch. In addition, the design of this program may vary according to the breed (*e.g.*, Rottweilers show increased susceptibility to viral gastroenteritis), habits and activity of the individual (participation in dog contests), coexistence with dogs of different ages, etc.

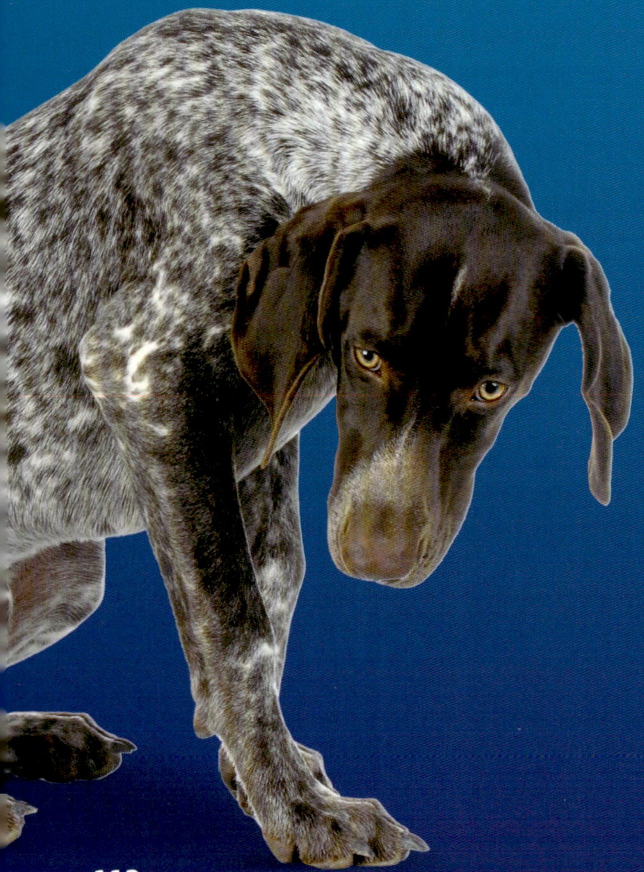

RECOMMENDATIONS FOR VACCINATION OF POPULATIONS

Vaccination guidelines within a health program to be used within a population must always be associated with good management and breeding practices of the animals. These guidelines should be consistent with the purpose of the population. Thus, in dog shelters and breeding kennels, the health criterion is closely linked to the economic limitations. However, when there is specific legislation for the inspection or management of facilities, such as in zoos or at veterinary border control posts, the objectives and prevention measures may vary, giving priority to health.

OBJECTIVES OF THE VACCINATION PROGRAM

The main objectives of a vaccination program are:

- To minimize the **risk of exposure, transmission of pathogens** and the **severity** and **clinical incidence of diseases**.
- **To achieve an optimal health status** of the animals.

Vaccination should always meet a criterion of usefulness, entail mechanisms that allow the observation and analysis of possible side effects, and should not exacerbate problems latent in the population.

VACCINATION PROGRAMS (individuals and populations)

GENERIC RECOMMENDATIONS

- Vaccinate only healthy and properly dewormed animals.
- Perform serology before vaccinating dogs with an unknown immune status.
- Do not use attenuated vaccines in pregnant or lactating females.
- Do not start a vaccination protocol prior to six weeks of age (it is advisable to wait till eight weeks).
- Use several vaccine doses at intervals of 2-3 weeks and avoid administering products with a large number of microbial strains in the primary vaccination of puppies.
- If different monovalent vaccines are going to be combined, pay special attention to the adjuvants and directions of the laboratory.
- Booster injection every 1-3 years. Longer interval with attenuated vaccines and shorter interval if there are risk factors (populations, contact with young animals, individual's specific habitat or activities, etc.).

SUGGESTIONS FOR VACCINE PROGRAMS DEPENDING ON THE DISEASE, AGE AND SITUATION

DISEASE (TYPE OF VACCINE)	NUMBER OF DOSIS PUPPIES[1]	NUMBER OF DOSIS ADULT DOGS	NUMBER OF DOSIS BREEDERS	INDICATIONS/ RISK FACTORS	PATHOGENIC LEVEL DISEASE
Canine distemper (attenuated)	3 doses, 2-3 week interval.	1 dose every 1-3 years.	1 annual dose.	All/contact with young animals, shows and contests.	High.
Canine parvoviral infections (attenuated)	3 doses, 2-3 week interval.	1 dose every 1-3 years.	1 annual dose.	All/contact with young animals.	High.
Canine coronaviral infections (inactivated)	2 doses, 2-3 week interval. 1st dose at 10-12 weeks old.	2 annual doses.	2 annual doses.	All/contact with young animals.	Low.
Infectious canine hepatitis (attenuated)	3 doses, 2-3 week interval.	1 dose every 1-3 years.	1 annual dose.	All/contact with young animals.	Moderate.
Canine leptospirosis (inactivated and subunit)	3 doses, 2-3 week interval.	2 annual doses.	2 annual doses.	All/populations.	Moderate.
Canine infectious respiratory disease (inactivated and attenuated)[2]	2 doses, 2-3 week interval. 1st dose at 10-12 weeks old.	1 annual dose.	1 annual dose.	All/contact with young animals, populations, shows and contests.	Low.
Rabies (inactivated)	1 dose, after 3 months old.	1 annual dose.	1 annual dose.	Mandatory vaccine[3].	Very high.
Infections by canine herpesvirus (subunit)	No.	No.	2 doses, 1st-2nd week after mating and 2 weeks before whelping.	Pregnant females.	Low in the bitch and high in litters.
Canine leishmaniosis (subunit)	3 doses, 3 week interval. 1st dose after 6 months old.	1 annual dose.	1 annual dose (do not administer to pregnant or lactating bitches).	Endemic regions.	Moderate.
Canine babesiosis (subunit of *B. canis*)	2 doses, 3-6 week interval. 1st dose after 5 months old.	2 annual doses (1 month prior to the tick season).	2 annual doses (do not administer to pregnant or lactating bitches).	Endemic regions and splenectomized animals.	Moderate-low.

[1] Unless otherwise mentioned, primary vaccination from eight weeks old.

[2] Vaccines against canine infectious respiratory disease may include vaccines against canine parainfluenza virus, canine adenovirus type 2 and *B. bronchiseptica*.

[3] Mandatory vaccination varies depending on the countries. Mandatory when traveling within countries of the European Union.

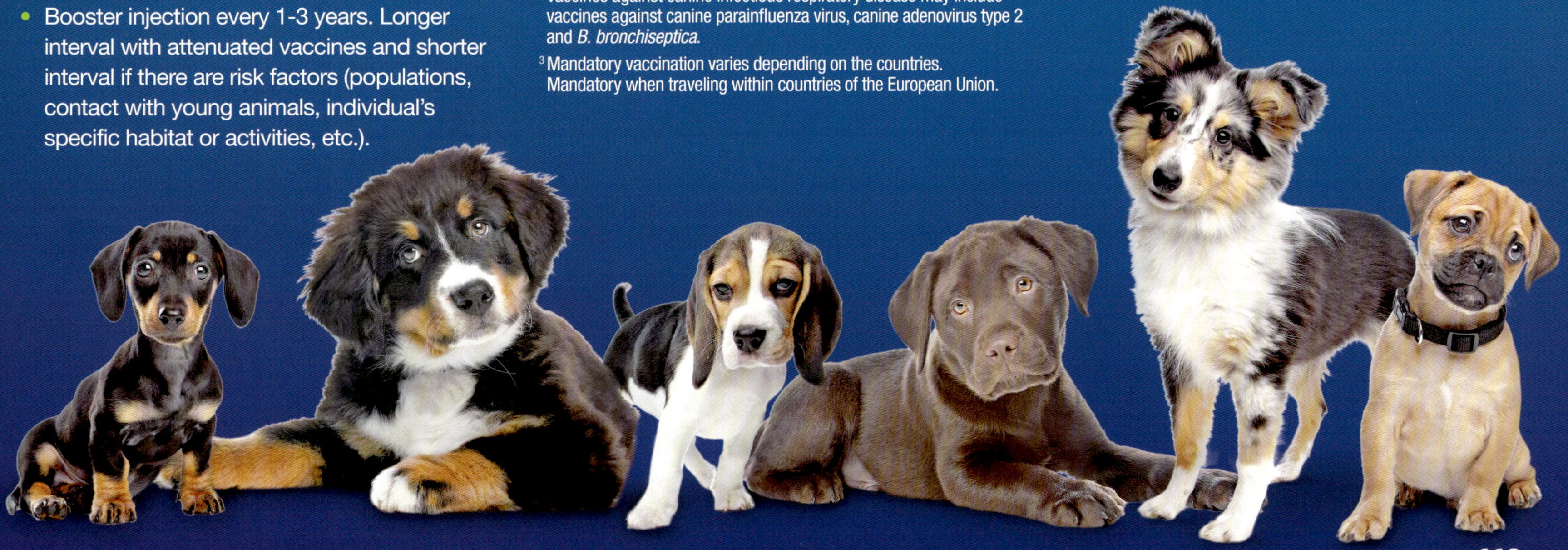

VACCINATION RECOMMENDATIONS FOR CATS

Preventable diseases by vaccination in the cat are feline panleukopenia, feline leukemia, feline infectious peritonitis, feline respiratory disease and rabies. In addition, a vaccine against feline immunodeficiency is marketed in some countries.

Vaccination is one more tool of sanitary programs that may be used both for individual cats and for feline populations (catteries, shelters, etc.). In cats it is especially crucial to combine this measure with others aimed at reducing stress.

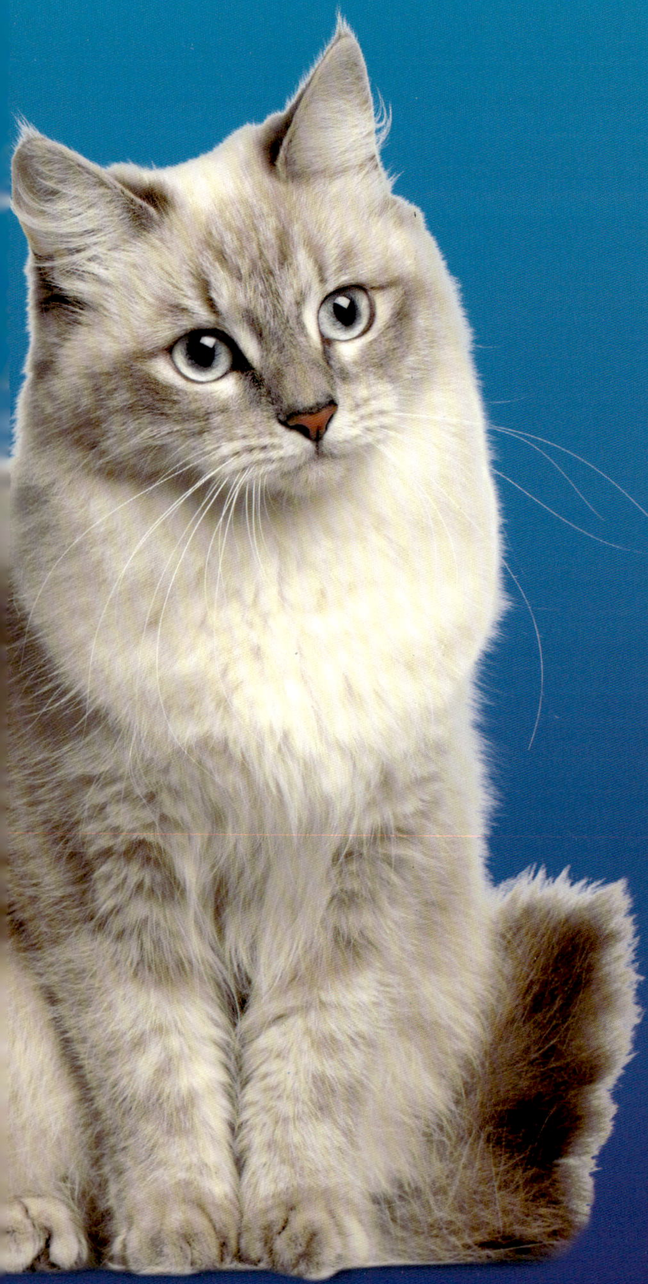

RECOMMENDATIONS FOR VACCINATION OF INDIVIDUALS

Individual vaccination guidelines in cats should be designed based on up-to-date information of the animal (age, breed, fitness, health and physiological states, etc.) and its surroundings.

The analysis of this information will allow for deciding:

- Against which **diseases** cats need to be protected. On the basis of their pathogenic category level and incidence in the geographical area where the animal lives.
- The choice of the **type of vaccine** (inactivated, subunit, attenuated or of recombinant vector). According to the characteristics of the animal to be protected.
- The **number of doses** and **administration interval**. Depending on the type of vaccine, age, health and physiological status of the cat.
- The use of **monovalent or polyvalent vaccines**. According to age, health and physiological status of the cat.
- The choice of the product with the strain that is most representative for the area where the animal resides, as there may be **important differences between strains** circulating in different geographical areas.
- The choice of the specific commercial product, once assessed the differences between equivalent vaccines, associated with the **titer or the concentration** of the microorganism or **the type of adjuvant**.

Immunization schedules must be flexible and be prescribed by vets. In cats, it is particularly appropriate to establish an individualized vaccination schedule.

The vaccine schedules will be different according to:

- Age and physiological status of the cat (young kitten, adult cat, pregnant queen).
- Breed (*e.g.*, increased susceptibility of Persian cats to feline infectious peritonitis).
- Activity of the cat (house-bound or allowed to roam).
- Contact with other individuals (very high contact, for example, for cats participating in contests, or limited contact).
- Coexistence with other individuals of different ages.

A good example of the effect of these factors on vaccination in cats is feline leukemia: it is highly advisable to vaccinate young kittens, but for adult animals it depends on whether they are home-bound or allowed to roam.

RECOMMENDATIONS FOR VACCINATION OF POPULATIONS

There are large differences in management, density, health plan, hygienic or therapeutic products, etc., between feline and canine populations. Unlike dogs, cat populations need:

- Greater reduction in stress, through toys and exercise.
- Lower population density.
- Design of specific facilities.
- Individualized vaccination and deworming guidelines.

The prevention schedules should conform to the main objective of the population.

There are vaccines that should be preferably used in populations, for example, attenuated vaccines for feline respiratory disease. Others, on the contrary, should be used according to the characteristics of individuals, such as the vaccine against feline infectious peritonitis in catteries and breeding colonies.

VACCINATION PROGRAMS (individuals and populations)

GENERIC RECOMMENDATIONS

- Vaccinate only healthy and properly dewormed cats.
- Evaluate a possible infection by feline leukemia virus in young animals prior to vaccination.
- Perform serology before vaccinating cats with an unknown immune status.
- Do not use attenuated or recombinant vector vaccines in pregnant or lactating queens.
- Do not start a vaccination protocol prior to six weeks of age (it is advisable to wait till 8-9 weeks).
- Use two vaccine doses with an interval of 3-5 weeks for the primary vaccination of kittens.
- Do not combine monovalent vaccines with other vaccines or immunological products.
- Booster injection every 1-3 years. Longer interval with attenuated vaccines and shorter interval if there are risk factors (populations, contact with young animals, individual's specific habitat or activities, etc.).

SUGGESTIONS FOR VACCINE PROGRAMS DEPENDING ON THE DISEASE, AGE AND SITUATION

DISEASE (TYPE OF VACCINE)	NUMBER OF DOSIS KITTENS[1]	NUMBER OF DOSIS ADULT CATS	NUMBER OF DOSIS BREEDERS	INDICATIONS/ RISK FACTORS	PATHOGENIC LEVEL OF DISEASE
Feline panleukopenia (attenuated)	2 doses, 3 week interval.	1 dose every 1-3 years.	1 annual or biannual dose.	All/contact with young animals, and populations.	Moderate, except for breeders and litters (high).
Feline respiratory disease (inactivated, subunit and attenuated)[2]	2 doses, 3 week interval.	1 dose every 1-3 years.	1 annual dose.	All/contact with young animals and populations.	Moderate in home-bound cats, low to moderate in populations and high in roaming animals (litters).
Feline leukemia (inactivated, subunit and recombinant vector)	2 doses, 3-5 week interval. Prior to 16 weeks old.	1 biannual dose.	1 biannual dose (do not use in pregnant or lactating queens).	All (use only in animals negative to p27 Ag)/ roaming.	High.
Rabies (inactivated and recombinant vector)	1 dose, after 3 months old.	1 annual dose.	1 annual dose.	Mandatory vaccine[3].	Very high.
Feline infectious peritonitis (attenuated)	2 doses, 3 week interval. 1st dose after 16 weeks old.	Variable.	1 annual dose.	Kittens and breeding colonies/ populations	Very high.

[1] Unless otherwise mentioned, primary vaccination from 8-9 weeks old.

[2] Vaccines against feline respiratory disease may include vaccines against feline rhinotracheitis virus, feline calicivirus and *Chlamydophyla felis*.

[3] Mandatory vaccination varies depending on the countries. Mandatory when traveling within countries of the European Union.

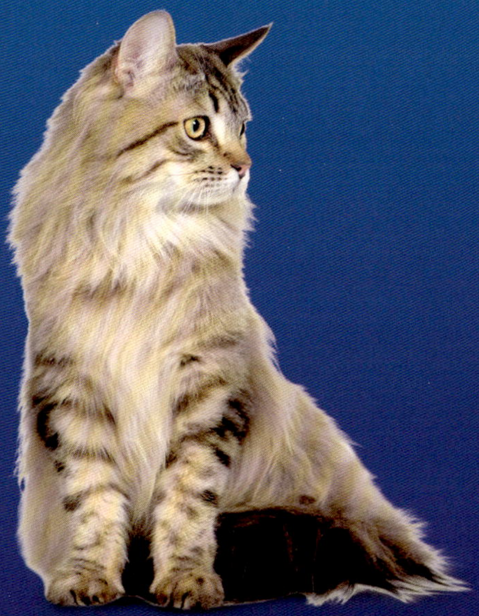

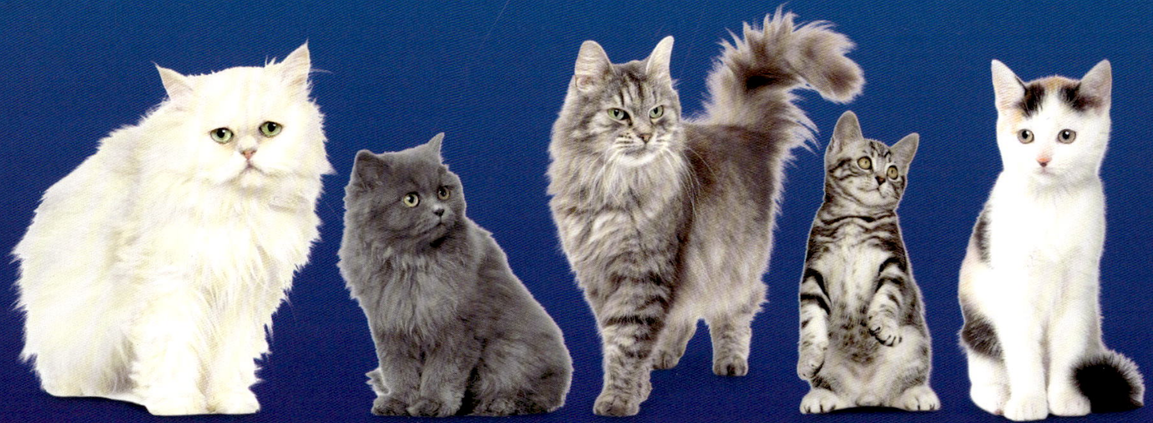

Abbreviations

Ab: antibody
ACTH: adreno corticotropic hormone
ADCC: antibody dependent cell-mediated cytotoxicity
Ag: antigen
ANA: antinuclear antibody
APC: antigen-presenting cell
B: B cell
BALT: bronchus-associated lymphoid tissue
BCR: B cell receptor
C3bR: receptor for the C3b molecule of complement
CAV: canine adenovirus
CBC: complete blood counts
CD: differentiation cluster
CD4+: helper T cells (Th)
CD8+: cytotoxic T cells (Tc and CTL)
CDC: Centers for Disease Control
CDR: complementary determining region
CLIP: class II associated invariant chain peptide
CNS: central nervous system
CPV: canine parvovirus
CSF: cerebrospinal fluid
CTL: cytolytic effector cell
DC: dendritic cell
DFA: direct fluorescent antibody assay
DIC: disseminated intravascular coagulation
dsDNA/RNA: double stranded DNA/RNA
E.M.: electron microscopy
ELISA: enzyme linked immunosorbent assay
Fab: antigen-binding fragment of an immunoglobulin
Fc: crystallizable fragment of an immunoglobulin
FcR: receptor for immunoglobulin Fc
FcεR: high affinity receptor for Ig E
FeLV: feline leukemia virus
FIP: feline infectious peritonitis
FIV: feline immunodeficiency virus
GALT: gut-associated lymphoid tissue
GI: gastrointestinal
HA: hemagglutination assay
HAI: inhibition of hemagglutination assay
H&E: hematoxylin & eosin
IC: immunochromatography
IEL: intraepithelial lymphocyte (γδ T cell)
IFA: indirect fluorescent antibody assay
IFN: interferon
Ig: immunoglobulin
IHC: immunohistochemistry
IL: interleukin
IP: immunoperoxidase
IV: intravenous
kd: kiloDalton
LPS: lipopolysaccharide
M: macrophage
MAC: membrane attack complex
MALT: mucosa-associated lymphoid tissue
MASP: mannose-associated serine protease
MAT: microagglutination test
MBL: mannose-binding lectin
MHC: major histocompatibility complex
NALT: nasal-associated lymphoid tissue
NK: natural killer cell
NO: nitric oxide
OIE: World Organization for Animal Health
PAMP: pathogen-associated molecular patterns
PCR: polymerase chain reaction
pIgR: polymeric immunoglobulin receptor
PMN: polymorphonuclear cells
PP: Peyer's patches
RAG: recombinant activating gene
ROS: reactive oxygen species
RT-PCR: reverse transcriptase-PCR
SC: subcutaneous
SCID: severe combined immunodeficiency
ssDNA/RNA: single stranded DNA/RNA
T: T cell
TAP: transporter-associated with antigen processing
Tc: cytotoxic T cell
TCR: T cell receptor
TD Ag: thymus dependent antigen
TGF-β: tumor growth factor
Th: helper T cell
TI Ag: thymus independent antigen
TLR: toll-like receptor
TNF: tumor necrosis factor
Treg: T regulatory lymphocyte
WB: Western blot
WHO: World Health Organization

Illustrator: Jacob Gragera

Photo credits:

SHUTTERSTOCK.COM
aastock: p. 63
Axel Bueckert: p. 105
cynoclub: p. 87 (1), p. 90 (2)
Daleen Loest: p. 73
Deep OV: p. 103 (3)
Dora Zett: p. 85 (1)
Dorottya Mathe: p. 68 (2)
Eric Isselee: p. 31 (2), p. 38, p. 47 (1, 2), p. 54, p. 61 (1), p. 70 (3), p. 72, p. 75 (1, 2), p. 76 (2), p. 77 (3), p. 79 (1, 2), p. 80 (4), p. 81 (2), p. 84, p. 89 (3), p. 91 (4), p. 95, p. 97, p. 100 (1), p. 107, p. 114, p. 115
Erik Lam: p. 39, p. 51, p. 113
Ermolaev Alexander: p. 69 (3)
Ewa Studio: p. 99 (2)
Ferenc Szelepcsenyi: p. 41
gillmar: p. 102 (1)
Hasloo Group Production Studio: p. 109 (2)
Hugo Felix: p. 52 (1)
Jagodka: p. 13, p. 104 (3)
karamysh: p. 92
Kirill Vorobyev: p. 90 (3)
kurhan: p. 106 (2)
Lebedinski Vladislav: p. 82
Liliya Kulianionak: p. 57, p. 111 (1)
Linn Currie: p. 14, p. 105
Mila Atkovska: p. 89
Nata Sdobnikova: p. 60
Nikolai Tsvetkov: p. 8 (2), p. 71, p. 111 (3)
ninaM: p. 87 (2)
Oksana Kuzmina: p. 62 (1), p. 98
Pinkcandy: p. 40
Sebastian Kaulitzki: p. 43
Sergey Lavrentev: p. 8 (1), p. 66, p. 67
steamroller_blues: p. 64
Steve Heap: p. 108 (2)
Susan Schmitz: p. 86 (2), p. 99 (1)
Tony Campbell: p. 100 (4)
urfin: p. 101 (3), p. 104 (4)
Utekhina Anna: p. 52 (2)
Vasiliy Koval: p. 93 (3)
vikiri: p. 31 (1)
Viorel Sima: p. 101 (2)
Willee Cole: p. 30, p. 80 (3), p. 112
Ysbrand Cosijn: p. 111 (2)
Zdorov Kirill Vladimirovich: p. 89 (2)

OTHERS
Guadalupe Miró: p. 83 (1, 2, 3, 4), p. 85 (2, 3, 4, 5), p. 86 (1), p. 87 (3)
Elena M. de Merlo: p. 93 (1)
Manuel Pizarro: p. 93 (2)

CDC
Dr. Fred Murphy, Sylvia Whitfield: p. 89 (2)
Dr. Daniel P. Perl: p. 91 (1, 2)
Dr. Hicklin: p. 91 (3)